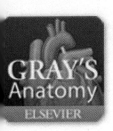

Introducing Gray's Anatomy for Students
for the iPad®!

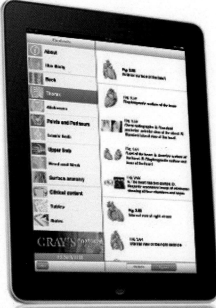

One of the world's best-selling, most readable anatomy textbooks is **now more accessible** than ever before! **Master anatomy** with interactive features and over 1000 innovative and beautiful full-color illustrations that make anatomy come alive!

- **Access and quickly search** the complete text and image library
- **View, save, pinch, zoom, or add notes** to illustrations and figures
- **Turn labels on and off**
- **Take it all with you** — anywhere, anytime on your iPad®

Gray's Atlas of Anatomy for the iPad®

A perfect companion to either the print or iPad version of *Gray's Anatomy for Students!* It presents a vivid visual depiction of human anatomy, correlated with appropriate clinical images and surface anatomy – essential for proper identification in the dissection lab or for course exams.

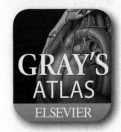

Gray's Anatomy Head and Neck for the iPad®

Taken directly from *Gray's Anatomy for Students*—it's an **ideal app for dental and other health care students** who want only content relevant to **head and neck anatomy!**

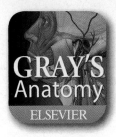

Order today in the iTunes® App Store!

iPad® and iTunes® are registered trademarks of Apple Inc.

Before we are Born

Essentials of Embryology and Birth Defects

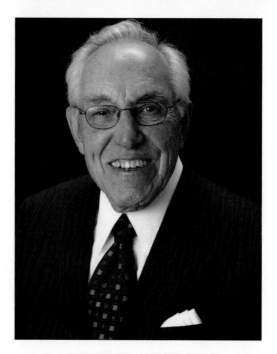

Keith L. Moore

Recipient of the inaugural Henry Gray/Elsevier Distinguished Educator Award in 2007—the American Association of Anatomists' highest award for excellence in human anatomy education at the medical/dental, graduate, and undergraduate levels of teaching; the **Honored Member Award of the American Association of Clinical Anatomists (1994)** for significant contributions to the field of clinically relevant anatomy; and of the **J.C.B. Grant Award of the Canadian Association of Anatomists (1984)** "in recognition of meritorious service and outstanding scholarly accomplishments in the field of anatomical sciences." In 2008 Professor Moore was inducted as a **Fellow of the American Association of Anatomists**. The rank of Fellow honors distinguished AAA members who have demonstrated excellence in science and in their overall contributions to the medical sciences.

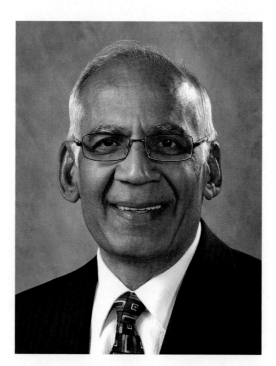

T.V.N. (Vid) Persaud

Recipient of the Henry Gray/Elsevier Distinguished Educator Award in 2010—the American Association of Anatomists' highest award for excellence in human anatomy education at the medical/dental, graduate, and undergraduate levels of teaching; the **Honored Member Award of the American Association of Clinical Anatomists (2008)** for significant contributions to the field of clinically relevant anatomy; and the **J.C.B. Grant Award of the Canadian Association of Anatomists (1991)** "in recognition of meritorious service and outstanding scholarly accomplishments in the field of anatomical sciences." In 2010 Professor Persaud was inducted as a **Fellow of the American Association of Anatomists**. The rank of Fellow honors distinguished AAA members who have demonstrated excellence in science and in their overall contributions to the medical sciences.

Before we are Born

Essentials of Embryology

and Birth Defects

8th Edition

Keith L. Moore,
MSc, PhD, FIAC, FRSM, FAAA
Professor Emeritus, Division of Anatomy, Department of Surgery
Faculty of Medicine, University of Toronto,
Former Professor and Head, Department of Anatomy, University of
Manitoba, Winnipeg, Manitoba, Canada
Former Professor and Chair, Department of Anatomy and
Cell Biology, University of Toronto, Toronto, Ontario, Canada

T.V.N. Persaud,
MD, PhD, DSc, FRCPath (Lond.), FAAA
Professor Emeritus and Former Head, Department of Human Anatomy
and Cell Science
Professor of Pediatrics and Child Health
Associate Professor of Obstetrics, Gynecology, and Reproductive Sciences,
Faculty of Medicine, University of Manitoba, Winnipeg, Manitoba,
Canada
Professor of Anatomy and Embryology, St. George's University, Grenada,
West Indies

Mark G. Torchia,
MSc, PhD
Associate Professor and Director of Development, Department of Surgery
Associate Professor, Department of Human Anatomy and Cell Sciences
Director, University Teaching Services, University of Manitoba,
Winnipeg, Manitoba, Canada

ELSEVIER
SAUNDERS

1600 John F. Kennedy Blvd.
Ste 1800
Philadelphia, PA 19103-2899

Notices

Knowledge and best practice in this field are constantly changing. As new research and experience
broaden our understanding, changes in research methods, professional practices, or medical
treatment may become necessary.

Practitioners and researchers must always rely on their own experience and knowledge in
evaluating and using any information, methods, compounds, or experiments described herein.
In using such information or methods they should be mindful of their own safety and the safety
of others, including parties for whom they have a professional responsibility.

With respect to any drug or pharmaceutical products identified, readers are advised to check
the most current information provided (i) on procedures featured or (ii) by the manufacturer of
each product to be administered, to verify the recommended dose or formula, the method and
duration of administration, and contraindications. It is the responsibility of practitioners, relying
on their own experience and knowledge of their patients, to make diagnoses, to determine dosages
and the best treatment for each individual patient, and to take all appropriate safety precautions.

To the fullest extent of the law, neither the Publisher nor the authors, contributors, or editors,
assume any liability for any injury and/or damage to persons or property as a matter of products
liability, negligence or otherwise, or from any use or operation of any methods, products,
instructions, or ideas contained in the material herein.

Previous editions copyrighted 2008, 2003, 1998, 1993, 1989, 1983, 1974

Library of Congress Cataloging-in-Publication Data
Moore, Keith L.
  Before we are born : essentials of embryology and birth defects / Keith L. Moore, T.V.N. Persaud,
Mark G. Torchia.—8th ed.
      p. ; cm.
  Includes bibliographical references and index.
  ISBN 978-1-4377-2001-3 (pbk. : alk. paper)   1. Embryology, Human.   2. Abnormalities,
Human.   I. Persaud, T.V.N.   II. Torchia, Mark G.   III. Title.
  [DNLM: 1. Embryonic Development.   2. Congenital Abnormalities.   3. Embryology—
methods.   4. Fetal Development.   QS 604]
  QM601.M757 2013
  612.6′4—dc23

                                                                                        2011022742

Executive Content Strategist: Madelene Hyde
Content Development Specialist: Christine Abshire
Publishing Services Manager: Pat Joiner-Myers
Project Manager: Marlene Weeks
Designer: Steven Stave

Printed in Canada

Last digit is the print number: 9   8   7   6   5   4   3   2   1

In Loving Memory of Marion

My best friend, wife, colleague, mother of our five children and grandmother of our nine grandchildren, for her love, unconditional support, and understanding. Wonderful memories keep you ever near our hearts.

—*KLM and family*

To Pam and Ron

I am grateful to my eldest daughter Pam, who assumed the office duties her mother previously carried out. She is also helpful in many other ways. I am also grateful to my son-in-law Ron Crowe, whose technical skills have helped me prepare the manuscript for this book.

—*KLM*

For Gisela

My lovely wife and best friend, for her endless support and patience; our three children—Indrani, Sunita, and Rainer (Ren)—and grandchildren (Brian, Amy, and Lucas).

—*TVNP*

For Barbara, Muriel, and Erik

You have never doubted my dreams and ideas, no matter how crazy they might be. Nothing could ever mean more to me than each of you. I also dedicate this book to my mother, Win; no words are sufficient to say thank you.

—*MGT*

For Our Students and Their Teachers

To our students: We hope you will enjoy reading this book, increase your understanding of human embryology, pass all of your exams, and be excited and well prepared for your careers in patient care, research, and teaching . You will remember some of what you hear; much of what you read; more of what you see, and almost all of what you experience and understand fully.

To their teachers: May this book be a helpful resource to you and your students. We appreciate the numerous constructive comments we have received over the years from both students and teachers. Your remarks have been invaluable to us in improving this book. Kindly keep on sending your suggestions by e-mail to: persaud@cc.umanitoba.ca (Dr. Vid Persaud).

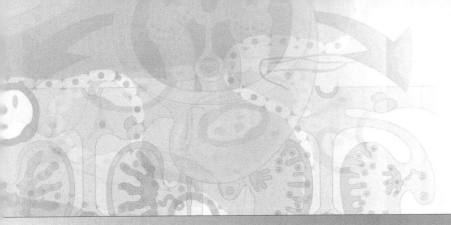

Contributors

David D. Eisenstat, MD, MA, FRCPC
Professor, Departments of Pediatrics and Medical Genetics, Faculty of Medicine and Dentistry, University of Alberta; Director, Division of Pediatric Hematology, Oncology, and Palliative Care, Department of Pediatrics, Stollery Children's Hospital and the University of Alberta; Inaugural Chair, Muriel and Ada Hole and Kids with Cancer Society Chair in Pediatric Oncology Research

Jeffrey T. Wigle, PhD
Principal Investigator, Institute of Cardiovascular Sciences, St. Boniface General Hospital Research Centre; Manitoba Research Chair and Associate Professor, Department of Biochemistry and Medical Genetics, University of Manitoba, Winnipeg, Manitoba, Canada

Preface

*B*efore *We Are Born* has been completely updated to reflect current understanding of human embryology. It provides medical and other students in the health professions with the essentials of normal and abnormal development. This concise work is a digest of our larger book, *The Developing Human: Clinically Oriented Embryology*, 9th edition, and is suited for a one-semester course and for review.

An important feature of this book is the **Clinically Oriented Questions**, which appear at the end of each chapter. In addition, available through Elsevier's *studentconsult.com* website are many helpful **clinical case studies** and questions with answers and explanations. These will benefit students preparing for USMLE Step 1 and similar examinations.

Accompanying this 8th edition of *Before We Are Born* is an innovative **set of 16 full-color animations** that will assist students in learning the complexities of embryological development. When one of the animations is especially relevant to the text, the 🎬 icon has been added in the margin. Also, many of the illustrations in the book have been improved with three-dimensional renderings and bold, effective color.

The teratology content has been updated because the study of abnormal development is required for understanding the causes of birth defects and how these may be prevented. *Molecular aspects of developmental biology* have been highlighted throughout the book, especially in areas that appear promising for clinical medicine and future research. We have also added a new chapter, contributed by Dr. Jeffrey T. Wigle and Dr. David D. Eisenstat, on the cellular and molecular basis of embryonic development.

Every chapter has been revised thoroughly to reflect new research findings and their clinical significance. The chapters are organized to present a clear, systematic, and logical approach to human prenatal development.

Keith L. Moore
Vid Persaud
Mark G. Torchia

Acknowledgments

Many colleagues and students have made invaluable contributions to this newest edition of BWAB. We are indebted to the following colleagues (listed alphabetically) for either critical reviewing of chapters, making suggestions for improvement of this book, or providing some of the new figures: Dr. Steve Ahing, Faculty of Dentistry, University of Manitoba, Winnipeg; Dr. Boris Kablar, Department of Anatomy and Neurobiology, Dalhousie University, Halifax; Dr. Albert Chudley, Departments of Pediatrics and Child Health, Biochemistry and Medical Genetics, University of Manitoba, Winnipeg; Dr. Blaine M. Cleghorn, Faculty of Dentistry, Dalhousie University, Halifax, NS; Dr. Frank Gaillard, Radiopaedia.org, Toronto, Ontario; Dr. Sylvia Kogan, Department of Ophthalmology, University of Alberta, Edmonton, AB; Dr. Deborah Levine, Beth Israel Deaconess Medical Center, Boston; Dr. Marios Loukas, St. George's University, Grenada; Professor Bernard J. Moxham, Cardiff School of Biosciences, Cardiff University, Cardiff, Wales; Dr. Stuart Morrison, Department of Radiology, Cleveland Clinic, Cleveland; Dr. Michael Narvey, Department of Pediatrics, University of Alberta, Edmonton, AB; Dr. Drew Noden, Department of Biomedical Sciences, Cornell University, College of Veterinary Medicine, Ithaca, NY; Dr. Shannon E. Perry, Professor Emeritus, San Francisco State University, San Francisco, CA; Professor T.S. Ranganathan, St. George's University, School of Medicine, Grenada; Dr. Gregory Reid, Department of Obstetrics, Gynecology and Reproductive Sciences, University of Manitoba, Winnipeg; Dr. L. Ross, Department of Neurobiology and Anatomy, University of Texas Medical School – Houston, TX; Dr. J. Elliott Scott, Departments of Oral Biology and Human Anatomy & Cell Science, University of Manitoba, Winnipeg; Dr. Gerald S. Smyser, Altru Health System, Grand Forks, North Dakota; Dr. Richard Shane Tubbs, Children's Hospital, University of Alabama at Birmingham, Alabama; Dr. Michael Wiley, Division of Anatomy, Department of Surgery, Faculty of Medicine, University of Toronto, Toronto, and Dr. Ed Uthman, Clinical pathologist, Houston/Richmond, Texas.

The new illustrations were prepared by Hans Neuhart, President of the Electronic Illustrators Group in Fountain Hills, AZ. We thank Ms. Madelene Hyde, Publisher, Elsevier; for her invaluable insights, advise and encouragement. We are especially thankful to Ms. Christine Abshire, our Developmental Editor, and her team at Elsevier. We are also grateful to Ms. Marlene Weeks, Project Manager-Books, Elsevier and Mr. Mike Ederer, Production Editor, Graphic World Publishing Services, for their help in the production of this book. This new edition of BWAB is the result of their dedication and technical expertise.

Keith L Moore
Vid Persaud
Mark G Torchia

Contents

Introduction to Human Development

H uman development begins when an **oocyte** (ovum) from a female is fertilized by a **sperm** (spermatozoon) from a male. Development involves many changes that transform a single cell, the **zygote**, into a multicellular human being. The term *conceptus* refers to the entire products of conception, which includes the embryo from fertilization onward and its membranes (e.g., placenta). Embryology is concerned with the origin and development of a human being from a zygote to birth. The stages of development before birth are shown in Figures 1-1 and 7-3.

IMPORTANCE OF AND ADVANCES IN EMBRYOLOGY

The study of prenatal stages and the mechanisms of human development help us understand the normal relationships of adult body structures and the causes of congenital anomalies. Much of the modern practice of obstetrics involves applied or **clinical embryology**. Because some children have birth defects, such as spina bifida or congenital heart disease, the significance of embryology is readily apparent to pediatricians. Advances in surgery, especially in procedures involving the prenatal and pediatric age groups, have made knowledge of human development more clinically significant.

Rapid advances in molecular biology have led to the use of sophisticated techniques (e.g., **recombinant DNA technology, chimeric models, transgenics, and stem cell manipulation**) in research laboratories to explore such diverse issues as the genetic regulation of morphogenesis, the temporal and regional expression of specific genes, and the mechanisms by which cells are committed to form the various parts of the embryo. For the first time, researchers are beginning to understand how, when, and where selected genes are activated and expressed in the embryo during normal and abnormal development.

TIMETABLE OF HUMAN PRENATAL DEVELOPMENT
1 TO 6 WEEKS

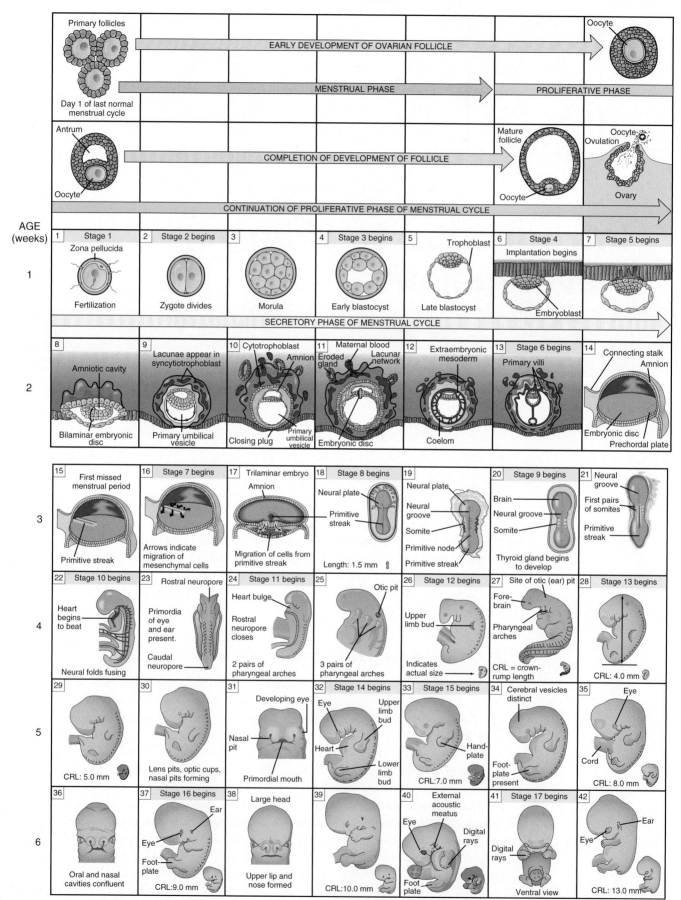

Figure 1–1 Early stages of human development. Development of an ovarian follicle containing an oocyte, ovulation, and the phases of the menstrual cycle are shown.

TIMETABLE OF HUMAN PRENATAL DEVELOPMENT

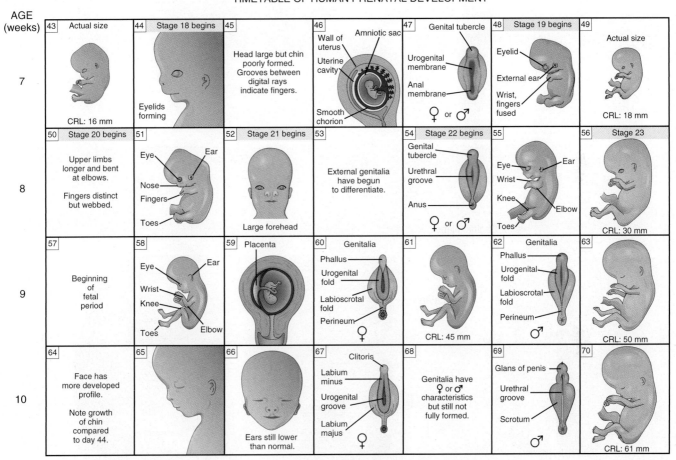

Figure 1–1, cont'd

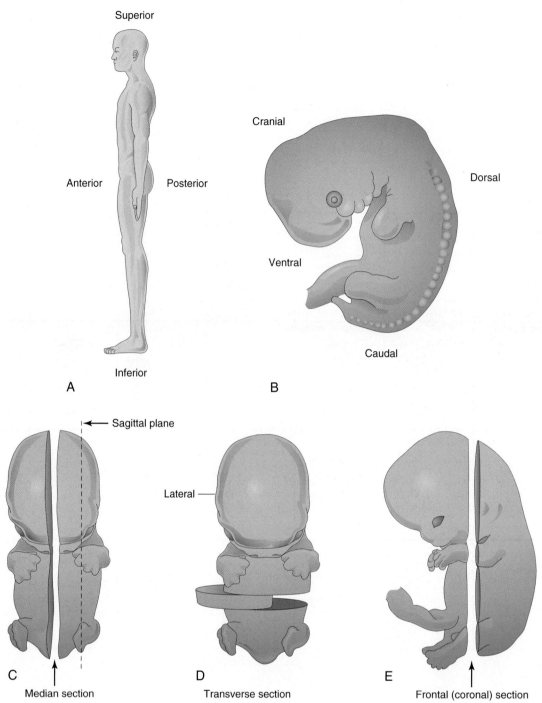

Figure 1–2 Illustrations of descriptive terms of position, direction, and planes of the body. **A,** Lateral view of an adult in the anatomical position. **B,** Lateral view of a 5-week embryo. **C** and **D,** Ventral views of a 6-week embryo. The median plane is an imaginary vertical plane of section that passes longitudinally through the body, dividing it into right and left halves. A sagittal plane refers to any plane parallel to the median plane. A transverse plane refers to any plane that is at right angles to both the median and the frontal planes. **E,** Lateral view of a 7-week embryo. A frontal (coronal) plane is any vertical plane that intersects the median plane at a right angle and divides the body into front (anterior, or ventral) and back (posterior, or dorsal) parts. In describing development, it is necessary to use words denoting the position of one part to another or to the body as a whole. For example, the vertebral column develops in the dorsal part of the embryo and the sternum in the ventral part of the embryo.

The critical role of genes, **signaling molecules,** receptors, and other molecular factors in regulating early embryonic development is rapidly being delineated. In 1995, Edward B. Lewis, Christiane Nüsslein-Volhard, and Eric F. Wieschaus were awarded the Nobel Prize in Physiology or Medicine for their discovery of genes that control embryonic development. Such discoveries are contributing to a better understanding of the causes of spontaneous abortion and congenital anomalies.

In 1997, Ian Wilmut and colleagues were the first to produce a mammal (a sheep dubbed **Dolly**) by cloning using the technique of somatic cell nuclear transfer. Since then, other animals have been cloned successfully from cultured differentiated adult cells. Interest in human cloning has generated considerable debate because of social, ethical, and legal implications. Moreover, there is concern that cloning may result in an increase in the number of infants born with birth defects and serious diseases.

Human embryonic stem cells are pluripotential and capable of developing into diverse cell types. The isolation and culture of human embryonic and other stem cells may hold great promise for the development of molecular therapies.

DESCRIPTIVE TERMS

In anatomy and embryology, special terms of position, direction, and various planes of the body are used. Descriptions of the adult are based on the *anatomical position*, the position in which the body is erect, the upper limbs are at the sides, and the palms are directed anteriorly (see Fig. 1-2A). The descriptive terms of position, direction, and planes used for embryos are shown in Figure 1-2B to E.

CLINICALLY ORIENTED QUESTIONS

1. What is the difference between the terms *conceptus* and *embryo*? What are the *products of conception*?

2. Why do we study human embryology? Does it have any practical value in medicine and other health sciences?

3. Physicians date a pregnancy from the first day of the last normal menstrual period, but the embryo does not start to develop until approximately 2 weeks later (see Fig. 1-1). Why do physicians use this terminology?

The answers to these questions are at the back of the book.

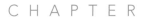
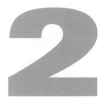

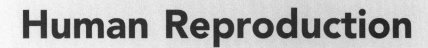

Human Reproduction

P uberty begins when secondary sex characteristics (e.g., pubic hair) appear, typically between the ages of 12 and 15 years in females and 13 and 16 years in males. **Menarche** (the time of the first menstrual period) may occur as early as 8 years of age. Puberty in females is largely completed by age 16 years. In males, puberty ends when the first mature sperms are formed.

REPRODUCTIVE ORGANS

Reproductive organs produce and transport germ cells (gametes) from the gonads (testes or ovaries) to the site of fertilization in the uterine tube (Fig. 2-1).

Female Reproductive Organs

Vagina
The vagina (see Fig. 2-1*A*) serves as the excretory passage for menstrual fluid, receives the penis (see Fig. 2-1*B*) during sexual intercourse, and forms the inferior part of the birth canal.

Uterus
The uterus is a thick-walled, pear-shaped organ (see Fig. 2-2*A* and *B*) and consists of two main parts:

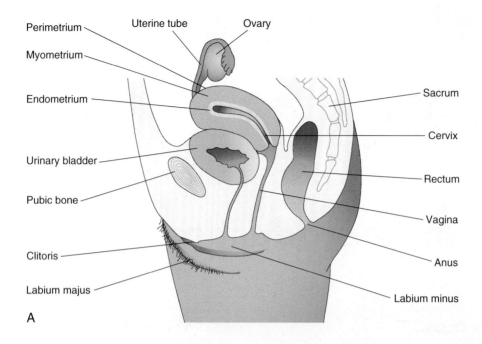

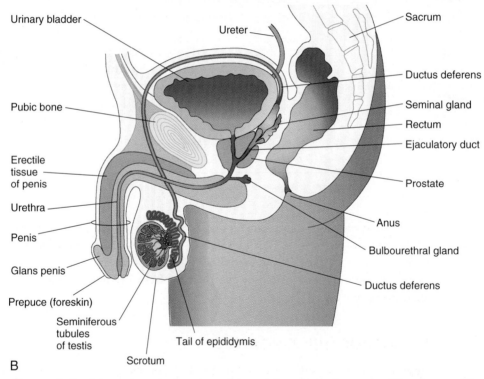

Figure 2–1   Schematic sagittal sections of the pelvic regions of a woman (**A**) and a man (**B**).

● The body, the expanded superior two thirds
● The cervix, the cylindrical inferior third

The **fundus of the uterus is** the rounded part of the uterine body that lies superior to the orifices of the uterine tubes. The **body of the uterus** narrows from the fundus to the **isthmus,** the constricted region between the body and the **cervix** (Fig. 2-2A). The lumen of the cervix, the **cervical canal,** has a constricted

opening, the *os (ostium),* at each end. The **internal os** communicates with the cavity of the body of the uterus, whereas the **external os** communicates with the vagina. The walls of the body of the uterus consist of three layers:

● **Perimetrium,** a thin external peritoneal layer
● **Myometrium,** a thick smooth muscle layer
● **Endometrium,** a thin internal layer

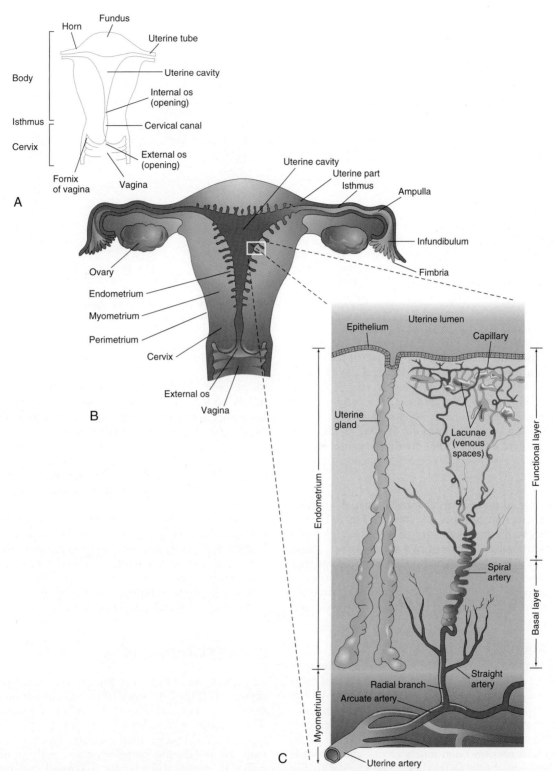

Figure 2–2 Female reproductive organs. **A,** Parts of the uterus. **B,** Diagrammatic frontal (coronal) section of the uterus, uterine tubes, and vagina. The ovaries are also shown. **C,** Enlargement of the area outlined in **B.** The functional layer of the endometrium is sloughed off during menstruation.

At the peak of its development, the endometrium is 4 to 5 mm thick. During the luteal (secretory) phase of the menstrual cycle (see Fig. 2-8), three layers of the endometrium can be distinguished microscopically (see Fig. 2-2*C*) into the following:

- A compact layer, consisting of densely packed connective tissue around the neck of the uterine glands
- A spongy layer, composed of edematous connective tissue containing the dilated, tortuous bodies of the uterine glands
- A basal layer, containing the blind ends of the uterine glands

The compact and spongy layers, known collectively as the *functional layer*, disintegrate and are shed at menstruation and after *parturition* (childbirth). The basal layer of the endometrium has its own blood supply and is not cast off during menstruation.

Uterine Tubes

The **uterine tubes**, measuring 10 cm long and 1 cm in diameter, extend laterally from the **horns of the uterus** (see Fig. 2-2*A*). Each tube opens into a horn of the uterus at its proximal end and into the peritoneal cavity at its distal end. *The uterine tube is divided into the following parts: the infundibulum, the ampulla, the isthmus, and the uterine part.* The tubes carry oocytes from the ovaries to the fertilization site in the ampulla (see Fig. 2-2*B*). The uterine tube then conveys the dividing zygote to the uterine cavity.

Ovaries

The **ovaries** are almond-shaped glands located on each side of the uterus that produce **oocytes** (see Fig. 2-1*A* and *B*). When released from the ovary at *ovulation*, the secondary oocyte passes into one of two *uterine tubes*. These tubes open into the *uterus*, which protects and nourishes the embryo and fetus until birth. The ovaries also produce estrogen and progesterone, the hormones responsible for the development of secondary sex characteristics and regulation of pregnancy.

Female External Sex Organs

The female external sex organs are known collectively as the **vulva** (Fig. 2-3). The **labia majora**, fatty external folds of skin, conceal the vaginal orifice, the opening of the vagina. Inside these labia are two smaller folds of mucous membrane, the **labia minora**. The **clitoris**, a small erectile organ, is situated at the superior junction of these folds. The vagina and urethra open into a cavity, the **vestibule** (the cleft between the labia minora). The vaginal orifice varies with the condition of the **hymen**, a fold of mucous membrane that surrounds the vaginal orifice.

Male Reproductive Organs

The male reproductive organs (see Fig. 2-1*B*) include the penis, testes, epididymis, ductus deferens (vas deferens), prostate, seminal glands, bulbourethral glands, ejaculatory ducts, and urethra. The two oval testes are located

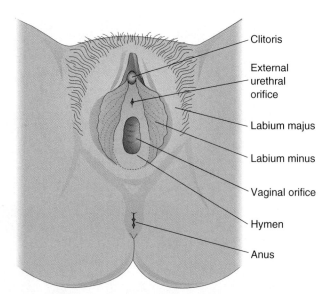

Figure 2–3 External female genitalia. The labia are spread apart to show the external urethral and vaginal orifices.

in the cavity of the **scrotum**. Each **testis** consists of many highly coiled **seminiferous tubules** that produce sperms. Immature sperms pass from the testis into a single, complexly coiled tube, the **epididymis**, where they are stored. From the epididymis, the **ductus deferens** carries the sperms to the ejaculatory duct. This duct descends into the pelvis, where it fuses with the ducts of the seminal glands to form the **ejaculatory duct**, which enters the urethra.

The **urethra** is a tube that leads from the urinary bladder through the penis to the outside of the body. Within the **penis**, *erectile tissue* surrounds the urethra. During sexual excitement, this tissue fills with blood, causing the penis to erect. **Semen** consists of sperms mixed with seminal fluid produced by the *seminal glands, bulbourethral glands,* and *prostate.*

GAMETOGENESIS

The sperm and oocyte are highly specialized gametes, or germ cells (Fig. 2-4). Each of these cells contains half the number of required chromosomes (i.e., 23 instead of 46). The number of chromosomes is reduced during a special type of cell division called **meiosis**. This type of cell division occurs during **gametogenesis** (formation of germ cells). In males, this process is termed **spermatogenesis**; in females, it is known as **oogenesis** (Fig. 2-5).

Meiosis

Meiosis consists of two meiotic cell divisions (Fig. 2-6), during which the chromosome number of the germ cells is reduced to half (23, the *haploid* number) the number present in other cells in the body (46, the *diploid* number).

During the **first meiotic division**, the chromosome number is reduced from diploid to haploid. Homologous

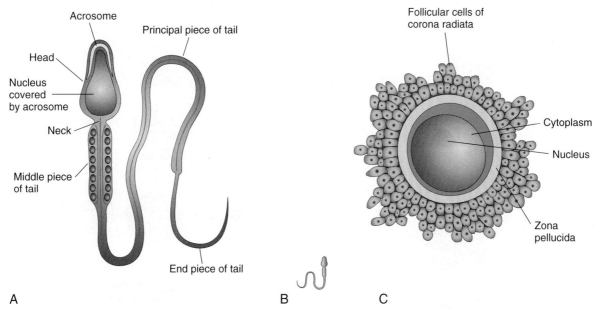

Figure 2–4 Male and female gametes or germ cells. **A,** The parts of a human sperm (×1250). The head, composed mostly of the nucleus, is partly covered by the acrosome, an organelle containing enzymes. **B,** A sperm drawn to approximately the same scale as the oocyte. **C,** A human secondary oocyte (×200), shown surrounded by the zona pellucida and corona radiata.

chromosomes (one from each parent) pair during prophase and then separate during anaphase, with one representative of each pair randomly going to each pole of the meiotic spindle. The spindle connects to the chromosome at the centromere (Fig. 2-6*B*). At this stage, they are double chromatid chromosomes. The X and Y chromosomes are not homologs; however, they have homologous segments at the tips of their short arms. They pair in these regions only. By the end of the first meiotic division, each new cell formed (secondary spermatocyte or secondary oocyte) has the haploid chromosome number of double chromatid chromosomes; therefore, each cell contains half the number of chromosomes of the preceding cell (primary spermatocyte or primary oocyte). This separation, or disjunction, of paired homologous chromosomes is the physical basis of segregation, or separation, of allelic genes during meiosis.

The **second meiotic division** follows the first division, without a normal interphase (i.e., without an intervening step of DNA replication). Each double chromatid chromosome divides, and each half, or *chromatid*, is randomly drawn to a different pole of the meiotic spindle; thus, the haploid number of chromosomes (23) is retained. Each daughter cell formed by meiosis has the reduced haploid number of chromosomes, with one representative of each chromosome pair (now a single chromatid chromosome).

Meiosis:

● Provides for *constancy of the chromosome number* from generation to generation by reducing the chromosome number from diploid to haploid, thereby producing haploid gametes.

● Allows *random assortment of maternal and paternal chromosomes* between the gametes.

● Relocates segments of maternal and paternal chromosomes by *crossing over of chromosome segments*, which "shuffles" the genes and produces a recombination of genetic material.

Spermatogenesis

Before puberty, primordial sperms (spermatogonia) remain dormant in the seminiferous tubules of the testes from the late fetal period. At puberty they begin to increase in number (see Fig. 2-5). After several mitotic cell divisions, the sperms grow and undergo gradual changes that transform them into **primary spermatocytes**—the largest germ cells in the seminiferous tubules. Each primary spermatocyte subsequently undergoes a reduction division—the *first meiotic division*—to form two haploid **secondary spermatocytes**, which are approximately half the size of primary spermatocytes. Subsequently, the secondary spermatocytes undergo a *second meiotic division* to form four haploid **spermatids**, which are approximately half the size of secondary spermatocytes. The spermatids are gradually transformed into four mature sperms during a process known as **spermiogenesis**. During this metamorphosis (change in form), the nucleus condenses, the acrosome forms, and most of the cytoplasm is shed and the tail forms. When spermiogenesis is complete, sperms enter the lumina (cavities) of the seminiferous tubules. The sperms then move to the **epididymis** (see Fig. 2-1*B*), where they are stored and become functionally mature. Spermatogenesis, including spermiogenesis, requires approximately 2 months for completion.

NORMAL GAMETOGENESIS

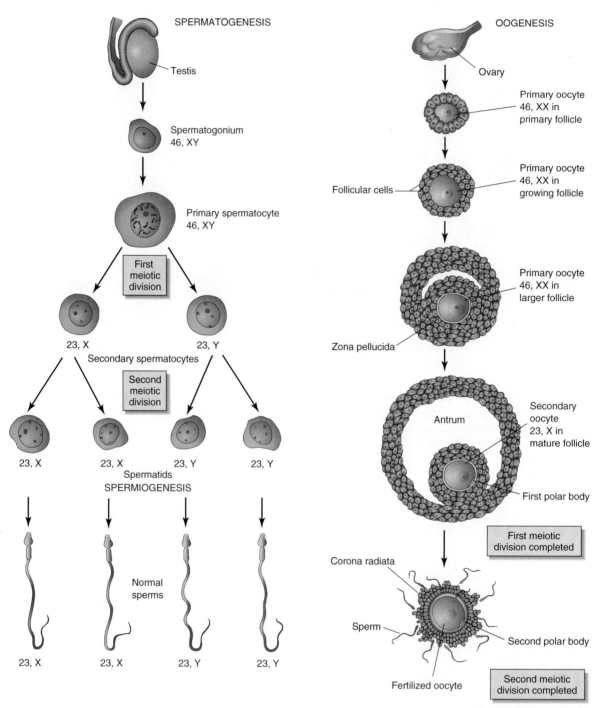

Figure 2–5   Normal gametogenesis: conversion of germ cells into gametes. The illustrations compare spermatogenesis and oogenesis. Oogonia are not shown in this figure because they differentiate into primary oocytes before birth. The chromosome complement of the germ cells is shown at each stage. The number designates the total number of chromosomes, including sex chromosome(s) (shown after the comma). Note: (1) After the two meiotic divisions, the diploid number of chromosomes, 46, is reduced to the haploid number, 23; (2) four sperms form from one primary spermatocyte, whereas only one secondary oocyte results from maturation of a primary oocyte; (3) the cytoplasm is conserved during oogenesis to form one large cell, the oocyte.

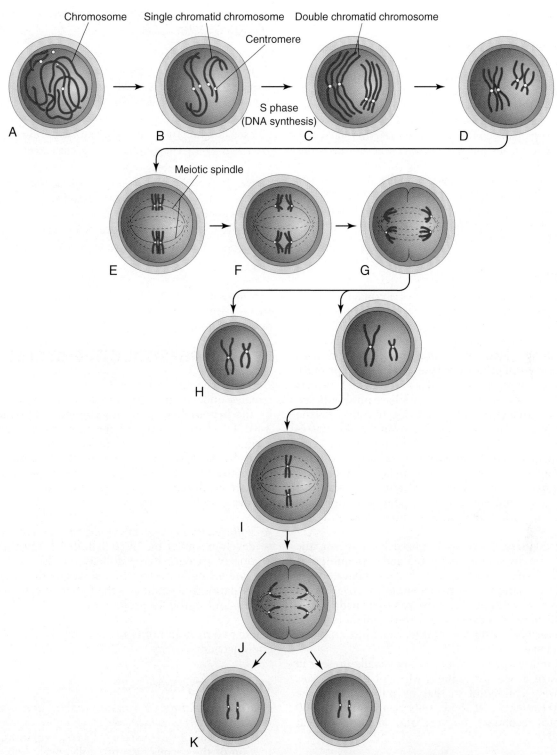

Figure 2–6 Diagrammatic representation of meiosis. Two chromosome pairs are shown. **A** to **D,** Stages of prophase of the first meiotic division. The homologous chromosomes approach each other and pair; each member of the pair consists of two chromatids. Observe the single crossover in one pair of chromosomes, resulting in the interchange of chromatid segments. **E,** Metaphase. The two members of each pair become oriented on the meiotic spindle. **F,** Anaphase. **G,** Telophase. The chromosomes migrate to opposite poles. **H,** Distribution of parental chromosome pairs at the end of the first meiotic division. **I** to **K,** Second meiotic division, which is similar to mitosis, except that the cells are haploid.

Spermiogenesis normally continues throughout the reproductive life of a male.

When ejaculated, the **mature sperms** are free-swimming, actively motile cells *consisting of a head and a tail* (see Fig. 2-4A). The neck of the sperm is the junction between the head and tail. The head of the sperm, forming most of the bulk of the sperm, contains the nucleus. The anterior two thirds of the head are covered by the **acrosome**, a cap-like organelle containing enzymes that facilitate sperm penetration during fertilization. The tail provides the motility of the sperm, assisting with its transport to the site of fertilization in the ampulla of the uterine tube. *The **tail of the sperm** consists of three parts:* the middle piece, principal piece, and end piece. The middle piece contains the energy-producing **mitochondria**, which fuel the lashing movements of the tail.

Oogenesis

Oogenesis refers to the sequence of events by which oogonia (primordial oocytes) are transformed into **oocytes**. This maturation process begins during the fetal period, but is not completed until after puberty (see Fig. 2-5). During early fetal life oogonia proliferate by mitosis and enlarge to form **primary oocytes**. At birth, all primary oocytes have completed the prophase of the *first meiotic division*. These oocytes remain in prophase until puberty. Shortly before ovulation, a primary oocyte completes the first meiotic division (see Fig. 2-5). Unlike the corresponding stage of spermatogenesis, the division of cytoplasm is unequal. The **secondary oocyte** receives almost all the cytoplasm, whereas the **first polar body** receives very little, causing it to degenerate after a short time. At ovulation, the nucleus of the secondary oocyte begins the *second meiotic division*, but progresses only to metaphase.

If the secondary oocyte is fertilized by a sperm, the second meiotic division is completed and a **second polar body** is also formed (see Fig. 2-5). The secondary oocyte released at ovulation is surrounded by a covering of amorphous material known as the **zona pellucida** and a layer of follicular cells called the **corona radiata** (see Fig. 2-4C). The **secondary oocyte** is large, being just visible to the unaided eye.

Up to 2 million primary oocytes are usually present in the ovaries of a newborn infant. Most of these oocytes regress during childhood so that by puberty, no more than 40,000 remain. Of these, only approximately 400 mature into secondary oocytes and are expelled at ovulation.

Comparison of Male and Female Gametes

Compared with sperms, the oocytes are massive, immotile (see Fig. 2-4B and C), and have an abundance of cytoplasm. In terms of sex chromosome constitution, **there are two kinds of normal sperms** (see Fig. 2-5): 22 autosomes plus either an X sex chromosome (i.e., 23, X) or a Y sex chromosome (23, Y). **There is only one kind of normal secondary oocyte:** 22 autosomes plus an X sex

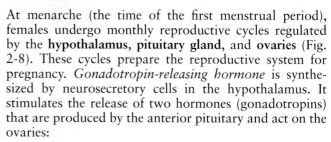

ABNORMAL GAMETOGENESIS

During gametogenesis, homologous chromosomes sometimes fail to separate—known as **nondisjunction**—and as a result, some gametes have 24 chromosomes and others only 22 (Fig. 2-7). If a gamete with 24 chromosomes unites with a normal one with 23 chromosomes, a zygote with 47 chromosomes results, as occurs in infants with **Down syndrome** (see Fig. 19-4). This condition is called **trisomy 21** because of the presence of three representatives of a particular chromosome instead of the usual two. If a gamete with only 22 chromosomes unites with a normal gamete, a zygote with 45 chromosomes results. This condition is known as **monosomy** because only one representative of the particular chromosomal pair is present. Embryos with monosomy usually die.

chromosome (i.e., 23, X). *The difference in sex chromosome complement forms the basis of primary sex determination.*

FEMALE REPRODUCTIVE CYCLES

At menarche (the time of the first menstrual period), females undergo monthly reproductive cycles regulated by the **hypothalamus, pituitary gland**, and **ovaries** (Fig. 2-8). These cycles prepare the reproductive system for pregnancy. *Gonadotropin-releasing hormone* is synthesized by neurosecretory cells in the hypothalamus. It stimulates the release of two hormones (gonadotropins) that are produced by the anterior pituitary and act on the ovaries:

● *Follicle-stimulating hormone (FSH)* stimulates the development of the ovarian follicles and the production of **estrogen** by the follicular cells.
● *Luteinizing hormone (LH)* serves as the "trigger" for ovulation and stimulates the follicular cells and corpus luteum to produce **progesterone**.

These two ovarian hormones also produce growth of the endometrium.

Ovarian Cycle

Follicle-stimulating hormone (FSH) and luteinizing hormone (LH) produce cyclic changes in the ovaries (development of the ovarian follicles, ovulation, and formation of the corpus luteum), collectively known as the **ovarian cycle**. During each cycle, FSH promotes growth of several primary follicles (Figs. 2-8 and 2-9); however, only one of them usually develops into a mature follicle and ruptures, expelling its oocyte (Fig. 2-10).

Follicular Development

Development of an ovarian follicle (Figs. 2-8 and 2-9) is characterized by:

● Growth and differentiation of a primary oocyte
● Proliferation of follicular cells

ABNORMAL GAMETOGENESIS

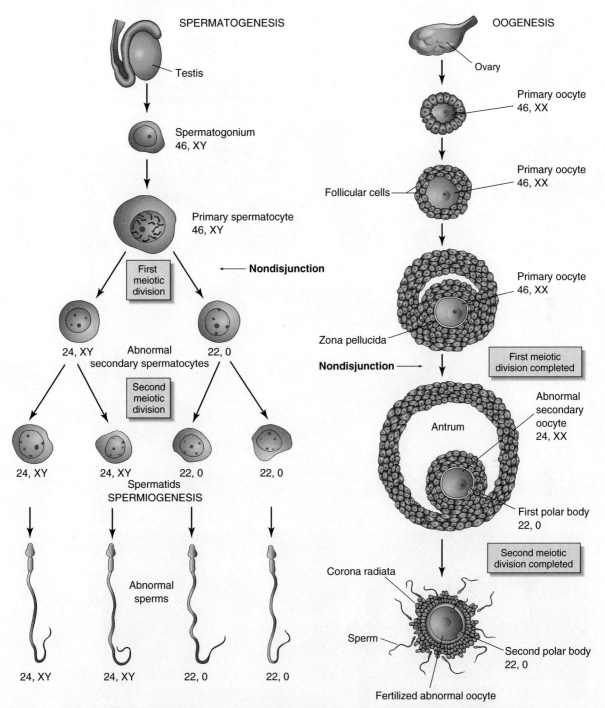

Figure 2–7 Abnormal gametogenesis. The illustrations show how nondisjunction, an error in cell division, results in an abnormal chromosome distribution in gametes. Although nondisjunction of sex chromosomes is illustrated, a similar defect may occur during the division of autosomes (any chromosomes other than sex chromosomes). When nondisjunction occurs during the first meiotic division of spermatogenesis, one secondary spermatocyte contains 22 autosomes plus an X and a Y chromosome, whereas the other one contains 22 autosomes and no sex chromosome. Similarly, nondisjunction during oogenesis may give rise to an oocyte with 22 autosomes and two X chromosomes (as shown) or one with 22 autosomes and no sex chromosome.

Figure 2–8 Illustrations of the interrelationships among the hypothalamus, pituitary gland, ovaries, and endometrium. One complete menstrual cycle and the beginning of another are shown.

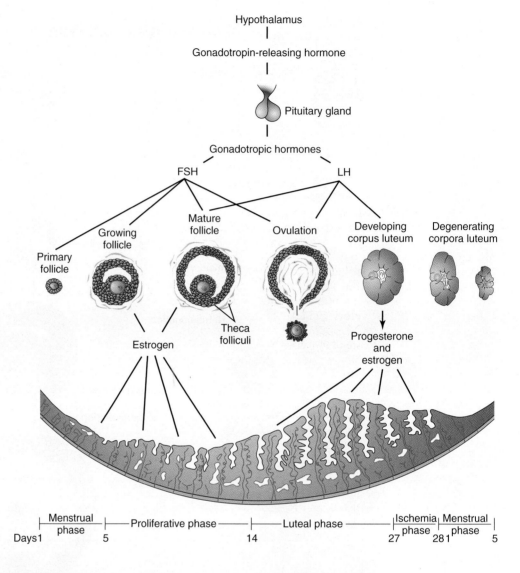

Hypothalamus

Gonadotropin-releasing hormone

Pituitary gland

Gonadotropic hormones

FSH   LH

Primary follicle

Growing follicle

Mature follicle

Ovulation

Developing corpus luteum

Degenerating corpora luteum

Theca folliculi

Estrogen

Progesterone and estrogen

| Menstrual phase | Proliferative phase | Luteal phase | Ischemia phase | Menstrual phase |

Days 1   5   14   27   28 1   5

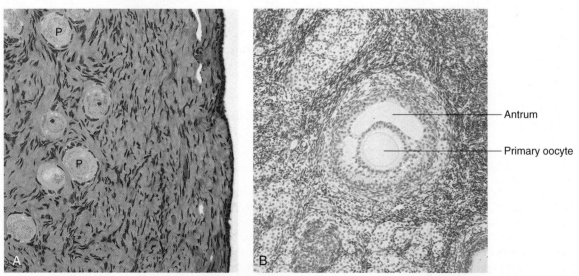

Figure 2–9 Photomicrographs of sections from adult human ovaries. **A,** Light micrograph of the ovarian cortex demonstrating primordial follicles *(P)*, which are primary oocytes surrounded by follicular cells (×270). **B,** Light micrograph of a secondary follicle. Observe the primary oocyte and antrum containing the follicular fluid (×132). *(From Gartner LP, Hiatt JL: Color Textbook of Histology, 2nd ed. Philadelphia, WB Saunders, 2001.)*

Antrum

Primary oocyte

- Formation of zona pellucida
- Development of a connective tissue capsule surrounding the follicle—the *theca folliculi*. Thecal cells are believed to produce an angiogenic factor that promotes growth of blood vessels that provide nutritive support for follicular development.

Ovulation

The follicular cells divide actively, producing a stratified layer around the oocyte (see Fig. 2-9*A* and *B*). Subsequently, fluid-filled spaces appear around the follicular cells, which coalesce to form a single cavity, the **antrum**, containing **follicular fluid**. When the antrum forms, the ovarian follicle is called a **secondary follicle** (see Fig. 2-9*B*). The primary oocyte is surrounded by follicular cells, called the **cumulus oophorus**, which projects into the enlarged antrum. The follicle continues to enlarge and soon forms a bulge on the surface of the ovary (Fig. 2-10*A*). A small, oval, avascular spot, the **stigma**, soon appears on this bulge. Before ovulation, the secondary oocyte and some cells of the cumulus oophorus detach from the interior of the distended follicle (see Fig. 2-10*B*).

Ovulation follows within 24 hours of a surge of LH production that appears to be the result of signaling molecules from the granulosa cells. This surge, elicited by the high estrogen level in blood (Fig. 2-11), appears to cause the stigma to rupture, expelling the secondary oocyte along with the follicular fluid (see Fig. 2-10*D*). Plasmins and matrix metalloproteinases also appear to have some control over stigma rupture.

The expelled secondary oocyte is surrounded by the **zona pellucida,** an acellular glycoprotein coat, and one or more layers of follicular cells, which are radially arranged to form the corona radiata (see Fig. 2-4*C*) and the cumulus oophorus.

Corpus Luteum

Shortly after ovulation, the ovarian follicle collapses (see Fig. 2-10*D*). Under the influence of LH, the walls of the follicle develop into a glandular structure, the **corpus luteum**, which secretes primarily progesterone, but also some estrogen.

If the oocyte is fertilized, the corpus luteum enlarges to form a *corpus luteum of pregnancy* and increases its hormone production. Degeneration of the corpus luteum is prevented by *human chorionic gonadotropin* (hCG) (see Chapter 4).

If the oocyte is not fertilized, the corpus luteum degenerates 10 to 12 days after ovulation. It is then called a *corpus luteum of menstruation*. The degenerated corpus luteum is subsequently transformed into white scar tissue in the ovary, forming the *corpus albicans*.

Menstrual Cycle

The menstrual cycle is the period during which the oocyte matures, is ovulated, and enters the uterine tube (Fig. 2-11). Estrogen and progesterone produced by the ovarian follicles and the corpus luteum cause cyclic changes in the endometrium of the uterus. These monthly changes in the uterine lining constitute the **menstrual cycle**. The average

MITTELSCHMERZ AND OVULATION

A variable amount of abdominal pain, called *mittelschmerz*, accompanies ovulation in some women. Mittelschmerz may be used as a sign of ovulation; however, there are better indicators, such as the slight drop in basal body temperature, followed by a sustained rise after ovulation.

ANOVULATION AND HORMONES

Some women do not ovulate because of an inadequate release of gonadotropins. In some of these women, ovulation can be induced by the administration of gonadotropins or an ovulatory agent, resulting in maturation of several ovarian follicles and multiple ovulations. The incidence of multiple pregnancy increases when ovulation is induced.

ANOVULATORY MENSTRUAL CYCLES

In anovulatory cycles, the endometrial changes are minimal; the proliferative endometrium develops as usual, but no ovulation occurs and no corpus luteum forms. Consequently, the endometrium does not progress to the luteal phase; it remains in the proliferative phase until menstruation begins. The estrogen in oral contraceptives, with or without progesterone, suppresses ovulation by acting on the hypothalamus and pituitary gland, inhibiting secretion of gonadotropin-releasing hormone, follicle-stimulating hormone, and luteinizing hormone.

menstrual cycle is 28 days (ranging from 23 to 35 days). Day 1 of the cycle corresponds to the day on which menstruation begins.

Phases of the Menstrual Cycle

The menstrual cycle is divided into three main phases for descriptive purposes only (see Fig. 2-11). In actuality, *the menstrual cycle is a continuous process*; each phase gradually passes into the next one. The reproductive cycles normally continue until the permanent cessation of the menses—**menopause**—which usually occurs between the ages of 48 and 55 years.

Menstrual Phase The first day of menstruation is the beginning of the menstrual phase. The functional layer of the uterine wall is sloughed off and discarded with the menstrual flow, which usually lasts 4 to 5 days. The menstrual flow, or **menses**, discharged through the vagina, consists of varying amounts of blood combined with

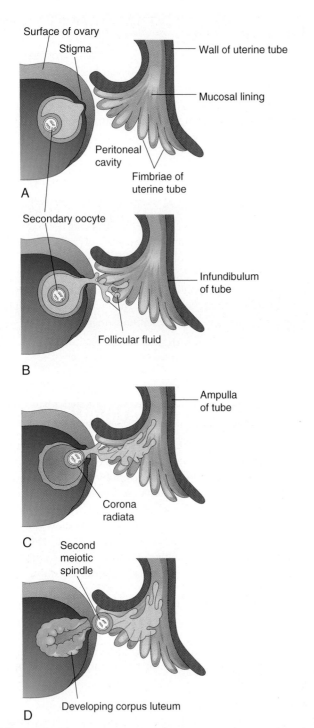

Figure 2–10 Diagrams **(A–D)** illustrating ovulation. When the stigma ruptures, the secondary oocyte is expelled from the ovarian follicle with the follicular fluid. After ovulation, the wall of the follicle collapses.

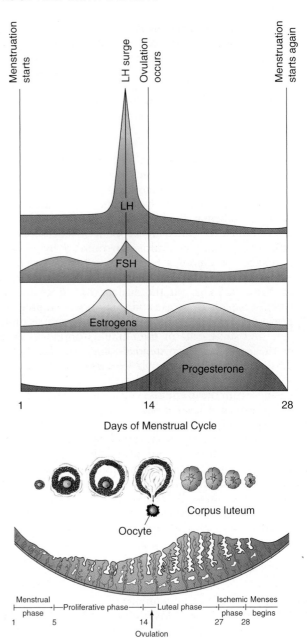

Figure 2–11 Blood levels of various hormones during the menstrual cycle. Follicle-stimulating hormone (FSH) stimulates the ovarian follicles to develop and produce estrogens. The level of estrogens rises to a peak just before the luteinizing hormone (LH) surge induces ovulation. Ovulation normally occurs within 24 hours after the LH surge. If fertilization does not occur, the blood levels of circulating estrogens and progesterone fall. This hormone withdrawal causes the endometrium to regress and menstruation to start again.

small pieces of endometrial tissue. After menstruation, the eroded endometrium is thin (see Fig. 2-11).

Proliferative Phase The proliferative phase, lasting approximately 9 days, coincides with growth of the ovarian follicles and is controlled by estrogen secreted by the follicles. There is a two- to three-fold increase in the

thickness of the endometrium during this time. Early during this phase, the surface epithelium of the endometrium regenerates. The glands increase in number and length, and the spiral arteries elongate (see Fig. 2-2C).

Luteal Phase The luteal (secretory) phase, lasting approximately 13 days, coincides with the formation, function, and growth of the corpus luteum. The progesterone produced by the corpus luteum stimulates the glandular epithelium to secrete a glycogen-rich, mucoid material. The glands become wide, tortuous, and saccular. The endometrium thickens because of the influence of progesterone and estrogen from the corpus luteum and the increase in fluid in the connective tissue.

If fertilization does not occur:

- The corpus luteum degenerates.
- Estrogen and progesterone levels decrease, and the endometrium enters an *ischemic phase.*
- Menstruation occurs.

Ischemia (reduced blood supply) of the spiral arteries occurs by constriction resulting from the decrease in the secretion of progesterone. Hormone withdrawal also results in the stoppage of glandular secretions, a loss of interstitial fluid, and a marked shrinking of the endometrium. As the spiral arteries constrict for longer periods, venous stasis and patchy ischemic necrosis (death) in the superficial tissues occur. Eventually, rupture of vessel walls follows, and blood seeps into the surrounding connective tissue. Small pools of blood form and break through the endometrial surface, resulting in bleeding into the uterus and vagina.

As small pieces of the endometrium detach and pass into the uterine cavity, the torn ends of the spiral arteries bleed into the uterine cavity, resulting in an accumulated loss of 20 to 80 mL of blood. Over 3 to 5 days, the entire compact layer and most of the spongy layer of the endometrium are discarded.

If fertilization occurs:

- Cleavage of the zygote and formation of the blastocyst occur.
- The blastocyst begins to implant on approximately the sixth day of the luteal phase.
- hCG maintains secretion of estrogens and progesterone by the corpus luteum.
- The luteal phase continues and menstruation does not occur.

During pregnancy, the menstrual cycles cease and the endometrium passes into a pregnancy phase. With the termination of pregnancy, the ovarian and menstrual cycles resume after a variable amount of time.

 ## TRANSPORTATION OF GAMETES

Oocyte Transport

During ovulation, the fimbriated (fringed) end of the uterine tube comes in close proximity to the ovary (see Fig. 2-10). The fingerlike processes of the tube, the *fimbriae,* move back and forth over the ovary. The sweeping action of the fimbriae and the fluid currents produced by them "sweep" the secondary oocyte into the funnel-shaped infundibulum of the tube (see Fig. 2-2B). The oocyte then passes into the ampulla of the tube, primarily as a result of waves of *peristalsis*—movements of the wall of the tube characterized by alternate contraction and relaxation.

Sperm Transport

During ejaculation, sperms are rapidly transported, from their storage site in the epididymis (see Fig. 2-1B) to the urethra by peristaltic contractions of the ductus deferens. Secretions from the *seminal glands, prostate,* and *bulbourethral glands* and the sperms form the **semen** (ejaculate). The number of sperms ejaculated ranges from 200 to 600 million. The sperms pass slowly through the cervical canal by movements of their tails. *Vesiculase,* an enzyme produced by the seminal glands, coagulates some of the *semen* and forms a vaginal plug that may prevent backflow of semen into the vagina. At the time of ovulation, the amount of cervical mucus increases and becomes less viscid, making it more favorable for sperm transport. *Prostaglandins* in the semen stimulate uterine motility and help to move the sperms through the uterus to the site of fertilization in the uterine tube.

The sperms move 2 to 3 mm per minute. They move slowly in the acid environment of the vagina, but more rapidly in the alkaline environment of the uterus. Approximately 200 sperms reach the fertilization site in the uterine tube.

SPERM COUNTS

Semen analysis is an important part of evaluating patients for infertility. Sperms account for less than 5% of the volume of semen. The remainder of the ejaculate consists of the secretions of the seminal glands (60%), prostate (30%), and bulbourethral glands (5%). The ejaculate of normal males usually contains more than 100 million sperms per milliliter of semen. Although there is much variation in individual cases, men whose semen contains a minimum of 20 million sperms per milliliter, or 50 million in the total specimen, are probably fertile. A man with less than 10 million sperms per milliliter of semen is likely to be sterile, especially when the specimen contains immotile and abnormal sperms. For potential fertility, at least 40% of sperms should be motile after 2 hours, and some should be motile after 24 hours. Male infertility may result from endocrine disorders, abnormal spermatogenesis, or obstruction of a genital duct (e.g., the ductus deferens). Male infertility is found in 30% to 50% of involuntary childless couples.

VASECTOMY

An effective method of contraception in males is **vasectomy**—excision of a segment of the ductus deferens (vas deferens). Two to 3 weeks after vasectomy, there are no sperms in the ejaculate, but the amount of seminal fluid is the same as before the procedure.

MATURATION OF SPERMS

Freshly ejaculated sperms are unable to fertilize oocytes. They must undergo a period of conditioning—**capacitation**—lasting approximately 7 hours. During this period, a glycoprotein coat and seminal proteins are removed from the surface of the sperm acrosome. *Capacitation and the acrosome reaction are regulated by src kinase, a tyrosine kinase.* Capacitated sperms show no morphologic changes, but they exhibit increased activity. Sperms are usually capacitated in the uterus or the uterine tubes by substances (including interleukin-6) secreted by these organs.

VIABILITY OF OOCYTES AND SPERMS

Oocytes in the uterine tube are usually fertilized within 12 hours of ovulation. In vitro observations have shown that oocytes cannot be fertilized after 24 hours, and they degenerate shortly thereafter. Most sperms probably do not survive for more than 24 hours in the female genital tract. Some sperms are captured in folds of the mucosa of the cervix and are gradually released into the cervical canal and pass through the uterus into the uterine tubes. Semen and oocytes can be stored frozen for many years to be used in assisted reproduction.

CLINICALLY ORIENTED QUESTIONS

1. There have been reports of a woman who claimed that she menstruated throughout her pregnancy. How could this happen?

2. If a woman forgets to take an oral contraceptive and then takes two, is she likely to become pregnant?

3. What is *coitus interruptus*? Some people believe that it is an effective method of birth control. Is this true?

4. What is the difference between spermatogenesis and spermiogenesis?

5. Some say that an intrauterine device (IUD) is a contraceptive. Is this correct?

The answers to these questions are at the back of the book.

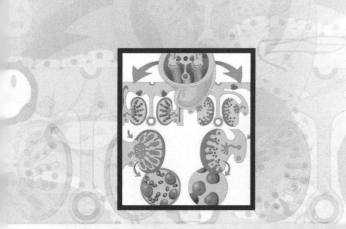

First Week of Development

A zygote, formed by the union of a **sperm** and an **oocyte**, is a highly specialized, totipotent cell. It contains chromosomes and genes derived from the mother and father. The zygote divides many times and is progressively transformed into a multicellular human being through cell division, migration, growth, and differentiation.

FERTILIZATION

The usual site of fertilization is in the ampulla of the uterine tube (see Fig. 2-2*B*). If the oocyte is not fertilized here, it slowly passes along the tube into the cavity of the uterus, where it degenerates and is resorbed.

Fertilization is a complex sequence of coordinated molecular events that begins with the contact between a sperm and an oocyte (Fig. 3-1) Fertilization ends with the intermingling of maternal and paternal chromosomes at metaphase of the first mitotic division of the **zygote** (see Fig. 2-5). Carbohydrate- and protein-binding molecules on the surface of the gametes are involved in sperm chemotaxis and gamete recognition, as well as in the process of fertilization.

Phases of Fertilization

The phases of fertilization follow (Figs. 3-1 and 3-2):

● Passage of a sperm through the corona radiata of the oocyte. Dispersal of the follicular cells of the corona radiata results mainly from the action of the enzyme *hyaluronidase*, which is released from the acrosome of the sperm. *Tubal mucosal enzymes* also appear to assist hyaluronidase. Additionally, movements of the tail of the sperm are important during penetration of the corona radiata.

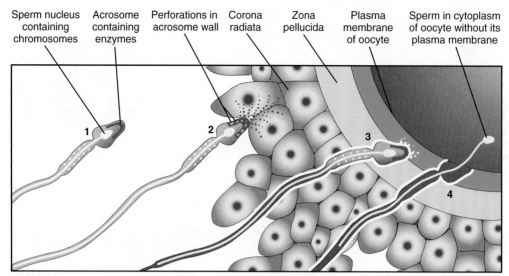

Sperm nucleus containing chromosomes · Acrosome containing enzymes · Perforations in acrosome wall · Corona radiata · Zona pellucida · Plasma membrane of oocyte · Sperm in cytoplasm of oocyte without its plasma membrane

Figure 3–1 Acrosome reaction and sperm penetration of an oocyte. *1*, Sperm during capacitation. *2*, Sperm undergoing the acrosome reaction. *3*, Sperm forming a path through the zona pellucida. *4*, Sperm entering the cytoplasm of the oocyte.

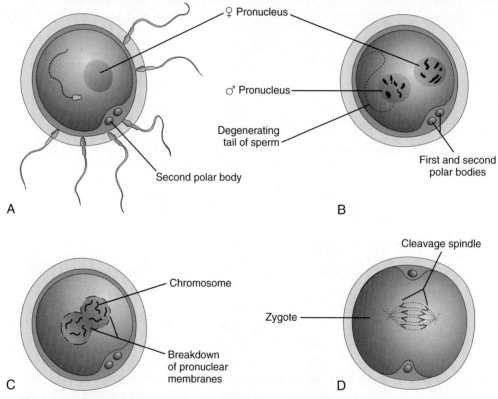

♀ Pronucleus · ♂ Pronucleus · Degenerating tail of sperm · Second polar body · First and second polar bodies · Chromosome · Breakdown of pronuclear membranes · Cleavage spindle · Zygote

A   B   C   D

Figure 3–2 Illustrations of fertilization. **A,** A sperm has entered the oocyte and the second meiotic division has occurred, resulting in the formation of a mature oocyte. The nucleus of the oocyte is now the female pronucleus. **B,** The sperm head has enlarged to form the male pronucleus. **C,** The pronuclei are fusing. **D,** The zygote has formed.

● Penetration of the zona pellucida. The formation of a pathway through the zona pellucida for the sperm results from the action of enzymes released from the acrosome. The proteolytic enzyme *acrosin* (as well as *esterases* and *neuraminidase*) appear to cause lysis of the zona pellucida, thereby forming a path for the sperm to follow to the oocyte.

● Fusion of the plasma cell membranes of the oocyte and sperm. Once the fusion occurs, the contents of cortical granules are released into the perivitelline space, resulting in changes in the zona pellucida. This change prevents other sperms from entering. The cell membranes break down at the area of fusion. The head and tail of the sperm then enter the cytoplasm of the

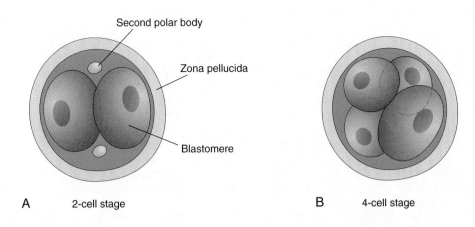

A   2-cell stage

Second polar body

Zona pellucida

Blastomere

B   4-cell stage

Figure 3–3 Illustrations showing cleavage of the zygote and formation of the blastocyst. **A–D** show various stages of cleavage. The period of the morula begins at the 12- to 32-cell stage and ends when the blastocyst forms. **E** and **F** show sections of blastocysts. The zona pellucida disappears by the late blastocyst stage (5 days). Although cleavage increases the number of blastomeres, note that each of the daughter cells is smaller than the parent cells. As a result, there is no increase in the size of the developing embryo until the zona pellucida degenerates.

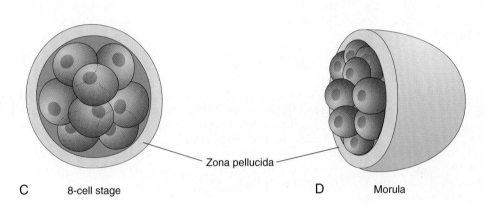

C   8-cell stage

Zona pellucida

D   Morula

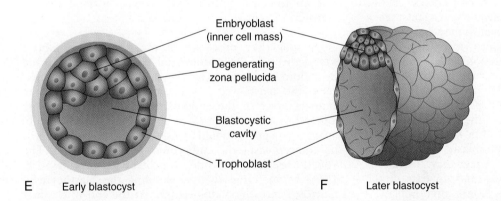

E   Early blastocyst

Embryoblast (inner cell mass)

Degenerating zona pellucida

Blastocystic cavity

Trophoblast

F   Later blastocyst

oocyte, but the plasma membrane and mitochondria of the sperm remains behind (see Figs. 3-1 and 3-2A).

- Completion of the second meiotic division of the oocyte. The oocyte completes the second meiotic division and forms a mature oocyte and a second polar body (see Fig. 3-2A). The nucleus of the mature oocyte becomes the female pronucleus.
- Formation of the male pronucleus. Within the cytoplasm of the oocyte, the nucleus of the sperm enlarges to form the male pronucleus. The tail of the sperm degenerates (see Fig. 3-2B). During growth, the male and female pronuclei replicate their DNA (Fig. 3-2C).
- Breakdown of the pronuclear membranes. Condensation of the chromosomes, arrangement of the

chromosomes for mitotic cell division, and the first cleavage division of the zygote occur (see Figs. 3-2D and 3-3A). The combination of 23 chromosomes in each pronucleus results in a zygote with 46 chromosomes.

Results of Fertilization

Fertilization:

- Stimulates the secondary oocyte to complete the second meiotic division, producing the second polar body

- Restores the normal diploid number of chromosomes (46) in the zygote
- Results in variation of the human species through mingling of maternal and paternal chromosomes
- Determines the chromosomal sex of the embryo; an X-bearing sperm produces a female embryo and a Y-bearing sperm produces a male embryo
- Causes metabolic activation of the oocyte, which initiates cleavage of the zygote

The zygote is genetically unique because half of its chromosomes come from the mother and half are derived from the father. This mechanism forms the basis for biparental inheritance and variation of the human species. Meiosis allows independent assortment of maternal and paternal chromosomes among the germ cells. Crossing over of chromosomes, by relocating segments of the maternal and paternal chromosomes, "shuffles" the genes, thereby producing a recombination of genetic material (see Fig. 2-6).

CLEAVAGE OF ZYGOTE

Cleavage consists of repeated mitotic divisions of the zygote, resulting in a rapid increase in the number of cells, now called **blastomeres**. Division of the zygote begins approximately 30 hours after fertilization. These blastomeres become smaller with each cleavage division (Fig. 3-3A to D). During cleavage, the zygote is still surrounded by the zona pellucida.

After the eight-cell stage, the blastomeres change their shape and tightly align themselves against each other—**compaction**. This phenomenon may be mediated by cell surface adhesion glycoproteins. Compaction permits greater cell-to-cell interaction and is a prerequisite for segregation of the internal cells that form the inner cell mass (see Fig. 3-3E). When there are 12 to 32 blastomeres, the conceptus is called a **morula**. The inner cells of the morula—the **embryoblast or inner cell mass**—are surrounded by a layer of flattened blastomeres that form the trophoblast. An immunosuppressant protein—the **early pregnancy factor**—is secreted by the trophoblastic cells and appears in the maternal serum within 24 to 48 hours after implantation. The early pregnancy factor forms the basis for a pregnancy test applicable during the first 10 days of development.

FORMATION OF BLASTOCYST

Shortly after the morula enters the uterus (approximately 4 days after fertilization), uterine fluid passes through the zona pellucida to form a fluid-filled space—the **blastocystic cavity**—inside the morula (see Fig. 3-3E). As fluid increases in the cavity, the blastomeres are separated into two parts:

- The trophoblast, the thin outer cells that give rise to the embryonic part of the placenta
- The embryoblast, a discrete group of blastomeres that is the primordium of the embryo

At this stage, the conceptus, or embryo, is called a **blastocyst**. The embryoblast now projects into the blastocystic cavity, and the trophoblast forms the wall of the blastocyst (see Fig. 3-3E and F). After the blastocyst has floated in the uterine fluid for approximately 2 days, the zona pellucida degenerates and disappears. Shedding of the zona pellucida has been observed in vitro. The shedding permits the blastocyst to increase rapidly in size. While floating freely in the uterine cavity, the blastocyst derives nourishment from secretions of the uterine glands.

Approximately 6 days after fertilization, the blastocyst attaches to the endometrial epithelium (Fig. 3-4A). As soon as it attaches to the epithelium, the trophoblast starts to proliferate rapidly and differentiate into two layers (Fig. 3-4B):

- The cytotrophoblast, the inner layer of cells
- The syncytiotrophoblast, the outer layer consisting of a multinucleate protoplasmic mass formed by the fusion of cells

The fingerlike processes of the syncytiotrophoblast extend through the endometrial epithelium and invade the endometrial connective tissue. By the end of the first week, the blastocyst is superficially implanted in the compact layer of the endometrium and is deriving its nourishment from the eroded maternal tissues. The highly invasive syncytiotrophoblast rapidly expands adjacent to the embryoblast—the **embryonic pole** (Fig. 3-4A). The syncytiotrophoblast produces proteolytic enzymes that erode the maternal tissues, enabling the blastocyst to "burrow" into the endometrium. At the end of the first week, a cuboidal layer of cells, called the **hypoblast**, appears on the surface of the embryoblast, facing the blastocystic cavity (see Fig. 3-4B).

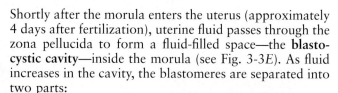

IN VITRO FERTILIZATION AND EMBRYO TRANSFER

The process of in vitro fertilization (IVF) of oocytes and transfer of either the dividing zygotes or a blastocyst into the uterus has provided an opportunity for many couples who are infertile. The first of these IVF babies was born in 1978. The steps involved in IVF and embryo transfer are summarized in Figure 3-5. The incidence of multiple pregnancies is higher with IVF than when pregnancy results from normal ovulation. The incidence of spontaneous abortion of transferred embryos is also higher with IVF.

The technique of **intracytoplasmic sperm injection** involves injecting a sperm directly into the cytoplasm of the mature oocyte. This procedure is invaluable in cases of infertility resulting from blocked uterine tubes or oligospermia (reduced number of sperms).

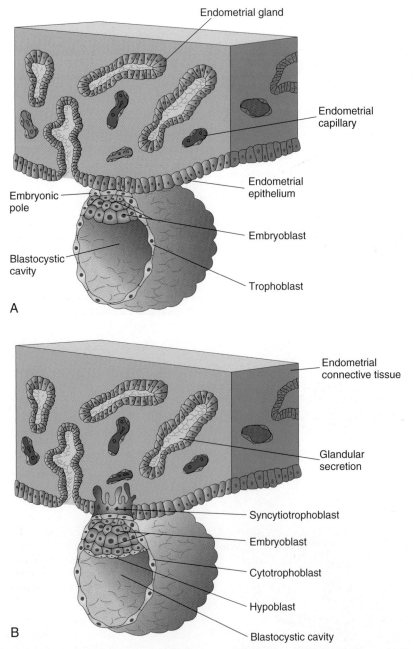

Figure 3–4 Attachment of the blastocyst to the endometrial epithelium during the early stages of its implantation. **A,** At 6 days, the trophoblast is attached to the endometrial epithelium at the embryonic pole of the blastocyst. **B,** At 7 days, the syncytiotrophoblast has penetrated the epithelium and has started to invade the endometrial connective tissue.

PREIMPLANTATION DIAGNOSIS OF GENETIC DISORDERS

Using currently available techniques, a cleaving zygote known to be at risk for a specific genetic disorder may be diagnosed before implantation during IVF. The sex of the embryo can be determined from a blastomere taken from a six- to eight-cell zygote and analyzed by DNA amplification of sequences from the Y chromosome. This procedure has been used to determine chromosomal sex in cases in which a male embryo would be at risk for a serious X-linked disorder. The polar body may also be tested for disorders when the mother is the carrier.

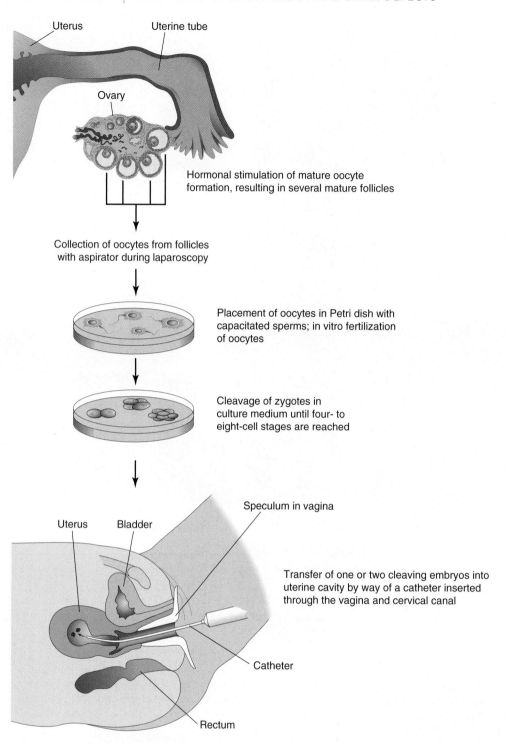

Figure 3–5 In vitro fertilization and embryo transfer procedures.

ABNORMAL EMBRYOS AND SPONTANEOUS ABORTIONS

Many early embryos abort spontaneously. The early implantation stages of the blastocyst are critical periods of development that may fail to occur because of inadequate production of progesterone and estrogen by the corpus luteum (see Fig. 2-8). Clinicians occasionally see a patient whose last menstrual period was delayed by several days and whose last menstrual flow was unusually profuse. Very likely, such patients have had an early spontaneous abortion. The overall early spontaneous abortion rate is believed to be approximately 45%. Early spontaneous abortions occur for a variety of reasons, an important one being the presence of **chromosomal abnormalities**.

CLINICALLY ORIENTED QUESTIONS

1. Although women do not commonly become pregnant after they are 48 years old, very elderly men may still be fertile. Why is this? Is there an increased risk of Down syndrome or other congenital anomalies in the child when the father is older than 50 years of age?

2. Are there oral contraceptives for men? If not, what is the reason?

3. Is a polar body ever fertilized? If so, does the fertilized polar body give rise to a viable embryo?

4. What is the most common cause of spontaneous abortion during the first week of development?

5. Could a woman have dissimilar twins as a result of one oocyte being fertilized by a sperm from one man and another one being fertilized by a sperm from another man?

6. When referring to a zygote, do the terms *cleavage* and *mitosis* mean the same thing?

7. How is the cleaving zygote nourished during the first week?

8. Is it possible to determine the sex of a cleaving zygote developing in vitro? If so, what medical reasons would there be for doing so?

The answers to these questions are at the back of the book.

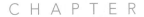

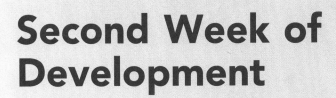

Second Week of Development

I mplantation of the blastocyst is completed during the second week of development. As this process takes place, changes occur, producing a bilaminar embryonic disc composed of two layers, the epiblast and hypoblast (Fig. 4-1A). The **embryonic disc** gives rise to germ layers that form all the tissues and organs of the embryo. Extraembryonic structures forming during the second week include the amniotic cavity, amnion, umbilical vesicle (yolk sac), connecting stalk, and chorionic sac.

Implantation of the blastocyst begins at the end of the first week and normally occurs in the endometrium, usually superiorly in the body of the uterus and slightly more often on the posterior than on the anterior wall. The actively erosive **syncytiotrophoblast** invades the endometrial connective tissue that supports the uterine capillaries and glands. As this occurs, the blastocyst slowly embeds itself in the endometrium. Syncytiotrophoblastic cells from this region displace endometrial cells in the central part of the implantation site. The endometrial cells undergo *apoptosis* (programmed cell death), which facilitates implantation. Proteolytic enzymes produced by the syncytiotrophoblast are involved in this process. The uterine connective tissue cells around the implantation site become loaded with glycogen and lipids. Some of these cells—**decidual cells**—degenerate adjacent to the penetrating syncytiotrophoblast. The syncytiotrophoblast engulfs these degenerating cells, providing a rich source of *embryonic nutrition*. As the blastocyst implants, more trophoblast contacts the endometrium and continues to differentiate into two layers (see Fig. 4-1A):

- The cytotrophoblast, a layer of mononucleated cells that is mitotically active. It forms new trophoblastic cells that migrate into the increasing mass of syncytiotrophoblast, where they fuse and lose their cell membranes.
- The syncytiotrophoblast, a rapidly expanding, multinucleated mass in which no cell boundaries are discernible.

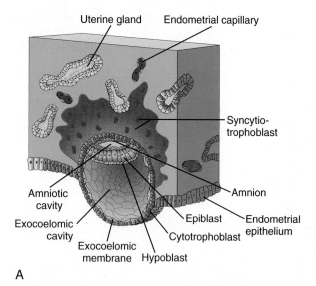

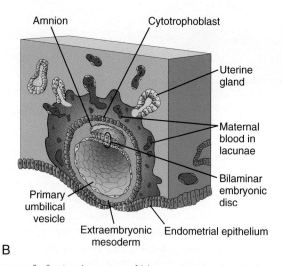

Figure 4–1 Implantation of blastocyst. The actual size of the conceptus is approximately 0.1 mm. **A,** Illustration of a section of a partially implanted blastocyst (approximately 8 days after fertilization). Note the slitlike amniotic cavity. **B,** Illustration of a section through a blastocyst at approximately 9 days.

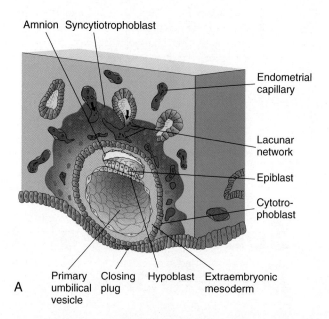

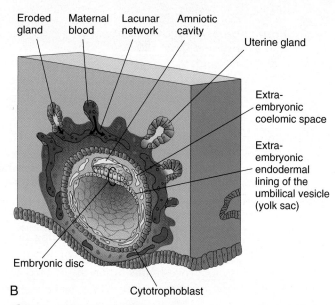

Figure 4–2 Illustration of sections of two implanted blastocysts at 10 days **(A)** and 12 days **(B)**.

The syncytiotrophoblast produces a hormone, **human chorionic gonadotropin (hCG)**, which enters the maternal blood in the lacunae in the syncytiotrophoblast (see Fig. 4-1B). hCG maintains the development of spiral arteries in the myometrium and formation of the syncytiotrophoblast. It also forms the basis for pregnancy tests. Highly sensitive radioimmunoassays are available for detecting hCG at the end of the second week even though the woman is probably unaware that she is pregnant.

FORMATION OF AMNIOTIC CAVITY AND EMBRYONIC DISC

As implantation of the blastocyst progresses, changes occurring in the embryoblast result in the formation of a flattened, almost circular, bilaminar plate of cells—the embryonic disc—consisting of two layers (Figs. 4-1A and 4-2B):

- The **epiblast**, the thicker layer, consists of high, columnar cells related to the amniotic cavity.
- The **hypoblast**, the thinner layer, consists of small, cuboidal cells adjacent to the exocoelomic cavity (the primordium of the umbilical vesicle).

Concurrently, a small cavity appears in the embryoblast, which is the primordium of the **amniotic cavity** (see Fig. 4-1A). Soon, amniogenic (amnion-forming) cells called *amnioblasts* separate from the epiblast and organize to form a thin membrane, the **amnion**, which encloses the amniotic cavity.

The epiblast forms the floor of the amniotic cavity and is continuous peripherally with the amnion. The hypoblast forms the roof of the **exocoelomic cavity** and is continuous with the cells that migrated from the hypoblast to form the **exocoelomic membrane**. This membrane surrounds the blastocystic cavity and lines the internal surface of the cytotrophoblast.

The exocoelomic membrane and cavity soon become modified to form the **primary umbilical vesicle** (the primary yolk sac). The embryonic disc then lies between the amniotic cavity and the primary umbilical vesicle (Fig. 4-1B). The outer layer of cells from the umbilical vesicle endoderm forms a layer of loosely arranged connective tissue, the **extraembryonic mesoderm** (Fig. 4-1B).

As the amnion, embryonic disc, and primary umbilical vesicle form, isolated cavities called **lacunae** appear in the syncytiotrophoblast (see Figs. 4-1B and 4-2). The lacunae are soon filled with a mixture of maternal blood from ruptured endometrial capillaries and cellular debris from eroded uterine glands. The fluid in the lacunae, sometimes called *embryotroph*, passes to the embryonic disc by diffusion. The communication of the eroded uterine vessels with the lacunae represents the *beginning of uteroplacental circulation*. When maternal blood flows into the lacunae, oxygen and nutritive substances become available to the extraembryonic tissues over the large surface of the syncytiotrophoblast. Oxygenated blood passes into the lacunae from the spiral endometrial arteries in the endometrium; deoxygenated blood is removed from the lacunae through endometrial veins.

The 10-day embryo is completely embedded in the endometrium (Fig. 4-2A). For approximately 2 more days, there is a defect in the endometrial epithelium that is filled by a **closing plug**, a fibrinous coagulum of blood. By day 12, an almost completely regenerated uterine epithelium covers the closing plug (Fig. 4-2B).

As the conceptus (the embryo and its membranes) implants, the endometrial connective tissue cells undergo a transformation known as the **decidual reaction** resulting from cAMP and progesterone signaling. The cells swell because of the accumulation of glycogen and lipid in their cytoplasm, and they are then known as *secretory decidual cells*. The primary function of the decidual reaction is to provide an immunologically privileged site for the conceptus.

In a *12-day embryo*, adjacent syncytiotrophoblastic lacunae have fused to form **lacunar networks** (Fig. 4-2B), the *primordia of the intervillous space of the placenta* (see Chapter 8). The endometrial capillaries around the implanted embryo become congested and dilated to form sinusoids, which are thin-walled terminal vessels that are larger than ordinary capillaries. The syncytiotrophoblast then erodes the sinusoids and maternal blood flows into the lacunar networks. The degenerated endometrial stromal cells and glands, together with the maternal blood, provide a rich source of material for *embryonic nutrition*. Growth of the bilaminar embryonic disc is slow compared with the growth of the trophoblast.

As changes occur in the trophoblast and endometrium, the extraembryonic mesoderm increases and isolated **extraembryonic coelomic spaces** appear within

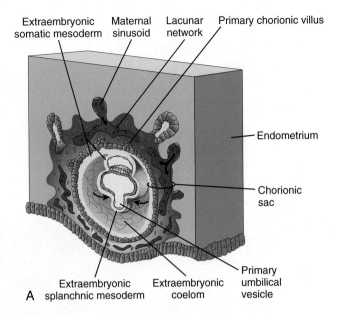

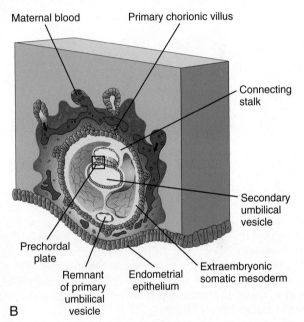

Figure 4–3 Sections of implanted embryos. **A,** At 13 days. Note the decrease in the relative size of the primary umbilical vesicle (yolk sac) and the appearance of primary chorionic villi. **B,** At 14 days. Note the newly formed secondary umbilical vesicle.

it (Fig. 4-2B). These spaces rapidly fuse to form a large, isolated cavity, the **extraembryonic coelom** (Fig. 4-3A). This fluid-filled cavity surrounds the amnion and the umbilical vesicle, except where they are attached to the **chorion** by the **connecting stalk**. As the extraembryonic coelom forms, the primary umbilical vesicle decreases in size and a smaller, **secondary umbilical vesicle** forms (Fig. 4-3B). During formation of the secondary umbilical vesicle, a large part of the primary umbilical vesicle is pinched off. The human umbilical vesicle (yolk sac) contains no yolk. It may have a role in the selective transfer of nutritive materials to the embryonic disc.

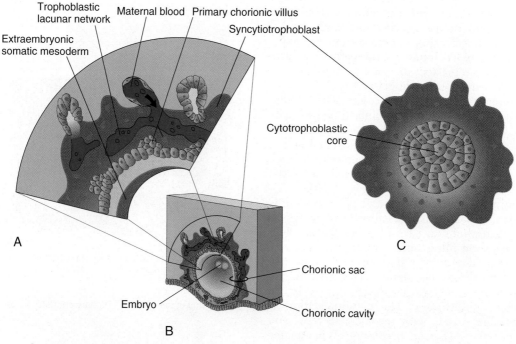

Figure 4–4   **A,** Illustration of a section of the wall of the chorionic sac. **B,** Illustration of a 14-day conceptus showing the chorionic sac and the chorionic cavity. **C,** Transverse section through a primary chorionic villus.

 DEVELOPMENT OF CHORIONIC SAC

The end of the second week is characterized by the appearance of **primary chorionic villi** (Figs. 4-3*A* and 4-4*A* and *C*). Proliferation of the cytotrophoblastic cells produces cellular extensions that grow into the overlying syncytiotrophoblast. The cellular projections form primary chorionic villi, the first stage in the development of the chorionic villi of the placenta. The extraembryonic coelom splits the extraembryonic mesoderm into two layers (Fig. 4-3*A* and *B*):

● The *extraembryonic somatic mesoderm*, which lines the trophoblast and covers the amnion

● The *extraembryonic splanchnic mesoderm*, which surrounds the umbilical vesicle

The growth of these cytotrophoblastic extensions is believed to be induced by the underlying **extraembryonic somatic mesoderm**. The extraembryonic somatic mesoderm and the two layers of trophoblast form the **chorion**. The chorion forms the wall of the chorionic sac (Fig. 4-3*A*). The embryo, amniotic sac, and umbilical vesicle are suspended in the **chorionic cavity** by the connecting stalk (Figs. 4-3*B* and 4-4*B*). Transvaginal ultrasonography (endovaginal sonography) is used to measure the diameter of the chorionic sac. This measurement is valuable for evaluating early embryonic development and pregnancy outcome.

EXTRAUTERINE IMPLANTATION SITES

Blastocysts may implant outside the uterus resulting in **ectopic pregnancies;** most ectopic implantations occur in the uterine tube (Figs. 2-2*B* and 4-5*A* and *B*). Ectopic tubal pregnancy occurs in approximately 1 in 200 pregnancies in North America. A woman with a tubal pregnancy has the usual signs and symptoms of pregnancy, but she may also experience abdominal pain (from distention of the uterine tube), abnormal bleeding, and irritation of the pelvic peritoneum.

The *causes of tubal pregnancy* are often related to factors that delay or prevent transport of the cleaving zygote to the uterus (e.g., blockage of the uterine tube). Ectopic tubal pregnancies usually result in rupture of the uterine tube and hemorrhage into the peritoneal cavity during the first 8 weeks, followed by death of the embryo.

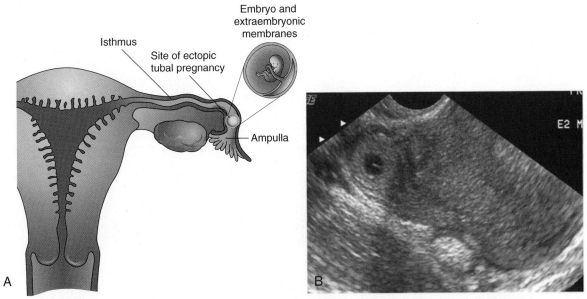

Figure 4–5 **A,** Coronal section of the uterus and uterine tube illustrating an ectopic pregnancy in the ampulla of the uterine tube. **B,** Endovaginal axial scan of the uterine fundus and isthmic portion of the right uterine tube The ring-like mass is a 4-week ectopic chorionic (gestational) sac in the tube *(arrow)* (*B, Courtesy E. A. Lyons, MD, Department of Radiology, Health Sciences Centre, University of Manitoba, Winnipeg, Manitoba, Canada.)*

INHIBITION OF IMPLANTATION

The administration of relatively *large doses of estrogen* ("morning-after pills") for several days, beginning shortly after unprotected sexual intercourse, usually does not prevent fertilization, but it often prevents implantation of the blastocyst. Normally, the endometrium progresses to the luteal phase of the menstrual cycle as the zygote forms, undergoes cleavage, and enters the uterus. A large amount of estrogen, however, disturbs the normal balance between estrogen and progesterone that is necessary to prepare the endometrium for implantation.

An **intrauterine device** inserted into the uterus through the vagina and cervix usually interferes with implantation by causing a local inflammatory reaction. Some intrauterine devices contain slow-release progesterone, which interferes with the development of the endometrium so that implantation does not usually occur. Copper-based IUDs appear to inhibit sperm tubal migration, while levonorgestrol-based IUDs alter the quality of cervical mucus and endometrial development.

CLINICALLY ORIENTED QUESTIONS

1. What is meant by the term *implantation bleeding*? Is this the same as *menses* (menstrual fluid)?
2. Can a drug taken during the first 2 weeks of pregnancy cause abortion of the embryo?
3. Can an ectopic pregnancy occur in a woman who has an intrauterine device?
4. Can a blastocyst that implants in the abdomen develop into a full-term fetus?

The answers to these questions are at the back of the book.

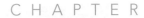

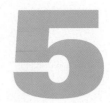

CHAPTER

5

Third Week of Development

R apid development of the embryo from the embryonic disc is characterized by the following:

- Appearance of the primitive streak
- Development of the notochord
- Differentiation of three germ layers

The third week of embryonic development occurs during the week of the first missed menstrual period, that is, the fifth week after the onset of the last normal menstrual period. Cessation of menstruation is usually an indication that conception has occurred. Approximately 3 weeks after conception, a normal pregnancy can be detected with ultrasonography (Fig. 5-1).

 GASTRULATION: FORMATION OF GERM LAYERS

Gastrulation is the process by which the bilaminar embryonic disc (Fig. 5-2*A* to *H*) is converted into a trilaminar embryonic disc. Each of the three germ layers (ectoderm, endoderm, and mesoderm) of the embryonic disc gives rise to specific tissues and organs (see Fig. 6-4). Gastrulation is the beginning of **morphogenesis** (development of the form and structure of various organs and parts of the body). This process begins with the formation of the **primitive streak** (see Fig. 5-2*B* and *C*).

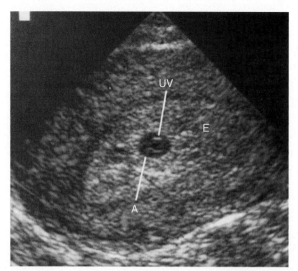

Figure 5–1 Endovaginal ultrasonogram of a conceptus 3 weeks after conception implanted in the posterior endometrium, showing the umbilical vesicle. The endometrium completely surrounds the conceptus. *A,* Amnion; *UV,* umbilical sac; *E,* endometrium. *(Courtesy E. A. Lyons, MD, Professor of Radiology, and Obstetrics and Gynecology, and Anatomy, Health Sciences Centre and University of Manitoba, Winnipeg, Manitoba, Canada.)*

 ## Primitive Streak

At the beginning of the third week, a thickened linear band of epiblast, the **primitive streak**, appears caudally in the median plane of the dorsal aspect of the embryonic disc (Fig. *5-2B*). The primitive streak results from proliferation and migration of cells of the epiblast to the median plane of the embryonic disc (Fig. *5-2D*). As the primitive streak elongates by the addition of cells to its caudal end, its cranial end proliferates to form the **primitive node** (Fig. *5-2E* and *F*). Concurrently, a narrow **primitive groove** develops in the primitive streak that ends in a small depression in the primitive node, the **primitive pit** (Fig. *5-2F*). As soon as the primitive streak appears, it is possible to identify the embryo's craniocaudal axis (cranial and caudal ends), dorsal and ventral surfaces, and right and left sides. Shortly after the primitive streak appears, cells leave its deep surface and form **mesoblast**, a loose network of embryonic connective tissue known as mesenchyme (Figs. *5-2H* and *5-3B* and *C*) that forms the supporting tissues of the embryo.

Under the influence of various embryonic growth factors, including BMP signaling, epiblast cells migrate through the primitive groove to become endoderm and mesoderm. Mesenchymal cells have the potential to proliferate and differentiate into diverse types of cells, such as fibroblasts, chondroblasts, and osteoblasts. *Recent studies indicate that signaling molecules (nodal factors) of the transforming growth factor β (TGF-β) superfamily induce the formation of mesoderm.*

The *primitive streak* actively forms **mesoderm** until the early part of the fourth week; thereafter, its production slows down. The streak diminishes in relative size and becomes an insignificant structure in the sacrococcygeal region of the embryo (Fig. *5-4A* to *D*).

 ## Notochordal Process and Notochord

Some mesenchymal cells migrate cranially from the primitive node and pit, forming a median cellular cord, the **notochordal process** (Figs. *5-2 G, 5-4B* to *D,* and *5-5A* to *C*). This process soon acquires a lumen, the **notochordal canal** (Fig. *5-5C* and *D*). The notochordal process grows cranially between the ectoderm and endoderm until it reaches the **prechordal plate**, a small, circular area of cells that is an important organizer of the head region (Fig. *5-2C*). The rod-like notochordal process can extend no farther because the prechordal plate is firmly attached to the overlying ectoderm. Fused layers of ectoderm and endoderm form the **oropharyngeal membrane** (Fig. *5-6C*) located at the future site of the oral cavity (mouth).

Some mesenchymal cells from the primitive streak and the notochordal process migrate laterally and cranially between the ectoderm and endoderm until they reach the margins of the embryonic disc. These mesenchymal cells are continuous with the extraembryonic mesoderm that covers the amnion and the umbilical vesicle (Fig. *5-2D* and *F*). Some cells from the primitive streak migrate cranially on each side of the notochordal process and around the prechordal plate. They meet cranially to form the cardiogenic mesoderm in the **cardiogenic area**, where the primordium of the heart begins to develop at the end of the third week. Caudal to the primitive streak there is a circular area—the **cloacal membrane**—that indicates the future site of the anus (Fig. *5-6D*).

The **notochord** is a cellular rod that:

- Further defines the axis of the embryo and gives it some rigidity
- Serves as the basis for the development of the axial skeleton (such as the bones of the head and vertebral column)
- Indicates the future site of the vertebral bodies

The **vertebral column** forms around the notochord, which extends from the oropharyngeal membrane to the primitive node. The notochord degenerates and disappears as the bodies of the vertebrae form, but parts of it persist as the *nucleus pulposus* of each intervertebral disc. The notochord functions as the primary inductor in the early embryo. It induces the overlying embryonic ectoderm to thicken and form the **neural plate** (see Figs. *5-4B* and *C* and *5-6A* to *C*), the primordium of the central nervous system.

Allantois

The **allantois** appears on approximately day 16 as a small, sausage-shaped diverticulum (outpouching) that extends from the caudal wall of the umbilical vesicle into the connecting stalk (see Fig. *5-5B, C,* and *D*). The allantois is involved with early blood formation and is associated with the urinary bladder as well.

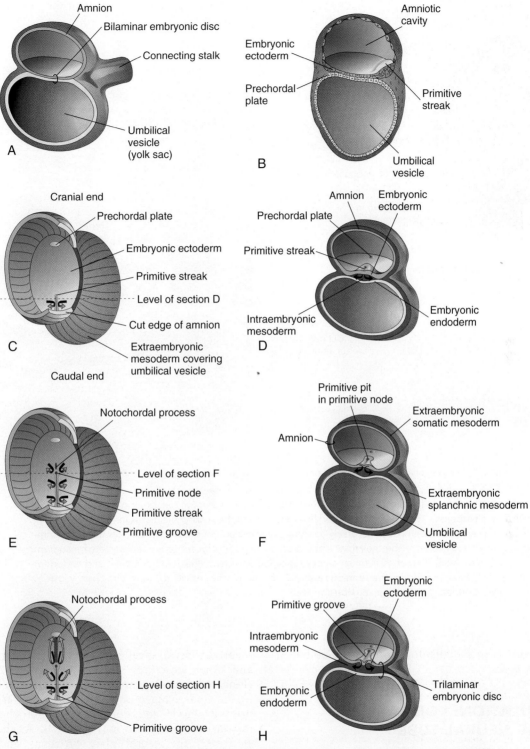

Figure 5–2 Formation of the trilaminar embryonic disc (days 15 to 16). The *arrows* indicate invagination and migration of the mesenchymal cells between the ectoderm and the endoderm. **C, E,** and **G,** Dorsal views of the embryonic disc early in the third week, exposed by removal of the amnion. **B, D, F,** and **H,** Transverse sections through the embryonic disc at the levels indicated.

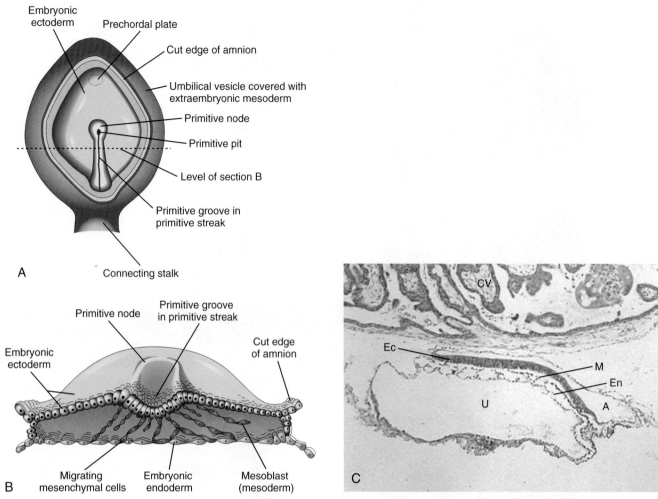

Figure 5–3 **A,** Dorsal view of a 16-day embryo. The amnion has been removed to expose the embryonic disc. **B,** Illustration of the cranial half of the embryonic disc during the third week. The disc has been cut transversely to show the migration of mesenchymal cells from the primitive streak to form the mesoblast that soon organizes to form the intraembryonic mesoderm. **C,** Sagittal section of a trilaminar embryo showing ectoderm *(Ec)*, mesoderm *(M)*, and endoderm *(En)*. Also visible are the amniotic sac *(A)*, the umbilical vesicle *(U)*, and chorionic villi *(CV)*. *(C, Courtesy Dr. E. Uthman, Houston/Richmond, Texas.)*

The blood vessels of the allantois become the umbilical arteries and veins.

NEURULATION: FORMATION OF THE NEURAL TUBE

The processes involved in the formation of the neural plate and neural folds and closure of these folds to form the neural tube constitute **neurulation**. These processes are completed by the end of the fourth week.

Neural Plate and Neural Tube

As the notochord develops, it induces the embryonic ectoderm over it to thicken and form an elongated plate of thickened neuroepithelial cells called the **neural plate** (Fig. 5-5C). The ectoderm of the neural plate

(neuroectoderm) gives rise to the central nervous system and other structures such as the retina. At first, the elongated neural plate corresponds precisely in length to the underlying notochord. It appears cranial to the primitive node and dorsal to the notochord and the mesoderm adjacent to it (Fig. 5-4B). As the notochord elongates, the neural plate broadens and eventually extends cranially as far as the **oropharyngeal membrane** (Fig. 5-4C).

On approximately day 18, the neural plate invaginates along its central axis to form a median longitudinal **neural groove** that has **neural folds** on each side (see Fig. 5-6F and G). The neural folds are particularly prominent at the cranial end of the embryo and are the first signs of brain development (Fig. 5-7C). By the end of the third week, the neural folds have begun to move together and fuse, converting the neural plate into a **neural tube** (Figs. 5-7F and 5-8). Neural

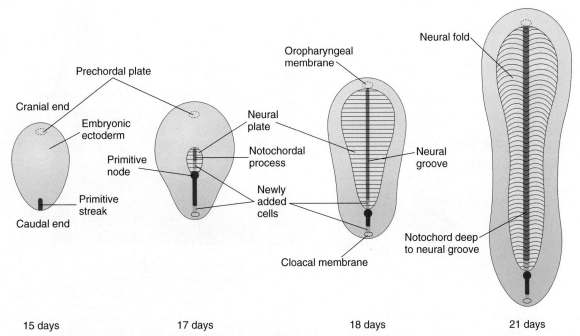

Figure 5–4 Dorsal views of the embryonic disc, showing how it lengthens and changes shape during the third week. The primitive streak lengthens by the addition of cells at its caudal end; the notochordal process lengthens by the migration of cells from the primitive node. At the end of the third week, the notochordal process is transformed into the notochord.

tube formation is a complex cellular and multifactorial process involving genes and extrinsic and mechanical factors.

The neural tube soon separates from the surface ectoderm (Fig. 5-8E). The free edges of the ectoderm fuse so that this layer becomes continuous over the neural tube and the back of the embryo. Subsequently, the surface ectoderm differentiates into the epidermis of the skin. Neurulation is completed during the fourth week (see Chapter 6).

Neural Crest Formation

As the neural folds fuse to form the neural tube, some neuroectodermal cells lying along the crest of each neural fold lose their epithelial affinities and attachments to neighboring cells (Fig. 5-8A to C). As the neural tube separates from the surface ectoderm, these **neural crest cells** migrate dorsolaterally on each side of the neural tube. They form a flattened irregular mass, the **neural crest**, between the neural tube and the overlying surface ectoderm (Fig. 5-8D and E). The neural crest soon separates into right and left parts that migrate in a wave to the dorsolateral aspects of the neural tube (see Fig. 5-8F). Neural crest cells also migrate widely within the mesenchyme. Neural crest cells differentiate into various cell types (see Fig. 6-4), including the spinal ganglia and the ganglia of the autonomic nervous system. The ganglia of cranial nerves V, VII, IX, and X are partially derived from neural crest cells. Neural crest cells also form the sheaths of the peripheral nerves and the pia mater and arachnoid mater.

DEVELOPMENT OF SOMITES

As the notochord and the neural tube form, the intra-embryonic mesoderm on each side of them proliferates to form a thick, longitudinal column of **paraxial mesoderm** (see Figs. 5-6G and 5-7B). Each column is continuous laterally with the **intermediate mesoderm**, which gradually thins into a layer of **lateral mesoderm**. The lateral mesoderm is continuous with the extraembryonic mesoderm that covers the umbilical vesicle and amnion (see Fig. 4-3B). Toward the end of the third week, the paraxial mesoderm differentiates and begins to divide into paired cuboidal bodies, **somites**, on each side of the developing neural tube (Fig. 5-7C and E). The somites form distinct surface elevations on the embryo and appear somewhat triangular on transverse section (Fig. 5-7D and F). Because the somites are so prominent during the fourth and fifth weeks, they are used as one of the criteria for determining an embryo's age (see Chapter 6 and Table 6-1).

The first pair of somites appears at the end of the third week (see Fig. 5-7C) near the cranial end of the notochord. Subsequent pairs form in a craniocaudal sequence. Somites give rise to most of the *axial skeleton* and the associated musculature, as well as to the adjacent dermis of the skin.

Somite formation from the paraxial mesoderm is preceded by expression of the forkhead transcription factors Fox C1 and C2. The craniocaudal segmental pattern of the somites is regulated by the Delta-Notch (Delta 1 and Notch 1) signaling pathway. A molecular oscillator, or clock, has been proposed as the mechanism responsible for the orderly sequencing of the somites.

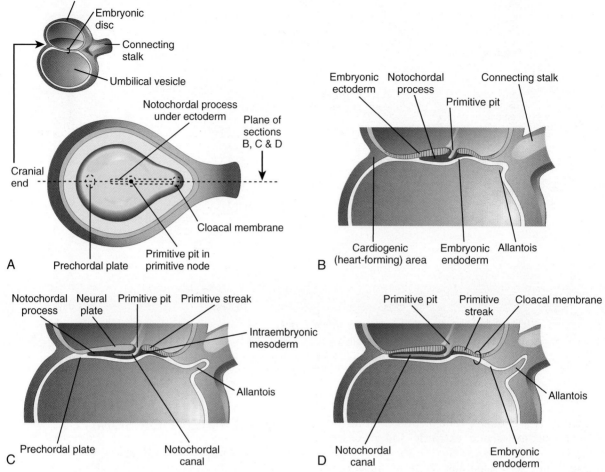

Figure 5–5 Illustrations of the development of the notochordal process. The small sketch at the upper left is for orientation. **A,** Dorsal view of the embryonic disc (at approximately 16 days), exposed by removal of the amnion. The notochordal process is shown as if it were visible through the embryonic ectoderm. **B, C,** and **D,** Median sections, at the same plane as shown in **A,** illustrating successive stages in the development of the notochordal process and canal. The stages shown in **C** and **D** occur at approximately 18 days.

DEVELOPMENT OF INTRAEMBRYONIC COELOM

The intraembryonic coelom (body cavity) first appears as small, isolated, coelomic spaces in the lateral mesoderm and cardiogenic (heart-forming) mesoderm (Fig. 5-6A to D). These spaces coalesce to form a single, horseshoe-shaped cavity—the **intraembryonic coelom** (see Fig. 5-7E and F). The coelom divides the lateral mesoderm into two layers:

- A somatic, or *parietal (somatopleure),* layer that is continuous with the extraembryonic mesoderm that covers the amnion
- A splanchnic, or *visceral (splancnopleure),* layer that is continuous with the extraembryonic mesoderm that covers the umbilical vesicle

The somatopleure and the overlying embryonic ectoderm form the body wall (Fig. 5-7F), whereas the

splancnopleure and the underlying embryonic endoderm form the wall of the gut. During the second month, the intraembryonic coelom is divided into three body cavities: the *pericardial cavity,* the *pleural cavities,* and the *peritoneal cavity* (see Chapter 9).

EARLY DEVELOPMENT OF CARDIOVASCULAR SYSTEM

At the end of the second week, embryonic nutrition is obtained from the maternal blood by diffusion through the chorion, extraembryonic coelom, and umbilical vesicle. The early formation of the cardiovascular system correlates with the urgent need for transportation of oxygen and nourishment to the embryo from the maternal circulation through the chorion.

At the beginning of the third week, blood vessel formation, or **vasculogenesis,** begins in the extraembryonic mesoderm of the umbilical vesicle and connecting stalk.

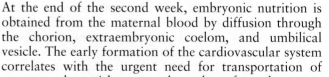

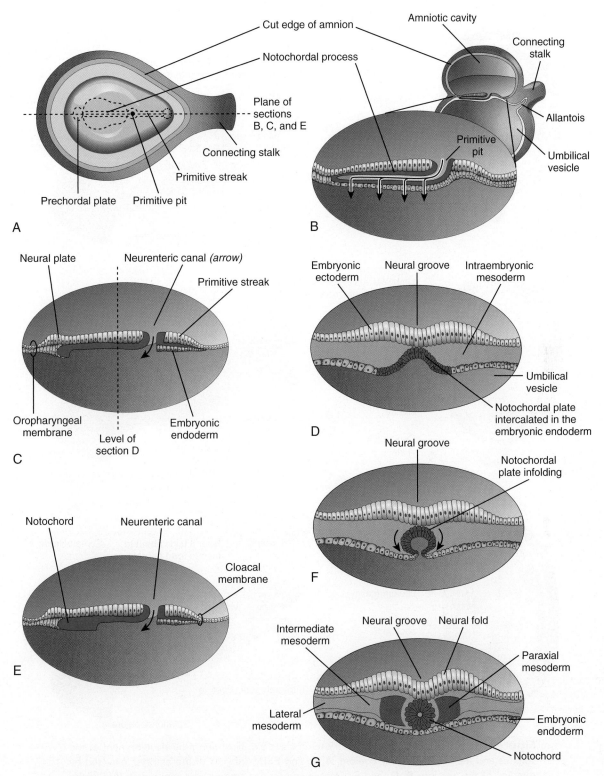

Figure 5–6 Development of the notochord by transformation of the notochordal process. **A,** Dorsal view of the embryonic disc (at approximately 18 days), exposed by removing the amnion. **B,** Three-dimensional median section of the embryo. **C** and **E,** Similar sections of slightly older embryos. **D, F,** and **G,** Transverse sections of the trilaminar embryonic disc shown in **C** and **E.**

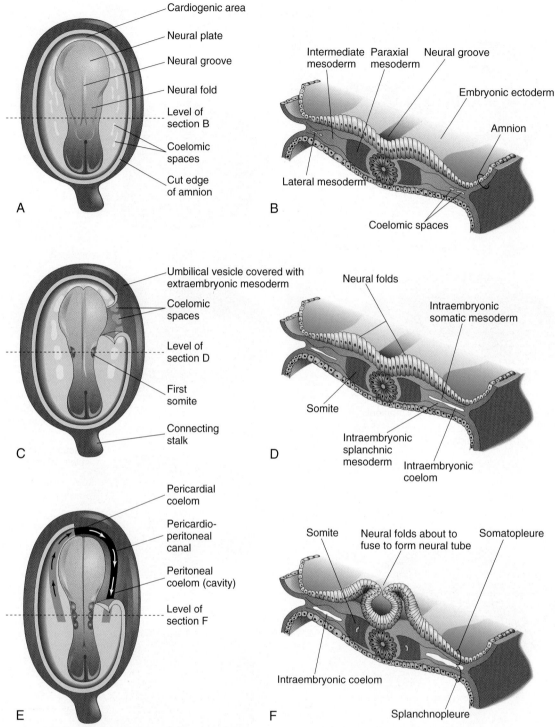

Figure 5–7 Illustrations of embryos 19 to 21 days old, illustrating the development of the somites and the intraembryonic coelom. **A, C,** and **E,** Dorsal view of the embryo, exposed by removal of the amnion. **B, D,** and **F,** Transverse sections through the embryonic disc at the levels shown. **A,** A presomite embryo of approximately 18 days. **C,** An embryo of approximately 20 days, showing the first pair of somites. A portion of the somatopleure on the right has been removed to show the isolated coelomic spaces in the lateral mesoderm. **E,** A three-somite embryo (approximately 21 days old), showing the horseshoe-shaped intraembryonic coelom, exposed on the right by removal of part of the somatopleure.

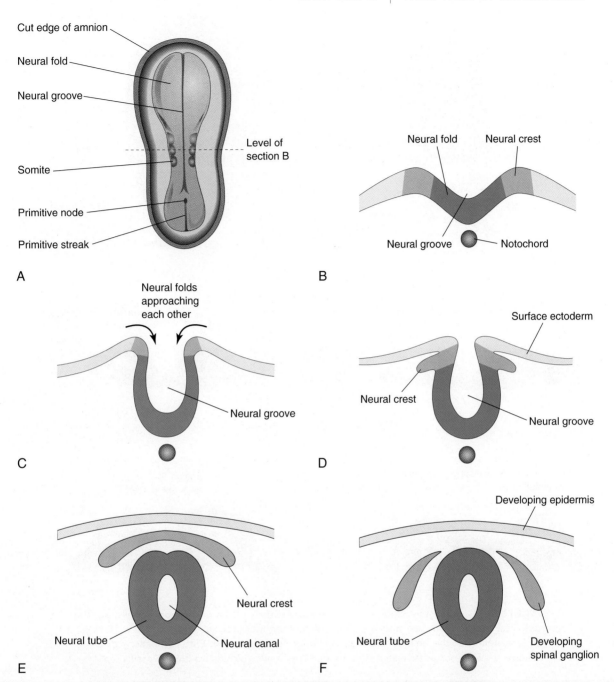

Figure 5–8 Diagrammatic transverse sections through progressively older embryos, illustrating the formation of the neural groove, neural tube, and neural crest up to the end of the fourth week.

Vasculogenesis begins in the chorion (Fig. 5-9A and B). Blood vessels develop approximately 2 days later. At the end of the third week, a primordial *uteroplacental circulation* has developed (Fig. 5-10).

Vasculogenesis and Angiogenesis

Blood vessel formation in the embryo and the extraembryonic membranes during the third week may be summarized as follows (Fig. 5-9C to F):

Vasculogenesis:

- Mesenchymal cells differentiate into endothelial cell precursors, or **angioblasts** (vessel-forming cells), that aggregate to form isolated angiogenic cell clusters known as **blood islands** (Fig. 5-9B and C).
- Small cavities appear within the blood islands by the confluence of intercellular clefts.
- Angioblasts flatten to form endothelial cells that arrange themselves around the cavities in the blood islands to form the primordial endothelium.

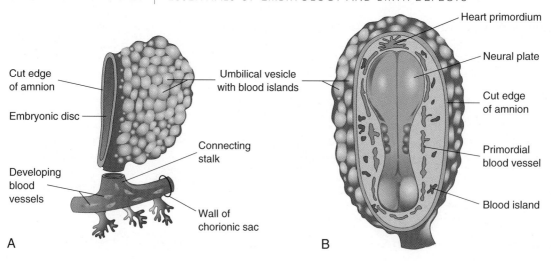

Cut edge of amnion

Embryonic disc

Developing blood vessels

Umbilical vesicle with blood islands

Connecting stalk

Wall of chorionic sac

A

Heart primordium

Neural plate

Cut edge of amnion

Primordial blood vessel

Blood island

B

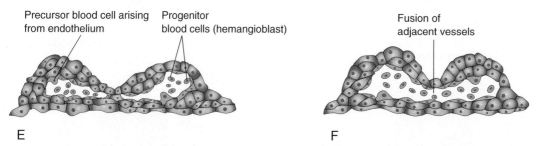

Blood island   Wall of umbilical vesicle

C

Lumen of primordial blood vessel   Primordial blood vessel   Endoderm of umbilical vesicle

D

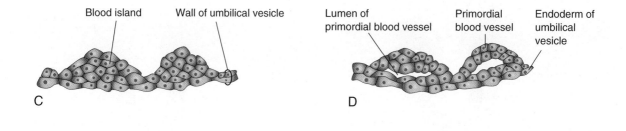

Precursor blood cell arising from endothelium   Progenitor blood cells (hemangioblast)

E

Fusion of adjacent vessels

F

Figure 5–9 Successive stages in the development of blood and blood vessels. **A,** The umbilical vesicle (yolk sac) and a portion of the chorionic sac (at approximately 18 days). **B,** Dorsal view of the embryo exposed by removing the amnion. **C** to **F,** Sections of blood islands, showing progressive stages in the development of blood and blood vessels.

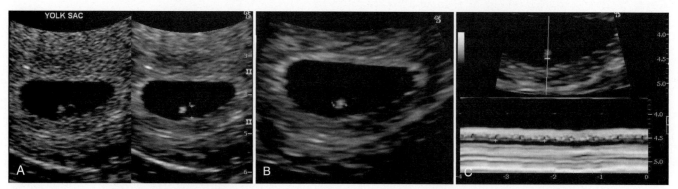

Figure 5–10 Endovaginal scan of a 4-week embryo. **A,** 2-mm secondary umbilical vesicle (calipers), **B,** Bright (echogenic) 2.4-mm, 4-week embryo (calipers). **C,** Cardiac activity of 116 beats/minute demonstrated with motion mode. Calipers used to encompass two beats. *(Courtesy E. A. Lyons, M.D., Professor of Radiology, and Obstetrics and Gynecology, and Anatomy, Health Sciences Centre and University of Manitoba, Winnipeg, Manitoba, Canada.)*

● These endothelium-lined cavities soon fuse to form networks of endothelial channels.

Angiogenesis:

● Vessels sprout by endothelial budding into adjacent nonvascularized areas and fuse with other vessels.

Blood cells develop from specialized endothelial cells of vessels (**hemangioblasts**) on the umbilical vesicle and allantois at the end of the third week (see Fig. 5-9E and F). Blood formation (**hematogenesis**) does not begin within the embryo until the fifth week. This process occurs first in various parts of the embryonic mesenchyme, chiefly the liver, and later, in the spleen, bone marrow, and lymph nodes. Fetal and adult erythrocytes are also derived from hematopoietic progenitor cells (hemangioblasts). The mesenchymal cells that surround the primordial endothelial blood vessels differentiate into muscular and connective tissue elements of the vessels.

The **heart and great vessels** form from mesenchymal cells in the heart primordium, or **cardiogenic area** (see Fig. 5-7A and 5-9B). Paired, endothelium-lined channels—endocardial **heart tubes**—develop during the third week and fuse to form a **primordial heart tube**. The tubular heart joins with blood vessels in the embryo, connecting stalk, chorion, and umbilical vesicle to form a **primordial cardiovascular system** (Fig. 5-11C). By the end of the third week, blood is flowing, and the heart begins to beat on day 21 or 22. Thus, the cardiovascular system is the first organ system to reach a primitive functional state. The embryonic heartbeat can be detected by Doppler ultrasonography during the fourth week, approximately 6 weeks after the last normal menstrual period (Fig. 5-10).

DEVELOPMENT OF CHORIONIC VILLI

Shortly after the **primary chorionic villi** are formed at the end of the second week, they begin to branch. Early in the third week, mesenchyme grows into the primary villi, forming a core of loose mesenchymal (connective) tissue (see Fig. 5-11A and B). The villi at this stage—**secondary chorionic villi**—cover the entire surface of the chorionic sac. Mesenchymal cells in the villi soon differentiate into both capillaries and blood cells (see Fig. 5-11 C and D). When capillaries are present, the villi are called **tertiary chorionic villi**. The capillaries in the chorionic villi fuse to form **arteriocapillary networks** that soon become connected with the embryonic heart through vessels that differentiate from the mesenchyme of the chorion and connecting stalk. By the end of the third week, embryonic blood begins to flow slowly through the capillaries in the chorionic villi. Oxygen and nutrients in the maternal blood in the intervillous space diffuse through the walls of the villi and enter the embryo's blood (Fig. 5-11C). Carbon dioxide and waste products diffuse from blood in the fetal capillaries through the wall of the villi into the maternal blood. Concurrently, cytotrophoblastic cells of the chorionic villi proliferate and extend through the syncytiotrophoblast to form a **cytotrophoblastic shell**, which gradually surrounds the chorionic sac and attaches it to the endometrium (see Fig. 5-11C).

Villi that attach to the maternal tissues through the cytotrophoblastic shell are called **stem chorionic villi** (anchoring villi). The villi that grow from the sides of the stem villi are called **branch chorionic villi** (terminal villi). It is through the walls of the branch villi that the main exchange of material between the blood of the mother and the embryo takes place. The branch villi are bathed in continually changing maternal blood in the **intervillous space**.

SACROCOCCYGEAL TERATOMA

Remnants of the primitive streak may persist and give rise to a large tumor known as a *sacrococcygeal teratoma* (Fig. 5-12). Because it is derived from pluripotent primitive streak cells, the tumor contains tissues derived from all three germ layers in incomplete stages of differentiation. Sacrococcygeal teratomas are the most common tumors in newborn infants and have an incidence of approximately 1 in 27,000 neonates. These tumors are usually surgically excised promptly, and the prognosis is good.

ABNORMAL NEURULATION

Disturbance of neurulation may result in severe abnormalities of the brain and spinal cord (see Chapter 16). **Neural tube defects** are among the most common congenital anomalies. Meroencephaly (anencephaly), or partial absence of the brain, is the most severe defect. Available evidence suggests that the primary disturbance affects the neuroectoderm. Failure of the neural folds to fuse and form the neural tube in the brain region results in meroencephaly, and in the lumbar region, spina bifida cystica (see Fig. 16-9).

ABNORMAL GROWTH OF TROPHOBLAST

Sometimes the embryo dies and the chorionic villi do not complete their development; that is, they do not become vascularized to form tertiary villi. These degenerating villi may form cystic swellings, called **hydatidiform moles**. These moles exhibit variable degrees of trophoblastic proliferation and produce excessive amounts of human chorionic gonadotropin. In 3% to 5% of such cases, these moles develop into malignant trophoblastic lesions, called **choriocarcinomas.** These tumors invariably metastasize (spread) by way of the blood to various sites, such as the lungs, vagina, liver, bone, intestine, and brain.

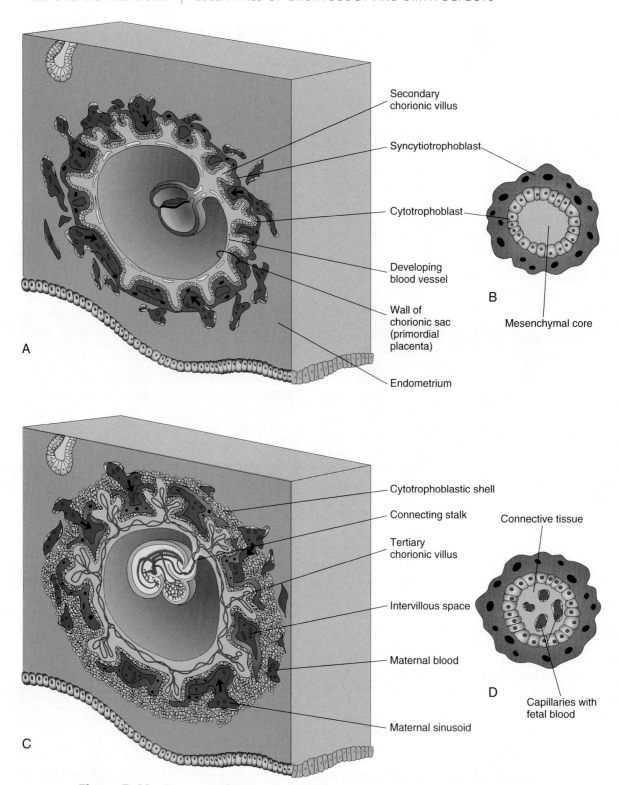

Figure 5–11   Illustrations of the development of the secondary chorionic villi into the tertiary chorionic villi. **A,** Sagittal section of an embryo (at approximately 16 days). **B,** Section of a secondary chorionic villus. **C,** Section of an embryo (at approximately 21 days). **D,** Section of a tertiary chorionic villus. By the end of the third week, a primordial uteroplacental circulation has developed.

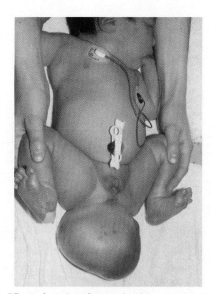

Figure 5–12 A female infant with a large sacrococcygeal teratoma that developed from remnants of the primitive streak. *(Courtesy A. E. Chudley, M.D., Section of Genetics and Metabolism, Department of Pediatrics and Child Health, Children's Hospital, University of Manitoba, Winnipeg, Manitoba, Canada.)*

CLINICALLY ORIENTED QUESTIONS

1. Can drugs and other agents cause congenital anomalies of the embryo if they are present in the mother's blood during the third week? If so, what organs would be most susceptible?

2. Are there increased risks for the embryo associated with pregnancies in women older than 40 years of age? If so, what are they?

The answers to these questions are at the back of the book.

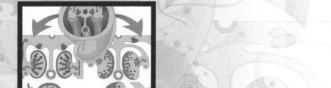

Development During Weeks Four to Eight

All major external and internal structures are established during the fourth to eighth weeks. By the end of this **organogenetic period**, all of the main organ systems have begun to develop. Exposure of embryos to teratogens (e.g., drugs) during this period may cause major congenital anomalies (see Chapter 19). As the tissues and organs form, the shape of the embryo changes so that, by the eighth week, the embryo has a distinctly human appearance.

FOLDING OF EMBRYO

A significant event in the establishment of body form is folding of the flat trilaminar embryonic disc into a somewhat cylindric embryo (Fig. 6-1). Folding results from rapid growth of the embryo, particularly the brain and the spinal cord. Folding at the cranial and caudal ends and at the sides of the embryo occurs simultaneously. Concurrently, a relative constriction occurs at the junction of the embryo and the umbilical vesicle. Head and tail folds cause the cranial and caudal regions to move ventrally as the embryo elongates (see Fig. 6-1A_2 to D_2).

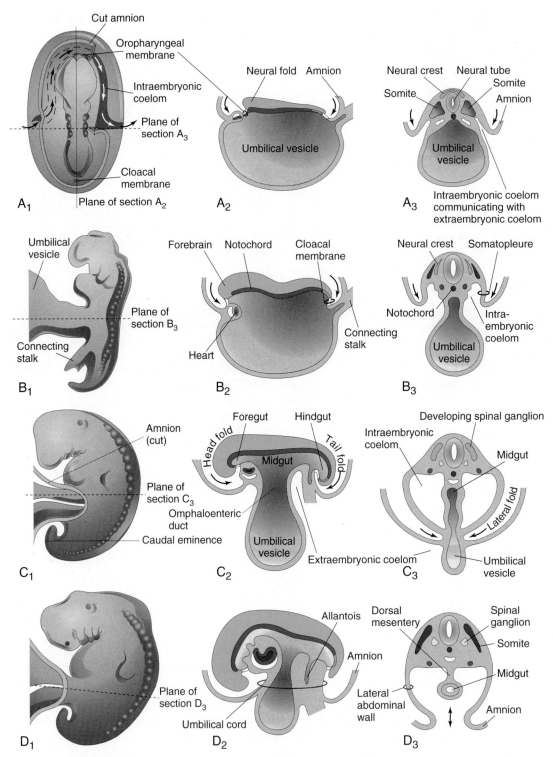

Figure 6–1 Folding of embryos during the fourth week. **A₁,** Dorsal view of an embryo early in the fourth week. Three pairs of somites are visible. The continuity of the intraembryonic coelom and the extraembryonic coelom is shown on the right side by removal of a part of the embryonic ectoderm and mesoderm. **B₁, C₁,** and **D₁,** Lateral views of embryos at 22, 26, and 28 days, respectively. **A₂, B₂, C₂,** and **D₂,** Sagittal sections at the plane shown in **A₁.** **A₃, B₃, C₃,** and **D₃,** Transverse sections at the levels indicated in **A₁** to **D₁.**

Head and Tail Folds

By the beginning of the fourth week, the neural folds in the cranial region form the **primordium of the brain**. Later, the developing forebrain grows cranially beyond the oropharyngeal membrane and overhangs the developing heart. Concomitantly, the primordial heart and the oropharyngeal membrane move onto the ventral surface of the embryo (Fig. 6-2). During lateral (longitudinal) folding, part of the endoderm of the umbilical vesicle is incorporated into the embryo as the **foregut** (Fig. 6-2C). The foregut lies between the brain and the heart, and the oropharyngeal membrane separates the foregut from the **stomodeum** (primordial mouth).

Folding of the caudal end of the embryo results primarily from growth of the distal part of the neural tube, the primordium of the spinal cord. As the embryo grows, the tail region projects over the **cloacal membrane** (future site of the anus) (Fig. 6-3B). During folding, part of the endodermal germ layer is incorporated into the embryo as the **hindgut** (see Fig. 6-3C). The terminal part of the hindgut soon dilates to form the **cloaca** (see Fig. 6-3B and C). The **connecting stalk** (primordium of the umbilical cord) is now attached to the ventral surface of the embryo, and the **allantois**— an endodermal diverticulum of the umbilical vesicle— is partially incorporated into the embryo (Fig. 6-1D_2 and 6-3C).

Lateral Folds

Folding of the sides of the embryo is thought to result from growth of the somites, which produces right and left **lateral folds** (Fig. 6-1A_3 to D_3). The lateral body wall folds toward the median plane, rolling the edges of the embryonic disc ventrally and forming a roughly cylindric embryo. As the abdominal walls form by fusion of the lateral folds, part of the endoderm germ layer is incorporated into the embryo as the **midgut**. Initially, there is a wide connection between the midgut and the umbilical vesicle (Fig. 6-1A_2). After lateral folding, the connection is reduced to an **omphaloenteric duct**, formerly called the yolk stalk (Fig. 6-1C_2). As the **umbilical cord** forms from the connecting stalk, ventral fusion of the lateral folds reduces the region of communication between the intraembryonic and extraembryonic coelomic cavities (Fig. 6-1C_2). As the amniotic cavity expands and obliterates most of the extraembryonic coelom, the amnion forms the epithelial covering of the umbilical cord (Fig. 6-1D_2).

 ## GERM LAYER DERIVATIVES

The three germ layers (ectoderm, mesoderm, and endoderm) formed during gastrulation give rise to the primordia of all tissues and organs (Fig. 6-4). The cells of each germ layer divide, migrate, aggregate, and differentiate in rather precise patterns as they form the various organ systems (organogenesis).

CONTROL OF EMBRYONIC DEVELOPMENT

Embryonic development results from genetic plans in the chromosomes. Knowledge of the genes that control human development is increasing exponentially. Most developmental processes depend on a precisely coordinated interaction of genetic and environmental factors. Several control mechanisms guide differentiation and ensure synchronized development, such as tissue interactions, regulated migration of cells and cell colonies, controlled proliferation, and apoptosis (programmed cell death). Each system of the body has its own developmental pattern, and most processes of morphogenesis are regulated by complex molecular mechanisms.

Embryonic development is essentially a process of growth and increasing complexity of structure and function. Growth is achieved by mitosis, together with the production of extracellular matrices, whereas complexity is achieved through morphogenesis and differentiation. The cells that make up the tissues of very early embryos are pluripotential; that is, depending on the circumstances, they are able to follow more than one pathway of development. This broad developmental potential becomes progressively restricted as tissues acquire the specialized features necessary for increased sophistication of structure and function. Such restriction presumes that choices must be made to achieve tissue diversification. Most evidence indicates that these choices are determined not as a consequence of cell lineage, but rather in response to cues from the immediate surroundings, including the adjacent tissues. As a result, the architectural precision and coordination that are often required for the normal function of an organ appear to be achieved by the interaction of its constituent parts during development.

The interaction of tissues during development is a recurring theme in embryology. The interactions that lead to a change in the course of development of at least one of the interactants are called **inductions**. Numerous examples of such inductive interactions can be found in the literature; for example, during the development of the eye, the optic vesicle induces the development of the lens from the surface ectoderm of the head. When the optic vesicle is absent, the eye does not develop. Moreover, if the optic vesicle is removed and placed in association with surface ectoderm that is not usually involved in eye development, lens formation can be induced. Clearly then, the development of a lens depends on the ectoderm acquiring an association with a second tissue. In the presence of the neuroectoderm of the optic vesicle, the surface ectoderm of the head follows a pathway of development that it would not otherwise have taken. Similarly, many of the morphogenetic tissue movements that play such important roles in shaping the embryo also provide for the changing tissue associations that are fundamental to inductive tissue interactions.

The fact that one tissue can influence the developmental pathway adopted by another tissue presumes that a signal passes between the two interactants. Analysis of the molecular defects in mutant strains that show abnormal tissue interactions during embryonic development and studies of the development of embryos with targeted

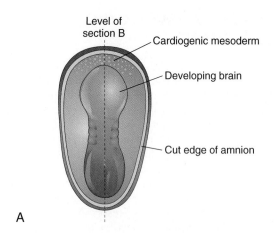

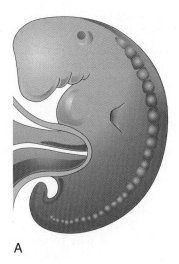

A

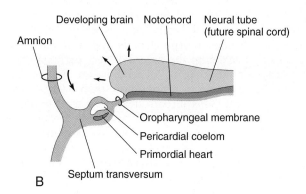

B

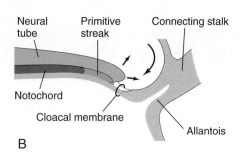

B

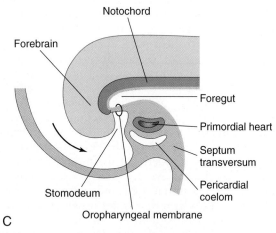

C

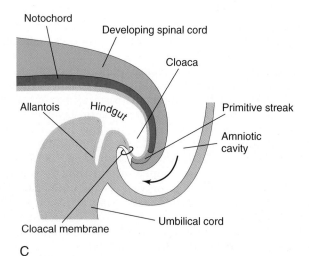

C

Figure 6–2 Folding of cranial end of the embryo. **A,** Dorsal view of an embryo at 21 days. **B,** Sagittal section of the cranial part of the embryo at the plane in **A,** showing the ventral movement of the heart. **C,** Sagittal section of an embryo at 26 days. Note that the septum transversum, heart, pericardial coelom, and oropharyngeal membrane have moved to the ventral surface of the embryo. Observe also that part of the umbilical vesicle is incorporated into the embryo as the foregut.

Figure 6–3 Folding of caudal end of the embryo. **A,** Lateral view of a 4-week embryo. **B,** Sagittal section of the caudal part of the embryo at the beginning of the fourth week. **C,** Similar section at the end of the fourth week. Note that part of the umbilical vesicle is incorporated into the embryo as the hindgut and that the terminal part of the hindgut has dilated to form the cloaca. Observe also the change in position of the primitive streak, allantois, cloacal membrane, and connecting stalk.

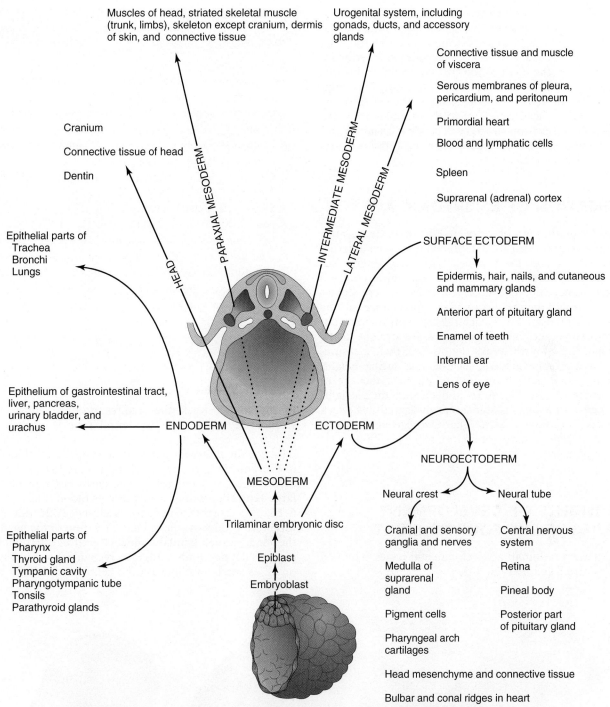

Figure 6–4 Illustration of derivatives of the three germ layers: ectoderm, endoderm, and mesoderm. Cells from these layers contribute to the formation of different tissues and organs; for example, the endoderm forms the epithelial lining of the gastrointestinal tract and the mesoderm gives rise to connective tissues and muscles.

gene mutations have begun to reveal the molecular mechanisms of induction. The mechanism of signal transfer appears to vary with the specific tissues involved. In some cases, the signal appears to take the form of a diffusible molecule that passes from the inductor to the reacting tissue. In other instances, the message appears to be mediated through a nondiffusible extracellular matrix that is secreted by the inductor and that comes into contact with the reacting tissue. In still other cases, the signal appears to require physical contact between the inducing tissue and the responding tissue. Regardless of the mechanism of intercellular transfer involved, the signal is translated into an intracellular message that influences the genetic activity of the responding cells.

To be competent to respond to an inducing stimulus, the cells of the reacting system must express the appropriate receptor for the specific inducing signal molecule, the components of the particular intracellular signal transduction pathway, and the transcription factors that mediate the particular response. Experimental evidence suggests that the acquisition of competence by the responding tissue is often dependent on its previous interactions with other tissues. For example, the lens-forming response of the head ectoderm to the stimulus provided by the optic vesicle appears to be dependent on a previous association of the head ectoderm with the anterior neural plate (see Chapter 20).

ESTIMATION OF EMBRYONIC AGE

Estimates of the age of recovered embryos (e.g., after spontaneous abortion) are determined from their external characteristics and measurements of their length (see Table 6-1). Size alone may be an unreliable criterion because some embryos undergo a progressively slower rate of growth before death. The appearance of the developing limbs is a very helpful criterion for estimating embryonic age. Because embryos are straight in the third and early fourth weeks (Fig. 6-5A), their measurements indicate the greatest length. The sitting height, or *crown–rump length*, is used to estimate the age of older embryos (see Fig. 6-5B and C). Standing height, or *crown–heel length*, is sometimes measured in 8-week embryos (see Fig. 6-5D). The *Carnegie Embryonic Staging System* is used internationally (see Table 6-1) for comparison.

HIGHLIGHTS OF DEVELOPMENT DURING WEEKS FOUR TO EIGHT

The criteria for estimating developmental stages in human embryos are listed in Table 6-1.

ULTRASONOGRAPHIC EXAMINATION OF EMBRYOS

Most women seeking obstetrical care have at least one ultrasonographic examination during their pregnancy for one or more of the following reasons:

* Estimation of gestational age for confirmation of clinical dating
* Evaluation of embryonic growth when intrauterine growth restriction (IUGR) is suspected
* Guidance during chorionic villus or amniotic fluid sampling
* Suspected ectopic pregnancy
* Possible uterine abnormality
* Detection of congenital anomalies

The size of an embryo in a pregnant woman can be estimated using ultrasonographic measurements. *Transvaginal* or *endovaginal ultrasonography* permits accurate measurement of crown–rump length in early pregnancy (Fig. 6-6).

Fourth Week

In the fourth week the somites produce conspicuous surface elevations and the neural tube is open at the rostral and caudal neuropores (Figs. 6-7A and 6-8A). By 24 days, the *pharyngeal arches* have appeared (Fig. 6-7A to C). The embryo now develops a curved shape because of the head and tail folds. The early heart produces a large ventral prominence and pumps blood (Figs. 6-9 and 6-10). The rostral neuropore is closed at 26 days. The **forebrain** produces a prominent elevation of the head and the long, curved **caudal eminence** (tail-like structure) is present. **Upper limb buds** are recognizable by day 26 or 27 as small swellings on the ventrolateral body walls

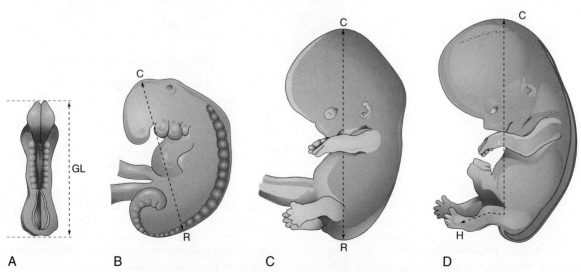

Figure 6–5 Methods used to measure the length of embryos. **A,** Greatest length (GL). **B** and **C,** Crown–rump length (CRL). **D,** Crown–heel length (CHL).

Table 6–1 Criteria for Estimating Developmental Stages in Human Embryos

AGE (days)	FIGURE REFERENCE	CARNEGIE STAGE	NUMBER OF SOMITES	LENGTH (mm)*	MAIN EXTERNAL CHARACTERISTICS†
20–21	6-1A₁ 6-8A	9	1–3	1.5–3.0	Flat embryonic disc. Deep neural groove and prominent neural folds. Head fold is evident.
22–23	6-8A, C	10	4–12	2.0–3.5	Embryo is straight or slightly curved. Neural tube is forming or has formed opposite somites, but is widely open at the rostral and caudal neuropores. First and second pairs of pharyngeal arches are visible.
24–25	6-9A	11	13–20	2.5–4.5	Embryo is curved owing to head and tail folds. Rostral neuropore is closing. Otic placodes are present. Optic vesicles have formed.
26–27	6-7D 6-10A	12	21–29	3.0–5.0	Upper limb buds appear. Rostral neuropore is closed. Caudal neuropore is closing. Three pairs of pharyngeal arches are visible. Heart prominence is distinct. Otic pits are present.
28–30	6-7E 6-11A	13	30–35	4.0–6.0	Embryo has C-shaped curve. Caudal neuropore is closed. Four pairs of pharyngeal arches are visible. Lower limb buds appear. Otic vesicles are present. Lens placodes are distinct.
31–32	6-12A	14	‡	5.0–7.0	Lens pits and nasal pits are visible. Optic cups are present.
33–36		15		7.0–9.0	Hand plates have formed; digital rays are present. Lens vesicles are present. Nasal pits are prominent. Cervical sinuses are visible.
37–40		16		8.0–11.0	Footplates have formed. Pigment is visible in the retina. Auricular hillocks are developing.
41–43	6-13A	17		11.0–14.0	Digital rays are clearly visible in hand plates. Auricular hillocks outline the future auricle of the external ear. Cerebral vesicles are prominent.
44–46		18		13.0–17.0	Digital rays are clearly evident in footplates. Elbow region is visible. Eyelids are forming. Notches are between the digital rays in the hands. Nipples are visible.
47–48		19		16.0–18.0	Limbs extend ventrally. Trunk is elongating and straightening. Midgut herniation is prominent.
49–51		20		18.0–22.0	Upper limbs are longer and are bent at the elbows. Fingers are distinct but webbed. Notches are between the digital rays in the feet. Scalp vascular plexus appears.
52–53		21		22.0–24.0	Hands and feet approach each other. Fingers are free and longer. Toes are distinct but webbed. Stubby caudal eminence (tail) is present.
54–55		22		23.0–28.0	Toes are free and longer. Eyelids and auricles of the external ears are more developed.
56	6-14A	23		27.0–31.0	Head is more rounded and shows human characteristics. External genitalia still have undifferentiated appearance. Midgut herniation is still present. Caudal eminence has disappeared.

*The embryonic lengths indicate the usual range. In stages 9 and 10, the measurement is greatest length; in subsequent stages, crown–rump measurements are given.
†Based on O'Rahilly R, Müller F: Developmental Stages in Human Embryos. Washington, DC, Carnegie Institute of Washington, 1987; and Gasser RF: Digitally Reproduced Embryonic Morphology DVDs. Computer Imaging Laboratory, Cell Biology and Anatomy, New Orleans, LA, Louisiana State University Health Sciences Center, 2002–2006.
‡At this stage and subsequent stages, the number of somites is difficult to determine and so is not a useful criterion.

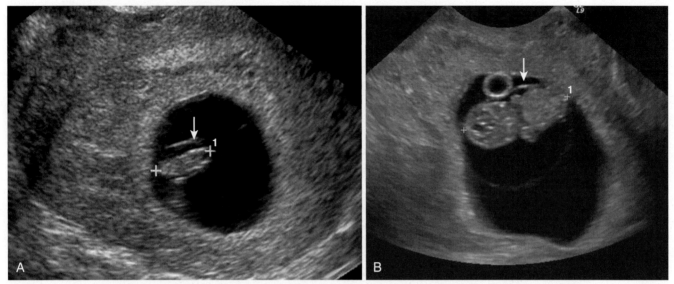

Figure 6–6 Endovaginal scan of embryos. **A,** Endovaginal scan of a 5-week embryo (CRL 10 mm, calipers) surrounded by the amniotic membrane *(arrow)*. **B,** Coronal scan of a 7-week embryo (CRL 22 mm, calipers). Amnion seen anterior *(arrow)*. Umbilical vesicle (yolk sac) anterior. *(Courtesy E. A. Lyons, M.D., Professor of Radiology and Obstetrics and Gynecology, Health Sciences Centre and University of Manitoba, Winnipeg, Manitoba, Canada.)*

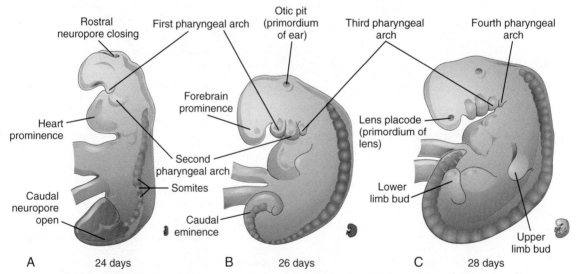

Figure 6–7 **A, B,** and **C,** Lateral views of older embryos, showing 16, 27, and 33 somites, respectively. The rostral neuropore is normally closed by 25 to 26 days, and the caudal neuropore is usually closed by the end of the fourth week.

(Fig. 6-11*A* and *B*). The **otic pits**, the primordia of the internal ears, are also visible. Ectodermal thickenings, called **lens placodes**, indicating the future lenses of the eyes, are visible on the sides of the head. The fourth pair of pharyngeal arches and the **lower limb buds** are visible by the end of the fourth week (see Fig. 6-7*C*). Rudiments of many organ systems, especially the cardiovascular system, are established.

Fifth Week

Changes in body form are minor during the fifth week compared with those that occurred during the fourth week. Growth of the head exceeds that of other regions (Fig. 6-12*A* and *B*), which is caused mainly by the rapid development of the brain and facial prominences. The face soon contacts the heart prominence. The *mesonephric ridges* indicate the site of the mesonephric kidneys.

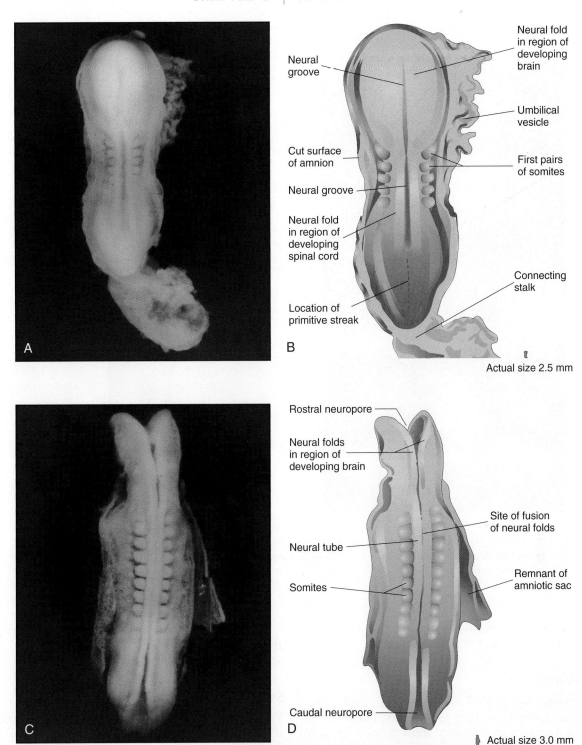

Neural fold in region of developing brain

Neural groove

Umbilical vesicle

Cut surface of amnion

First pairs of somites

Neural groove

Neural fold in region of developing spinal cord

Connecting stalk

Location of primitive streak

B

Actual size 2.5 mm

Rostral neuropore

Neural folds in region of developing brain

Site of fusion of neural folds

Neural tube

Somites

Remnant of amniotic sac

Caudal neuropore

D

Actual size 3.0 mm

Figure 6–8 **A,** Dorsal view of a five-somite embryo at Carnegie stage 10, approximately 22 days, showing the neural folds and the neural groove. The neural folds in the cranial region have thickened to form the primordium of the brain. **B,** Illustration of the structures shown in **A.** Most of the amniotic and chorionic sacs have been cut away to expose the embryo. **C,** Dorsal view of a 10-somite embryo at Carnegie stage 10, approximately 23 days. The neural folds have fused opposite the somites to form the neural tube (primordium of the spinal cord in this region). The neural tube is in open communication with the amniotic cavity at the cranial and caudal ends through the rostral and caudal neuropores, respectively. **D,** Diagram of the structures shown in **C.**

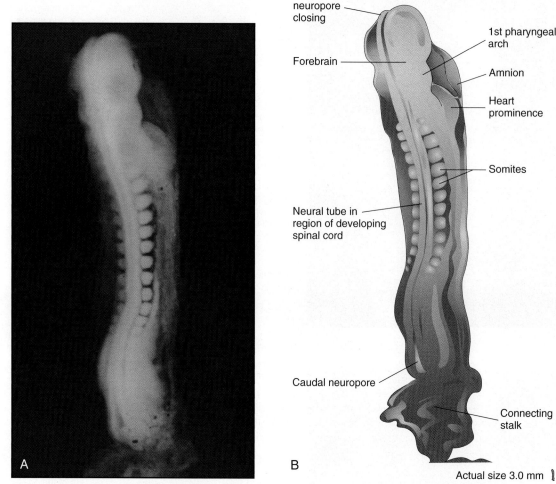

Figure 6–9   **A,** Dorsal view of a 13-somite embryo at Carnegie stage 11, approximately 24 days. The rostral neuropore is closing, but the caudal neuropore is wide open. **B,** Illustration of the structures shown in **A.** The embryo is curved because of folding of the cranial and caudal ends.

The mesonephric kidneys are the primordia of the permanent kidneys (see Fig. 6-12A and B).

Sixth Week

It has been reported that embryos in the sixth week show spontaneous movements, such as twitching of the trunk and limbs. Embryos at this stage show reflex responses to touch. The primordia of the digits—the **digital rays**—begin to develop (Fig. 6-13A and B). Development of the lower limbs occurs 4 to 5 days later than that of the upper limbs. Several small swellings—**auricular hillocks**—develop and contribute to the formation of the *auricle*, the shell-shaped part of the external ear. The eyes are now obvious largely because retinal pigment has formed. The head is much larger relative to the trunk and is bent over the large **heart prominence**. This head position results from bending in the cervical (neck) region. The trunk then begins to straighten. During the sixth week, the *intestines enter the extraembryonic coelom in the proximal part of the umbilical cord.* This **umbilical herniation**

is a normal event in the embryo, occurring because the abdominal cavity is too small at this stage to accommodate the rapidly growing intestines.

Seventh Week

The limbs undergo considerable change during the seventh week. Notches appear between the digital rays in the **hand plates**, partially separating the future digits. Communication between the primordial gut and the umbilical vesicle is now reduced to a relatively slender duct, the *omphaloenteric duct.*

Eighth Week

At the beginning of this final week of the embryonic period, the digits of the hand are separated, but noticeably webbed. Notches are clearly visible between the digital rays of the feet. The **scalp vascular plexus** has appeared and forms a characteristic band around the head.

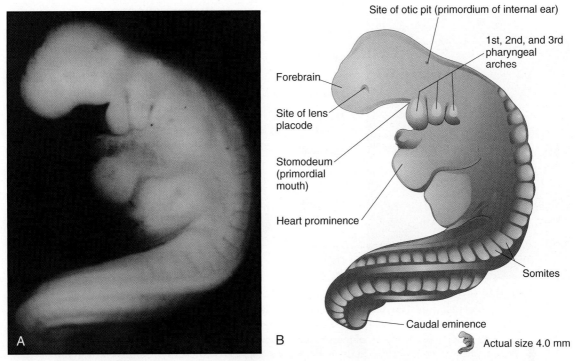

Figure 6–10 **A,** Lateral view of a 27-somite embryo at Carnegie stage 12, approximately 26 days. The embryo is very curved, especially its long, tail-like caudal eminence. The lens placode is the primordium of the lens of the eye. The otic pit indicates early development of the internal ear. **B,** Illustration of the structures shown in **A.** The rostral neuropore is closed, and three pairs of pharyngeal arches are present. (**A,** From Nishimura H, Semba H, Tanimura T, Tanaka O: Prenatal Development of the Human with Special Reference to Craniofacial Structures: An Atlas. Washington, DC, National Institutes of Health, 1977.)

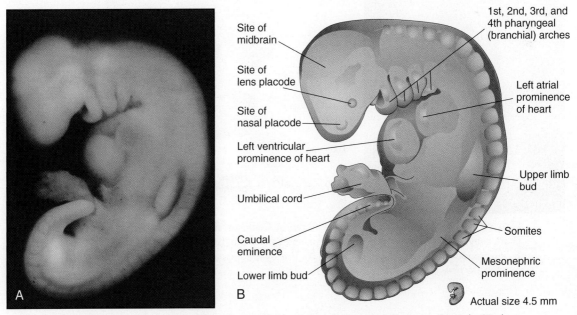

Figure 6–11 **A,** Lateral view of an embryo at Carnegie stage 13, approximately 28 days. The primordial heart is large and is divided into a primordial atrium and a ventricle. The rostral and caudal neuropores are closed. **B,** Illustration of the structures shown in **A.** The embryo has a characteristic C-shaped curvature, four pharyngeal arches, and upper and lower limb buds. (**A,** From Nishimura H, Semba H, Tanimura T, Tanaka O: Prenatal Development of the Human with Special Reference to Craniofacial Structures: An Atlas. Washington, DC, National Institutes of Health, 1977.)

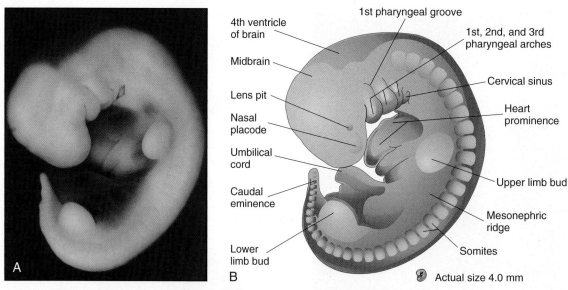

Figure 6–12 **A,** Lateral view of an embryo at Carnegie stage 14, approximately 32 days. The second pharyngeal arch has overgrown the third arch, forming a depression known as the *cervical sinus*. The mesonephric ridge indicates the site of the mesonephric kidney, an interim functional kidney. **B,** Illustration of the structures shown in **A.** The upper limb buds are paddle-shaped, whereas the lower limb buds are flipper-like. (**A,** *From Nishimura H, Semba H, Tanimura T, Tanaka O: Prenatal Development of the Human with Special Reference to Craniofacial Structures: An Atlas. Washington, DC, National Institutes of Health, 1977.*)

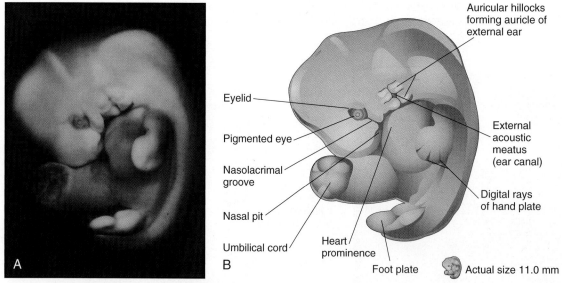

Figure 6–13 **A,** Lateral view of an embryo at Carnegie stage 17, approximately 42 days. Digital rays are visible in the hand plate, indicating the future site of the digits (fingers). **B,** Illustration of the structures shown in **A.** The eye, auricular hillocks, and external acoustic meatus are now clearly discernible.

At the end of the fetal period, the digits have lengthened and are separated (Fig. 6-14*A* and *B*). *Coordinated limb movements first occur during this week.* Primary ossification begins in the femur. All evidence of the tail-like caudal eminence has disappeared by the end of the eighth week. The hands and feet each approach each other ventrally. At the end of the eighth week, the embryo has visually distinct human characteristics; however, the head is still disproportionately large, constituting almost half of the embryo. The neck region is established. The eyelids are closing, and by the end of the eighth week, they begin to unite by epithelial fusion.

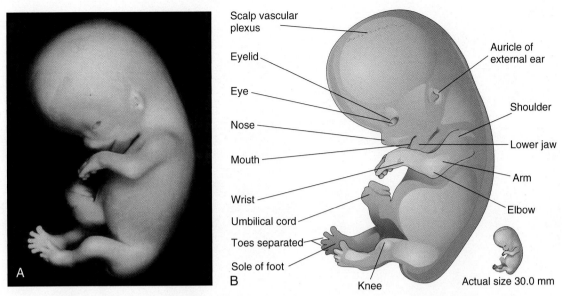

Figure 6–14 **A,** Lateral view of an embryo at Carnegie stage 23, approximately 56 days. **B,** Illustration of the structures shown in **A.** (**A,** *From Nishimura H, Semba H, Tanimura T, Tanaka O: Prenatal Development of the Human with Special Reference to Craniofacial Structures: An Atlas. Washington, DC, National Institutes of Health, 1977.*)

The intestines are still in the proximal portion of the umbilical cord. The auricles of the external ears begin to assume their final shape, but are still low-set on the head. Although sex differences exist in the appearance of the external genitalia, they are not distinctive enough to permit accurate sex identification.

CLINICALLY ORIENTED QUESTIONS

1. There is little apparent difference between an 8-week embryo and a 9-week fetus. Why do embryologists give them different names?

2. When does the embryo become a human being?

3. Can the sex of embryos be determined by ultrasonographic study? What other methods can be used to determine sex?

The answers to these questions are at the back of the book.

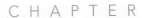

Fetal Period:
The Ninth Week to Birth

Development during the fetal period is concerned primarily with body growth and differentiation of tissues, organs, and systems. Rudimentary organ systems have formed during the embryonic period. The rate of body growth during the fetal period is rapid, and fetal weight gain is phenomenal during the terminal weeks (Table 7-1). Ultrasonographic measurements of the crown-rump length (CRL) can be used to determine fetal size and probable age (Fig. 7-1). The intrauterine period may be divided into days, weeks, or months (Table 7-2), but confusion arises if it is not stated whether the age is calculated from the last normal menstrual period (LNMP) or from the fertilization age. *Unless otherwise stated, fetal age in this book is calculated from the estimated time of fertilization, and months refer to calendar months.* Clinically, the gestational period is divided into three **trimesters**, each lasting 3 months. Various measurements and external characteristics are useful for estimating fetal age (see Table 7-1). Measurement of the CRL (crown- rump length) is the method of choice for estimating fetal age until the end of the *first trimester*.

HIGHLIGHTS OF FETAL PERIOD

There is not a formal staging system for the fetal period; however, it is helpful to consider the main changes that occur in terms of periods of 4 to 5 weeks.

Table 7–1   Criteria for Estimating Fertilization Age during the Fetal Period

AGE (weeks)	CROWN–RUMP LENGTH (mm)*	FOOT LENGTH (mm)*	FETAL WEIGHT (g)†	MAIN EXTERNAL CHARACTERISTICS
Previable Fetus				
9	50	7	8	Eyelids are closing or have closed. Head is rounded. External genitalia are still not distinguishable as male or female. Intestinal herniation is present.
10	61	9	14	Intestine is in the abdomen. Early fingernail development.
12	87	14	45	Sex is distinguishable externally. Well-defined neck.
14	120	20	110	Head is erect. Lower limbs are well developed. Early toenail development.
16	140	27	200	Auricles of the ears stand out from the head.
18	160	33	320	Vernix caseosa covers the skin. Fetal movement (quickening) is felt by the mother.
20	190	39	460	Head and body hair (lanugo) are visible.
Viable Fetus‡				
22	210	45	630	Skin is wrinkled and red.
24	230	50	820	Fingernails are present. Lean body.
26	250	55	1000	Eyes are partially open. Eyelashes are present.
28	270	59	1300	Eyes are open. Most fetuses have scalp hair. Skin is slightly wrinkled.
30	280	63	1700	Toenails are present. Body is filling out. Testes are descending.
32	300	68	2100	Fingernails extend to fingertips. Skin is smooth.
36	340	79	2900	Body is usually plump. Lanugo is almost absent. Toenails extend to the toe tips. Flexed limb; firm grasp.
38	360	83	3400	Prominent chest; breasts protrude. Testes in the scrotum or palpable in the inguinal canals. Fingernails extend beyond fingertips.

*These measurements are averages, and dimensional variations increase with age.

†These weights refer to fetuses that have been fixed for approximately 2 weeks in 10% formalin. Fresh specimens usually weigh approximately 5% less.

‡There is no sharp limit of development, age, or weight at which a fetus automatically becomes viable or beyond which survival is ensured, but experience has shown that it is uncommon for an infant to survive if its weight is less than 500 g or if its fertilization age or developmental age is less than 22 weeks.

Table 7–2   Comparison of Gestational Time Units

REFERENCE POINT	CALENDAR			LUNAR MONTHS
	DAYS	WEEKS	MONTHS	
Fertilization	266	38	8.75	9.5
Last normal menstrual period	280	40	9.25	10

Nine to Twelve Weeks

At the beginning of the ninth week, *the head constitutes half of the CRL of the fetus* (Fig. 7-1). Subsequently, growth in body length accelerates rapidly, and by the end of 12 weeks, the CRL has more than doubled (Table 7-1). At 9 weeks, the face is broad, the eyes are widely separated, the ears are low set, and the eyelids are fused. Early in the ninth week, the legs are short and the thighs are relatively small. By the end of 12 weeks, the upper limbs have almost reached their final relative lengths, but the lower limbs are still slightly shorter than their final relative lengths. The *external genitalia* of males and females are not in their mature fetal form until the 12th week. Intestinal coils are clearly visible in the proximal end of

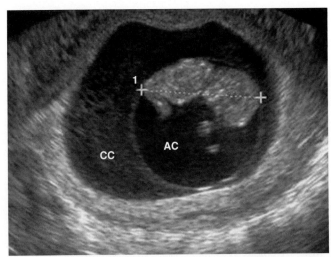

Figure 7–1   Endovaginal scan of a 9-week embryo with a CRL of 41.7 mm (calipers). Amniotic cavity (*AC*). Chorionic cavity (*CC*) has low level echoes normally while the AC is echo-free. (*Courtesy E. A. Lyons, M.D., Professor of Radiology, and Obstetrics and Gynecology, and Anatomy, University of Manitoba, Health Sciences Centre, Winnipeg, Manitoba, Canada.*)

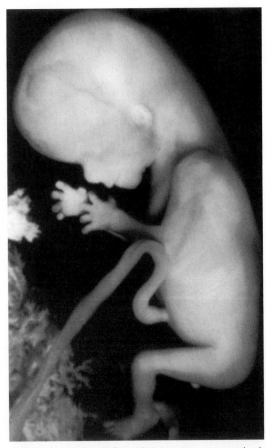

Figure 7–2   An 11-week fetus that was spontaneously aborted. Its chorionic and amniotic sacs have been removed (×1.5). Note that the head is relatively large. (*Courtesy Jean Hay, retired, University of Manitoba, Winnipeg, Manitoba, Canada.*)

the umbilical cord until the middle of the 10th week. By the 11th week, *the intestines have returned to the abdomen* (Fig. 7-2).

Urine formation begins between the 9th and 12th weeks, and urine is discharged through the urethra into the amniotic fluid. The fetus reabsorbs some of this fluid after swallowing it. Fetal waste products in blood are transferred to the maternal circulation by passing across the placental membrane (see Chapter 8).

Thirteen to Sixteen Weeks

Growth is very rapid during the 13th to 16th weeks (Figs. 7-3 and 7-4; see Table 7-1). By 16 weeks, the head is relatively small compared with that of the 12-week fetus, and the lower limbs have lengthened. *Limb movements*, which first occur at the end of the embryonic period, become coordinated by the 14th week, but are too slight to be felt by the mother. However, these movements are visible during ultrasonographic examinations. By the beginning of the 16th week, the bones are clearly visible on ultrasound images. *Slow eye movements* occur at 14 weeks. Scalp hair patterning is also determined during this period. By 16 weeks, the ovaries are differentiated and contain in them primordial ovarian follicles that have oogonia. By 16 weeks, the eyes face anteriorly rather than anterolaterally.

Seventeen to Twenty Weeks

Growth slows down during weeks 17 to 20, but the fetus still increases its CRL by approximately 50 mm (Figs. 7-3 and 7-5; see Table 7-1). Fetal movements—**quickening**—are commonly felt by the mother. The skin is now covered with a greasy material called **vernix caseosa**, which consists of dead epidermal cells and a fatty secretion from

the fetal sebaceous glands. The vernix caseosa protects the delicate fetal skin from abrasions, chapping, and hardening that could result from exposure to the amniotic fluid. Fetuses are usually completely covered with fine, downy hair called *lanugo*, which helps to hold the vernix caseosa on the skin. Eyebrows and head hair are also visible. *Brown fat* forms during weeks 17 through 20 and is the site of heat production, particularly in the newborn. This specialized adipose tissue produces heat by oxidizing fatty acids. By 18 weeks, the uterus is formed in female fetuses. By this time, many *primordial ovarian follicles* containing oogonia have formed. In male 20-week fetuses, the testes have begun to descend, but they are still located on the posterior abdominal wall.

Twenty-One to Twenty-Five Weeks

Substantial weight gain occurs during weeks 21 to 25 and the fetus is better proportioned. At 21 weeks, rapid eye movements begin; *blink-startle responses* have been reported at 22 to 23 weeks. By 24 weeks, the secretory epithelial cells (type II pneumocytes) in the interalveolar walls of the lung have begun to secrete *surfactant*, a surface-active lipid that maintains the patency of the

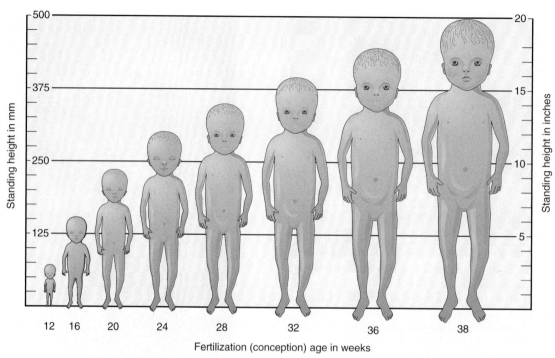

Figure 7–3   Diagram, drawn to scale, showing progressive fetal growth.

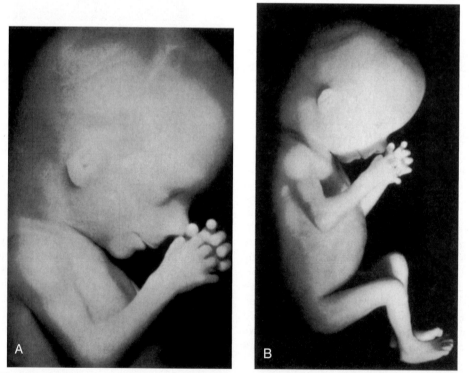

Figure 7–4   A 13-week fetus. **A,** An enlarged photograph of the head and shoulders (×2). **B,** Actual size. *(Courtesy Jean Hay, retired, University of Manitoba, Winnipeg, Manitoba, Canada.)*

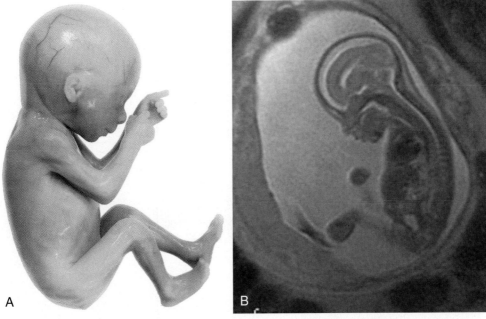

Figure 7–5 **A,** A 17-week fetus (actual size). Fetuses at this age are unable to survive if born prematurely, mainly because the respiratory system is immature. *(From Moore KL, Persaud TVN, Shiota K: Color Atlas of Clinical Embryology, 2nd ed. Philadelphia, WB Saunders, 2000).* **B,** Magnetic resonance imaging scan of an 18-week-old normal fetus (20 weeks gestational age). *(Courtesy Deborah Levine, M.D., Director of Obstetric and Gynecologic Ultrasound, Department of Radiology, Beth Israel Deaconess Medical Center, Boston, MA.)*

developing alveoli of the lungs. Although a 22- to 25-week fetus born prematurely may survive initially if given intensive care support, the fetus may die because its respiratory system is still immature. Infants born before 26 weeks of gestation have a high risk of neurodevelopmental (functional) disability. *Fingernails* are also present by 24 weeks.

Twenty-Six to Twenty-Nine Weeks

At 26 to 29 weeks, a fetus often survives if born because the lungs have developed sufficiently to provide adequate gas exchange. In addition, the central nervous system has matured to the stage at which it can direct rhythmic breathing movements and control body temperature. The greatest neonatal mortality occur in low–birth weight infants (weighing 2500 g or less) and especially in very low–birth weight infants (weighing 1500 g or less). *The eyelids are open at 26 weeks,* and lanugo and head hair are well developed. Toenails are visible, and considerable subcutaneous fat is now present, smoothing out many of the skin wrinkles.

Thirty to Thirty-Eight Weeks

The *pupillary light reflex of the eyes* can be elicited by 30 weeks. Usually, by the end of this period, the skin is pink and smooth, and the upper and lower limbs have a chubby appearance. Fetuses 32 weeks and older usually survive if born. Fetuses at 35 weeks have a firm grasp and exhibit a spontaneous orientation to light. As term

approaches (37–38 weeks), the nervous system is sufficiently mature to carry out some integrative functions. Most fetuses during this "finishing period" are plump (Fig. 7-6). By 36 weeks, the circumferences of the head and the abdomen are approximately equal. Growth slows as the time of birth approaches (Fig. 7-7). Most fetuses weigh approximately 3400g at term. A fetus adds approximately 14 g of fat daily during the last weeks of gestation. The chest is prominent, and the breasts protrude slightly in both sexes.

Expected Date of Delivery

The expected date of delivery of a fetus is 266 days, or 38 weeks, after fertilization (i.e., 280 days, or 40 weeks, after the LNMP) [see Table 7-2]. Approximately 12% of babies are born 1 to 2 weeks after the expected time of birth

FACTORS INFLUENCING FETAL GROWTH

The fetus requires substrates for growth and the production of energy. Gases and nutrients pass freely to the fetus from the mother through the placental membrane (see Chapter 8). **Glucose** is a primary source of energy for fetal metabolism and growth; **amino acids** are also required. **Insulin,** which is required for the metabolism of glucose, is secreted by the fetal pancreas. Insulin, human growth hormone, and some small polypeptides (e.g.,

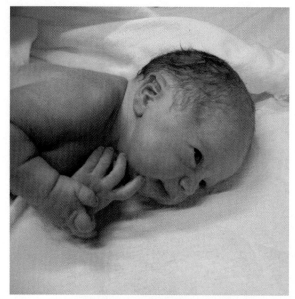

Figure 7–6 A healthy male newborn infant at 36 weeks gestational age. *(Courtesy of Michael and Michele Rice.)*

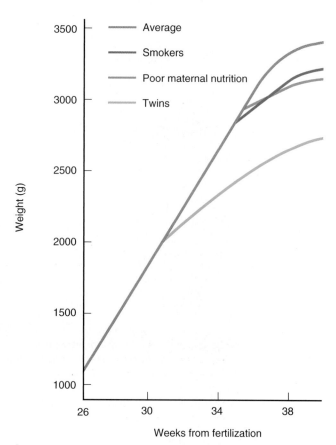

Figure 7–7 Graph showing the rate of fetal growth during the last trimester. After 36 weeks, the growth rate deviates from the straight line. The decline, particularly after full term (38 weeks), probably reflects inadequate fetal nutrition caused by placental changes. *(Adapted from Gruenwald P: Growth of the human fetus. I. Normal growth and its variation. Am J Obstet Gynecol 94:1112, 1966.)*

insulin-like growth factor I) are believed to stimulate fetal growth.

Many factors—maternal, fetal, and environmental—may affect prenatal growth. In general, factors operating throughout pregnancy, such as *cigarette smoking* and *consumption of alcohol,* tend to produce intrauterine growth restriction (IUGR) and small infants, whereas factors operating during the last trimester (e.g., maternal malnutrition) usually produce underweight infants with normal length and head size. Severe maternal malnutrition resulting from a poor-quality diet is known to cause reduced fetal growth (see Fig. 7-7).

Neonates (newborns) resulting from twin, triplet, and other multiple pregnancies usually weigh considerably less than infants resulting from a single pregnancy (see Fig. 7-7). It is evident that the total requirements of two or more fetuses exceed the nutritional supply available from the placenta during the third trimester.

Repeated cases of IUGR in one family indicate that recessive genes may be the cause of the abnormal growth. In recent years, structural and numeric chromosomal aberrations have also been shown to be associated with cases of restricted fetal growth. IUGR is pronounced in infants with trisomy 21 (Down syndrome) (see Chapter 19).

PROCEDURES FOR ASSESSING FETAL STATUS

Ultrasonography

Ultrasonography is the primary imaging modality in the evaluation of the fetus because of its wide availability, low cost, and lack of known adverse effects (Fig. 7-8). Placental and fetal size, multiple births, abnormalities of placental shape, and abnormal presentations can also be

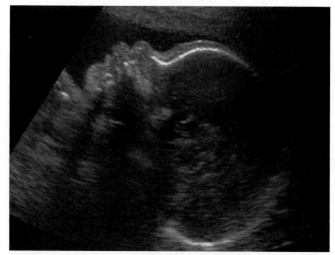

Figure 7–8 Ultrasonogram (axial scan) of a 25-week fetus showing the facial profile. *(Courtesy E. A. Lyons, M.D., Professor of Radiology, Obstetrics and Gynecology, and Anatomy, University of Manitoba, Health Sciences Centre, Winnipeg, Manitoba, Canada.)*

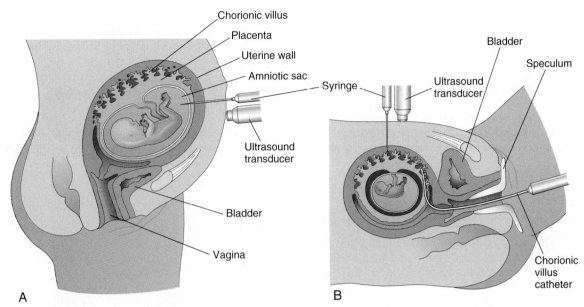

Figure 7–9 **A,** Illustration of the technique of amniocentesis. Using ultrasonographic guidance, a needle is inserted through the mother's abdominal and uterine walls into the amniotic sac. A syringe is attached and amniotic fluid is withdrawn for diagnostic purposes. **B,** Illustration of chorionic villus sampling. Two sampling approaches are shown—one through the anterior abdominal wall and amniotic sac using a needle, and one through the vagina and cervical canal using a malleable chorionic villus catheter.

determined. Many developmental defects can also be detected prenatally by ultrasonography.

Diagnostic Amniocentesis

Diagnostic amniocentesis is a common invasive prenatal diagnostic procedure (Fig. 7-9A) typically performed during the second trimester. For prenatal diagnosis, amniotic fluid is sampled by insertion of a hollow needle through the mother's anterior abdominal and uterine walls and into the amniotic sac. A syringe is then attached to the needle and amniotic fluid is withdrawn. The procedure is relatively devoid of risk, especially when performed by an experienced physician using ultrasonography as a guide for outlining the position of the fetus and the placenta.

Chorionic Villus Sampling

Biopsy of chorionic villi (see Fig. 7-9B) is performed to detect chromosomal abnormalities, inborn errors of metabolism, and X-linked disorders. Chorionic villus sampling can be performed as early as 7 weeks after fertilization. The rate of fetal loss is approximately 1%, slightly more than the risk associated with amniocentesis. The major advantage of chorionic villus sampling over amniocentesis is that it allows fetal chromosomal sampling to be performed several weeks earlier.

Cell Cultures

Fetal sex and chromosomal aberrations can also be determined by studying the sex chromosomes in cultured fetal cells obtained during amniocentesis. These cultures are

commonly performed when an autosomal abnormality, such as occurs in Down syndrome, is suspected. Inborn errors of metabolism and enzyme deficiencies in fetuses can also be detected by studying cell cultures.

Percutaneous Umbilical Cord Blood Sampling

For chromosomal analysis, blood samples may be obtained from the umbilical vessels by **percutaneous umbilical cord blood sampling**. Ultrasonographic scanning is used to outline the location of the vessels. Percutaneous umbilical cord blood sampling is often performed approximately 20 weeks after the LNMP to obtain samples for chromosomal analysis when ultrasonographic or other examinations have shown characteristics of birth defects

Magnetic Resonance Imaging

When fetal treatment, such as surgery, is planned, computed tomography and magnetic resonance imaging (MRI) may be used. MRI has the advantage of not requiring ionizing radiation to produce images. These studies can provide additional information about a fetal abnormality detected ultrasonographically.

Fetal Monitoring

Continuous fetal heart rate monitoring in high-risk pregnancies is routine and provides information about the oxygenation of the fetus. *Fetal distress*, as indicated by an abnormal heart rate or rhythm, suggests that the fetus is in jeopardy.

Alpha Fetoprotein Assay

Alpha fetoprotein, a glycoprotein that is synthesized in the fetal liver and umbilical vesicle, escapes from the fetal circulation into the amniotic fluid in fetuses with open neural tube defects, such as spina bifida with myeloschisis (see Chapter 19). Alpha fetoprotein can also enter the amniotic fluid from open ventral wall defects, as occurs with gastroschisis and omphalocele (see Chapter 13). Alpha fetoprotein can also be measured in maternal serum.

 CLINICALLY ORIENTED QUESTIONS

1. Some say that the mature embryo twitches and that a first-trimester fetus moves its limbs. Is this true? If so, can the mother feel her baby kicking at this time?

2. Some reports suggest that vitamin supplementation around the time of conception will prevent neural tube defects, such as spina bifida. Is there scientific proof to support this statement?

3. Can the fetus be injured by the needle during amniocentesis? Is there a risk of inducing an abortion or causing maternal or fetal infection?

The answers to these questions are at the back of the book.

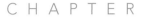

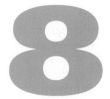

Placenta and Fetal Membranes

T he fetal part of the placenta and fetal membranes separate the embryo or fetus from the endometrium. The chorion, amnion, umbilical vesicle (yolk sac), and allantois constitute the fetal membranes. An interchange of substances (e.g., nutrients and oxygen) occurs between the maternal and fetal blood through the placenta. The vessels in the umbilical cord connect the placental circulation with the fetal circulation.

PLACENTA

The placenta is a **fetomaternal organ** that has two components:

- A **fetal part** that develops from part of the chorionic sac
- A **maternal part** that is derived from the endometrium (inner layer of uterine wall)

The placenta and umbilical cord function as a *transport system* for substances passing between the mother and the fetus. Nutrients and oxygen pass from the maternal blood through the placenta to the fetal blood, and waste materials and carbon dioxide pass from the fetal blood through the placenta to the maternal blood. The placenta and fetal membranes perform the following functions and activities: protection, nutrition, respiration, excretion, and hormone production. Shortly after birth, the placenta and fetal membranes are expelled from the uterus as the *afterbirth*.

Decidua

The *decidua* is the gravid (pregnant) endometrium, the functional layer of the endometrium in a pregnant woman that separates from the remainder of the uterus after *parturition* (childbirth).

Three regions of the decidua are named according to their relation to the implantation site (Fig. 8-1):

- Decidua basalis—the part of the decidua deep to the conceptus that forms the maternal part of the placenta
- Decidua capsularis—the superficial part of the decidua overlying the conceptus
- Decidua parietalis—the remaining intervening parts of the decidua

In response to increasing progesterone levels in the maternal blood, the connective tissue cells of the decidua enlarge to form pale-staining **decidual cells**. These cells enlarge as glycogen and lipid accumulate in their cytoplasm. The cellular and vascular changes in the decidua that result from pregnancy are referred to as the **decidual reaction**. Many decidual cells degenerate near the chorionic sac in the region of the syncytiotrophoblast and, together with maternal blood and uterine secretions, provide a rich source of nutrition for the embryo. Decidual regions, clearly recognizable during ultrasonography, are important in diagnosing early pregnancy.

Development of Placenta

Early placental development is characterized by the rapid proliferation of the trophoblast and development of the chorionic sac and chorionic villi. By the end of the third week, the anatomic arrangements necessary for physiologic exchanges between the mother and the embryo have been established. By the end of the fourth week, a complex vascular network develops in the placenta, allowing maternal-embryonic exchanges of gases, nutrients, and metabolic waste products. Chorionic villi cover the entire chorionic sac until the beginning of the eighth week (Figs. 8-1*D* and 8-2). As this sac grows, the villi associated with the decidua capsularis are compressed, reducing the blood supply to them. These villi soon degenerate, producing a relatively avascular bare area, the **smooth chorion**. As these villi disappear, those associated with the decidua basalis rapidly increase in number, branch profusely, and enlarge (Fig. 8-3). This bushy part of the chorionic sac is known as the **villous chorion** or **chorion frondosum** (Figs. 8-1*E* and 8-4).

Fetomaternal Junction

The fetal part of the placenta (villous chorion) is attached to the maternal part of the placenta (decidua basalis) by the **cytotrophoblastic shell**, the external layer of trophoblastic cells on the maternal surface of the placenta (see Fig. 8-5). The chorionic villi, which are attached firmly to the decidua basalis through the cytotrophoblastic shell, anchor the chorionic sac to the decidua basalis. Endometrial arteries and veins pass freely through gaps in the

ULTRASONOGRAPHY OF THE CHORIONIC SAC

The size of the chorionic sac is useful in determining the gestational age of embryos in pregnant women with uncertain menstrual histories. Growth of the chorionic sac is extremely rapid between the 5th and 10th weeks of development. Modern ultrasound devices permit detection of the chorionic sac when it has a median diameter of 2 to 3 mm (Fig. 8-4). Chorionic sacs with this diameter indicate a gestational age of approximately 32 days.

cytotrophoblastic shell and open into the intervillous space.

The **shape of the placenta** is determined by the shape of the persistent area of chorionic villi (Fig. 8-1*F*). Usually this is a circular area, giving the placenta a discoid shape. As the chorionic villi invade the decidua basalis during placental formation, decidual tissue is eroded to enlarge the intervillous space. This erosion produces several wedge-shaped areas of decidua—**placental septa**—that project toward the **chorionic plate** (Fig. 8-5). The placental septa divide the fetal part of the placenta into irregular convex areas called **cotyledons** (Fig. 8-3). Each cotyledon consists of two or more stem villi and many **branch villi**.

The **decidua capsularis**, the layer overlying the implanted chorionic sac, forms a capsule over the external surface of the sac (Fig. 8-1*A* to *D*). As the conceptus enlarges, the decidua capsularis bulges into the uterine cavity and becomes greatly attenuated. Eventually, parts of the decidua capsularis make contact and fuse with the **decidua parietalis**, thereby slowly obliterating the uterine cavity (Fig. 8-1*E* and *F*). By 22 to 24 weeks, reduced blood supply to the decidua capsularis causes it to degenerate and disappear.

Intervillous Space

The intervillous space of the placenta contains maternal blood, which is derived from the lacunae that developed in the syncytiotrophoblast during the second week of development (see Fig. 4-1*C*). This large, blood-filled space results from the coalescence and enlargement of these lacunar networks. The intervillous space of the placenta is divided into compartments by the *placental septa*; however, free communication occurs between the compartments because the septa do not reach the **chorionic plate** (Fig. 8-5), the part of the chorion associated with the placenta. Maternal blood enters the intervillous space from the **spiral arteries** in the decidua basalis; these arteries pass through gaps in the cytotrophoblastic shell and discharge blood into the intervillous space. This large space is drained by endometrial veins that also penetrate the cytotrophoblastic shell. The numerous **branch villi**, arising from **stem villi**, are continuously showered with maternal blood as it circulates through the intervillous space. The blood in this space carries oxygen and nutritional materials that are necessary for fetal growth and

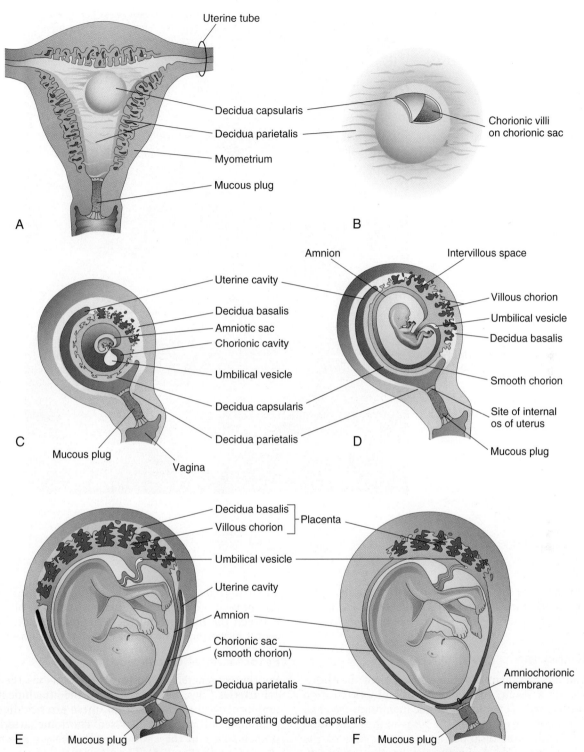

Figure 8–1 Development of placenta and fetal membranes. **A,** Coronal section of the uterus showing elevation of the decidua capsularis and the expanding chorionic sac at 4 weeks. **B,** Enlarged illustration of the implantation site. The chorionic villi were exposed by cutting an opening in the decidua capsularis. **C to F,** Sagittal sections of the gravid (pregnant) uterus from the 5th to 22nd weeks, showing the changing relationship of the fetal membranes to the decidua. In **F,** the amnion and the chorion are fused with each other and with the decidua parietalis, thereby obliterating the uterine cavity.

Figure 8–2 Lateral view of a spontaneously aborted embryo at Carnegie stage 14, approximately 32 days. The chorionic and amniotic sacs have been opened to show the embryo.

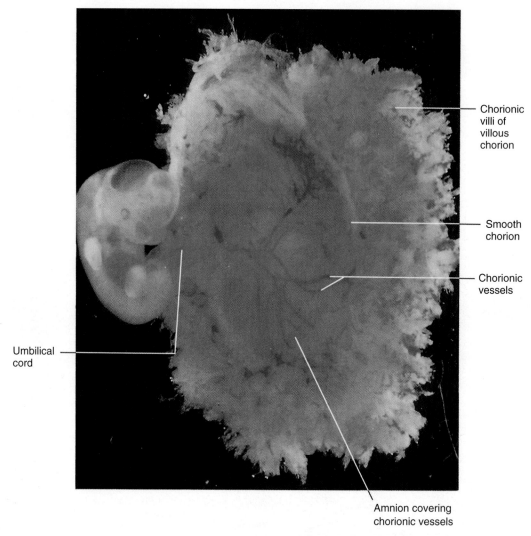

Chorionic villi of villous chorion

Smooth chorion

Chorionic vessels

Umbilical cord

Amnion covering chorionic vessels

development. The maternal blood also contains fetal waste products, such as carbon dioxide, salts, and products of protein metabolism.

Amniochorionic Membrane

The amniotic sac enlarges more quickly than the chorionic sac. As a result, the amnion and smooth chorion soon fuse to form the amniochorionic membrane (see Fig. 8-1F). This composite membrane fuses with the decidua capsularis and, after disappearance of this part of the decidua, adheres to the decidua parietalis. *It is the amniochorionic membrane that ruptures during labor.* Preterm rupture of this membrane is the most common event leading to premature labor. When the amniochorionic membrane ruptures, the amniotic fluid escapes through the cervix and vagina.

Placental Circulation

The many *branch chorionic villi* provide a large surface area where materials may be exchanged across the very thin **placental membrane** interposed between the fetal

and maternal circulations (Fig. 8-6B and C). It is through the branch villi that the main exchange of material between the mother and the fetus takes place. The placental membrane consists of extrafetal tissues.

Fetoplacental Circulation

Poorly oxygenated blood leaves the fetus via the **umbilical arteries** (Figs. 8-5 and 8-7). At the attachment of the umbilical cord to the placenta, these arteries divide into a number of radially disposed **chorionic arteries** that branch freely in the chorionic plate before entering the chorionic villi (Fig. 8-5). The blood vessels form an extensive **arteriocapillary venous system** within the chorionic villi (Fig. 8-6A) that brings the fetal blood extremely close to the maternal blood (Fig. 8-7). This system provides a very large surface area for the exchange of metabolic and gaseous products between the maternal and fetal blood. Normally, no intermingling of fetal and maternal blood occurs. The well-oxygenated fetal blood in the fetal capillaries passes into thin-walled veins that follow the chorionic arteries to the site of attachment of the umbilical cord, where they converge to form the **umbilical vein**. This large vessel carries oxygen-rich blood to the fetus.

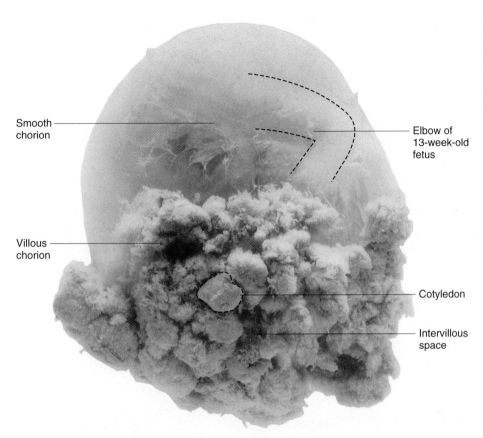

Figure 8-3 A human chorionic sac containing a 13-week fetus. The villous chorion is where chorionic villi persist and form the fetal part of the placenta. In situ, the cotyledons were attached to the decidua basalis and the intervillous space was filled with maternal blood.

Smooth chorion

Elbow of 13-week-old fetus

Villous chorion

Cotyledon

Intervillous space

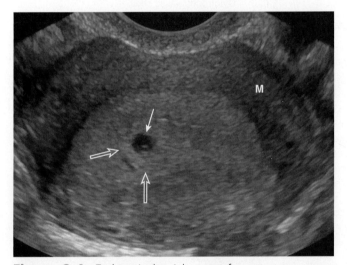

Figure 8-4 Endovaginal axial scan of a pregnant uterus showing a 3-week chorionic sac *(arrow)* in the posterior endometrium (decidua). There is a bright (echogenic) ring of chorionic villi *(open arrows)* around the sac. *M,* Myometrium. *(Courtesy E. A. Lyons, M.D., Professor of Radiology, Obstetrics and Gynecology, and Anatomy, University of Manitoba, Health Sciences Centre, Winnipeg, Manitoba, Canada.)*

Maternal-Placental Circulation

The maternal blood enters the intervillous space through 80 to 100 **spiral arteries** in the decidua basali (Fig. 8-5). The entering blood is at considerably higher pressure than that in the intervillous space, so it spurts toward the

chorionic plate. As the pressure dissipates, the blood flows slowly around the branch villi, allowing an exchange of metabolic and gaseous products with the fetal blood. The blood eventually returns through the endometrial veins to the maternal circulation (Fig. 8-7). Reductions of uteroplacental circulation result in **fetal hypoxia** (decreased level of oxygen) and IUGR (intrauterine growth restriction). The intervillous space of the mature placenta contains approximately 150 ml of blood that is replenished three or four times each minute.

Placental Membrane

The **placental membrane (placental barrier)** consists of the extrafetal tissues that separate the maternal and fetal blood. Until approximately 20 weeks, *the placental membrane consists of four layers* (Fig. 8-6B): syncytiotrophoblast, cytotrophoblast, connective tissue of the villus, and endothelium of the fetal capillaries.

After the 20th week, microscopic changes occur in the branch villi that result in the cytotrophoblast becoming attenuated in many villi. Eventually, cytotrophoblastic cells disappear over large areas of the villi, leaving only thin patches of syncytiotrophoblast. As a result, the placental membrane at full term consists of only three layers in most places (Fig. 8-6C). In some areas, the placental membrane becomes markedly thinned. At these sites, the syncytiotrophoblast comes in direct contact with the endothelium of the fetal capillaries to form a *vasculosyncytial placental membrane.*

Only a few substances, endogenous or exogenous, are unable to pass through the placental membrane. The

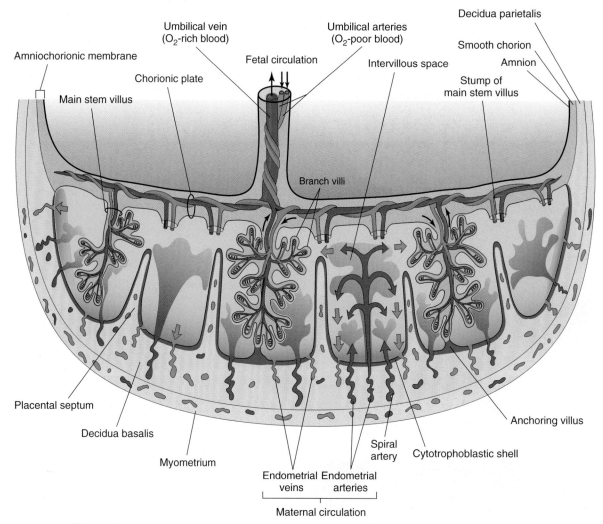

Figure 8–5   Illustration of a transverse section through a full-term placenta, showing (1) the relation of the villous chorion (fetal part of placenta) to the decidua basalis (maternal part of placenta); (2) the fetal placental circulation; and (3) the maternal placental circulation. Maternal blood flows into the intervillous spaces in funnel-shaped spurts from the spiral arteries, and exchanges occur with the fetal blood as the maternal blood flows around the branch villi. The inflowing arterial blood pushes venous blood out of the intervillous space and into the endometrial veins. Note that the umbilical arteries carry poorly oxygenated fetal blood (shown in *blue*) to the placenta and that the umbilical vein carries oxygenated blood (shown in *red*) to the fetus. Only one stem villus is shown in each cotyledon, but the stumps of those that have been removed are indicated. *Arrows* indicate direction of maternal (*red* and *blue*) and fetal (*black*) blood flow.

membrane acts as a true barrier only when the molecule or organism has a certain size, configuration, and charge. *Most drugs and other substances in the maternal plasma pass through the placental membrane and are found in the fetal plasma* (Fig. 8-7).

During the third trimester, numerous nuclei in the syncytiotrophoblast of the villi aggregate to form **syncytial knots** (*nuclear aggregations*) (Fig. 8-6C). These knots continually break off and are carried from the intervillous space into the maternal circulation; some may lodge in capillaries of the maternal lungs, where they are rapidly destroyed by local enzyme action. Toward the end of pregnancy, **fibrinoid material** also forms on the surfaces of the villi.

The placenta has three main functions:

- Metabolism
- Transport of gases and nutrients
- Endocrine secretion

Placental Metabolism

The placenta synthesizes glycogen, cholesterol, and fatty acids, which serve as sources of nutrients and energy for the embryo or fetus. Many of the metabolic activities of the placenta are critical for its other two major activities: transport and endocrine secretion.

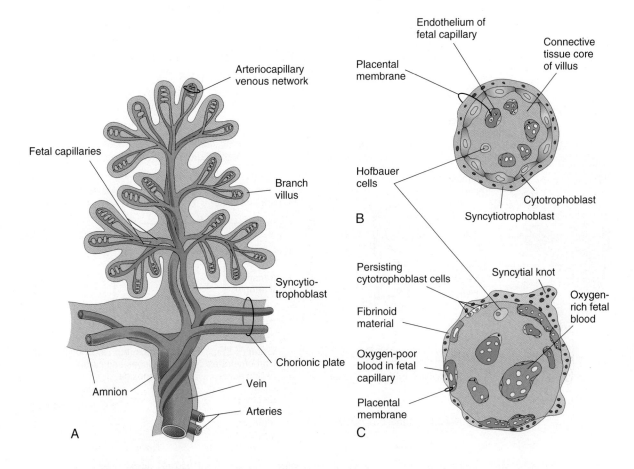

Figure 8–6 **A**, Illustration of a stem chorionic villus showing its arteriocapillary-venous system. The arteries carry poorly oxygenated fetal blood and waste products from the fetus, whereas the vein carries oxygenated blood and nutrients to the fetus. **B** and **C**, Sections through a branch villus at 10 weeks' gestation and at full term, respectively. The placental membrane, composed of extrafetal tissues, separates the maternal blood in the intervillous space from the fetal blood in the capillaries in the villi. Note that the placental membrane becomes very thin at full term. Hofbauer cells are believed to be phagocytic cells.

Placental Transport

The transport of substances in both directions between the placenta and the maternal blood is facilitated by the large surface area of the placental membrane. Almost all materials are transported across the placental membrane by one of the following four main **transport mechanisms**: simple diffusion, facilitated diffusion, active transport, and pinocytosis.

Passive transport by simple diffusion is usually characteristic of substances moving from areas of higher to lower concentration until equilibrium is established. *Facilitated diffusion* requires a transporter but no energy.

Active transport against a concentration gradient requires energy. This mechanism of transport may involve carrier molecules that temporarily combine with the substances to be transported. *Pinocytosis* is a form of endocytosis in which the material being engulfed is a small amount of extracellular fluid. Some proteins are transferred very slowly through the placenta by pinocytosis.

Transfer of Gases

Gases, such as oxygen, carbon dioxide, and carbon monoxide, cross the placental membrane by simple diffusion. *Interruption of oxygen transport for several minutes endangers the survival of the embryo or fetus.* The efficiency of the placental membrane approaches that of the lungs for gas exchange. The quantity of oxygen reaching the fetus is generally flow-limited, rather than diffusion-limited; hence, fetal hypoxia results primarily from factors that diminish either uterine blood flow or fetal blood flow through the placenta. Nitrous oxide, an inhalation analgesic and anesthetic, also readily crosses the placenta.

Nutritional Substances

Water is rapidly exchanged by simple diffusion and in increasing amounts as pregnancy advances. *Glucose* produced by the mother and the placenta is quickly transferred to the embryo or fetus by facilitated diffusion. Very small amounts of maternal cholesterol, triglycerides, and phospholipids are transferred. Although free fatty acids

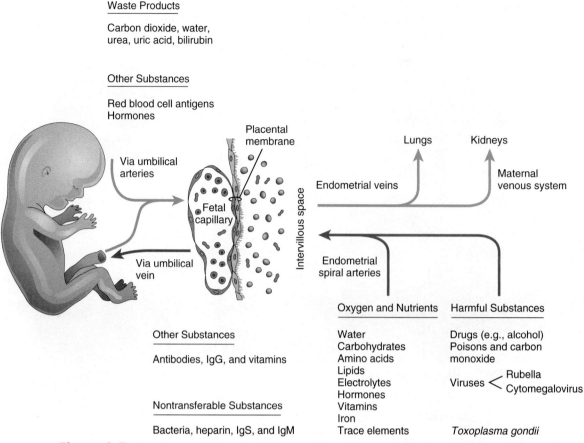

Figure 8–7   Transfer across the placental membrane. The extrafetal tissues, across which transport of substances between the mother and the fetus occurs, collectively constitute the placental membrane. *IgG*, Immunoglobulin G; *IgM*, immunoglobulin M; *IgS*, immunoglobulin S.

are transported, the amount transferred appears to be relatively small. *Amino acids* cross the placenta to the fetus in high concentrations by active transport. *Vitamins* cross the placental membrane and are essential for normal development. A maternal protein, *transferrin*, crosses the placental membrane and carries iron to the embryo or fetus. The placental surface contains special receptors for this protein.

Hormones

Protein hormones do not reach the embryo or fetus in significant amounts, except for a slow transfer of thyroxine and triiodothyronine. Unconjugated *steroid hormones* cross the placental membrane relatively freely. Testosterone and certain synthetic progestins also cross the placenta.

Electrolytes

Electrolytes are freely exchanged in significant quantities, each at its own rate. When a mother receives intravenous fluids with electrolytes, they also pass to the fetus and affect the fetal water and electrolyte status.

Maternal Antibodies

The fetus produces only small amounts of antibodies because of its immature immune system. Some passive immunity is conferred on the fetus by placental transfer of maternal antibodies. Only immunoglobulin G is transferred across the placenta (receptor-mediated transcytosis). *Maternal antibodies confer fetal immunity* for diseases such as diphtheria, smallpox, and measles; however, no immunity is acquired to pertussis (whooping cough) or chickenpox.

Waste Products

Urea and uric acid pass through the placental membrane by simple diffusion. Conjugated bilirubin (which is fat soluble) is easily transported by the placenta and is quickly cleared.

Drugs and Drug Metabolites

Most drugs and drug metabolites cross the placenta by simple diffusion. Drugs taken by the mother can affect the embryo or fetus, directly or indirectly, by interfering with maternal or placental metabolism. Some drugs cause major birth defects (see Chapter 19). *Fetal drug addiction* may occur after maternal use of drugs such as heroin, and newborn infants may experience withdrawal symptoms. Most drugs used for the management of labor readily cross the placental membrane. Depending on their dose and timing in relation to delivery, these drugs may cause respiratory depression of the newborn infant. Neuromuscular blocking agents, such as succinylcholine, that might be used during operative obstetrics, cross the placenta in only very small amounts. All sedatives and analgesics affect the fetus to some degree. Inhaled anesthetics can also cross the placental membrane and affect fetal breathing if used during parturition.

Infectious Agents

Cytomegalovirus, rubella, and coxsackie viruses, as well as viruses associated with variola, varicella, measles, and poliomyelitis, may pass through the placental membrane and cause *fetal infection*. In some cases, as with the **rubella virus**, severe congenital anomalies may result (see Chapter 19). Maternal infection with *Treponema pallidum* causes fetal syphilis and *Toxoplasma gondii* produces destructive changes in the brain and eyes of the fetus.

Placental Endocrine Synthesis and Secretion

Using precursors derived from the fetus, the mother, or both, the *syncytiotrophoblast* of the placenta synthesizes protein and steroid hormones. **Protein hormones** synthesized by the placenta include the following:

● Human chorionic gonadotropin (hCG)
● Human chorionic somatomammotropin, or human placental lactogen
● Human chorionic thyrotropin
● Human chorionic corticotropin

The glycoprotein hCG, similar to luteinizing hormone, is first secreted by the syncytiotrophoblast during the second week. The *hCG maintains the corpus luteum*, preventing the onset of menstrual periods. The concentration of hCG in the maternal blood and urine rises to a maximum by the eighth week and then declines. The placenta also plays a major role in the production of **steroid hormones** (i.e., progesterone and estrogens). Progesterone is essential for the maintenance of pregnancy.

HEMOLYTIC DISEASE OF THE NEWBORN

Small amounts of fetal blood may pass to the maternal blood through microscopic breaks in the placental membrane. If the fetus is Rh-positive and the mother is Rh-negative, the fetal cells may stimulate the formation of anti-Rh antibody by the mother's immune system. This antibody passes to the fetal blood and causes hemolysis of fetal Rh-positive blood cells and anemia in the fetus. Some fetuses with hemolytic disease of the newborn, or fetal erythroblastosis, do not make a satisfactory intrauterine adjustment. They may die unless delivered early or given intraperitoneal, or intravenous transfusions of packed Rh-negative blood cells to maintain the fetus until after birth. Hemolytic disease of the newborn is relatively uncommon now because Rh immunoglobulin given to the mother usually prevents development of this disease in the fetus.

Uterine Growth during Pregnancy

The uterus of a nonpregnant woman lies in the pelvis. It increases in size during pregnancy to accommodate the growing fetus. As the uterus enlarges, it increases in weight and its walls become thinner. During the first trimester the uterus expands out of the pelvic cavity, and by 20 weeks, it usually reaches the level of the umbilicus. By 28 to 30 weeks, the uterine fundus reaches the epigastric region, the area between the xiphoid process of the sternum and the umbilicus.

PARTURITION

Parturition (childbirth) is the process during which the fetus, placenta, and fetal membranes are expelled from the mother (Fig. 8-8). **Labor** is the *sequence of uterine contractions* that results in dilation of the cervix and delivery of the fetus and placenta from the uterus. The factors that trigger labor are not completely understood, but several hormones are related to the initiation of contractions. The fetal hypothalamus secretes **corticotrophin-releasing hormone**, stimulating the pituitary gland to produce **adrenocorticotrophic hormone (ACTH)**. ACTH causes the suprarenal (adrenal) cortex to secrete **cortisol**, which is involved in the synthesis of estrogens.

Peristaltic contractions of the uterine smooth muscle are elicited by **oxytocin**, which is released by the maternal neurohypophysis of the pituitary gland. This hormone is administered clinically when it is necessary to induce labor. Oxytocin also stimulates the release of **prostaglandins** that, in turn, stimulate myometrial contractility by sensitizing the myometrial cells to oxytocin. Estrogens also increase myometrial contractile activity and stimulate the release of oxytocin and prostaglandins.

Stages of Labor

Labor is a continuous process, but clinically it is divided into three stages:

● **Dilation** begins with *progressive dilation of the cervix* (Fig. 8-8A and B), and ends with complete dilation of the cervix. During this phase, regular contractions of the uterus occur less than 10 minutes apart. The average duration of the first stage is approximately 12 hours for first pregnancies (primigravidas) and approximately 7 hours for women who have had a child previously (multigravidas).
● **Expulsion** begins when the cervix is fully dilated and ends with delivery of the infant (Fig. 8-8C to E). During this stage, the *fetus descends through the cervix and vagina*. As soon as the fetus is outside the mother, it is called a *newborn infant*, or *neonate*. The average duration of this stage is 50 minutes for primigravidas and 20 minutes for multigravidas.
● **Placental separation** begins as soon as the infant is born and *ends with the expulsion of the placenta and fetal membranes* (Fig. 8-8F to H). A hematoma forms deep to the placenta, separating it from the uterine wall. The placenta and fetal membranes are then

Figure 8–8 Illustrations of parturition. **A** and **B,** The cervix is dilating during the first stage of labor. **C** to **E,** The fetus is passing through the cervix and vagina during the second stage of labor. **F** and **G,** As the uterus contracts during the third stage of labor, the placenta folds and pulls away from the uterine wall. Separation of the placenta results in bleeding and the formation of a large hematoma (mass of blood). Pressure on the abdomen facilitates placental separation. **H,** The placenta is expelled and the uterus contracts.

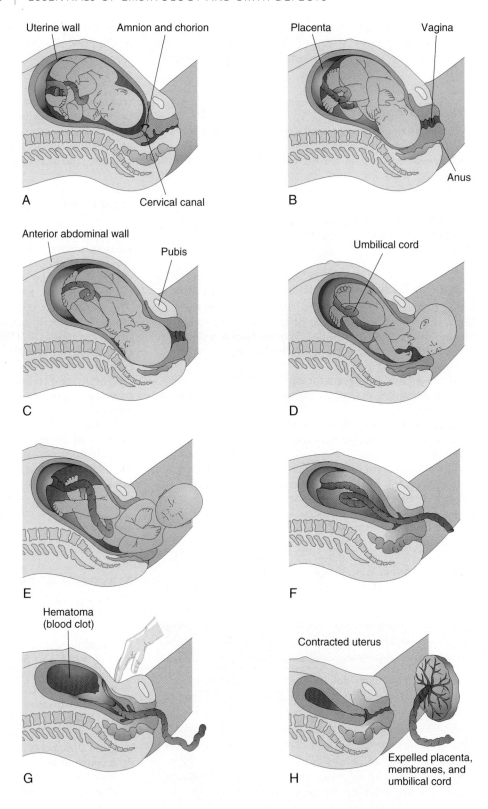

expelled. Contractions of the uterus constrict the spiral arteries, preventing excessive uterine bleeding. The duration of this stage is approximately 15 minutes. A retained or **adherent placenta**—one not expelled within 1 hour of delivery—is a cause of postpartum bleeding.

Placenta and Fetal Membranes after Birth

The placenta is commonly discoid, with a diameter of 15 to 20 cm and a thickness of 2 to 3 cm (Fig. 8-9). The margins of the placenta are continuous with the ruptured amniotic and chorionic sacs.

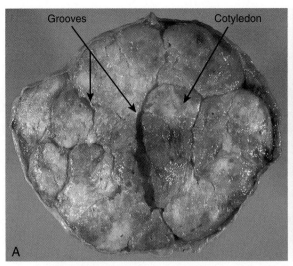
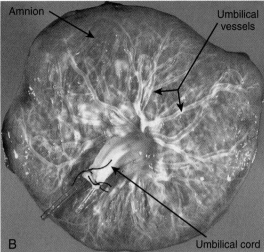

Figure 8–9 Placentas and fetal membranes after birth, shown approximately one third their actual size. **A,** Maternal surface, showing cotyledons and the grooves around them. Each convex cotyledon consists of a number of main stem villi with their many branch villi. The grooves were occupied by the placental septa when the maternal and fetal parts of the placenta were together (see Fig. 8-5). **B,** Fetal surface showing blood vessels running in the chorionic plate deep to the amnion and converging to form the umbilical vessels at the attachment of the umbilical cord.

Variations in Placental Shape

As the placenta develops, chorionic villi usually persist only where the villous chorion is in contact with the decidua basalis. When villi persist elsewhere, several variations in placental shape occur, such as **accessory placenta** (Fig. 8-10). Examination of the placenta, prenatally by ultrasonography or postnatally by gross and microscopic study, may provide clinical information about the causes of placental dysfunction, intrauterine growth restriction, fetal distress and death, and neonatal illness. Postnatal placental examination can also determine whether the expelled placenta is intact. Retention of cotyledons or an accessory placenta in the uterus causes postpartum uterine hemorrhage.

PLACENTAL ABNORMALITIES

Abnormal adherence of the chorionic villi to the myometrium of the uterine wall is called *placenta accreta* (Fig. 8-11). When chorionic villi penetrate the myometrium all the way to the perimetrium (peritoneal covering), the abnormality is called *placenta percreta*. Third-trimester bleeding is the most common presenting sign of these placental abnormalities. After birth, the placenta does not separate from the uterine wall, and attempts to remove it may cause severe hemorrhage that is difficult to control. When the blastocyst implants close to or overlying the internal os of the uterus, the abnormality is called *placenta previa*. Late pregnancy bleeding can result from this placental abnormality. In such cases, the fetus is delivered by cesarean section because the placenta blocks the cervical canal.

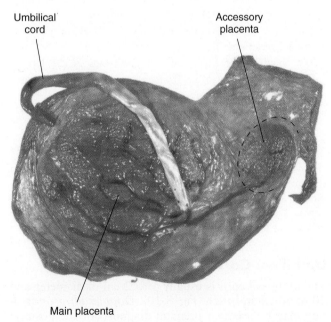

Figure 8–10 Maternal surface of a full-term placenta and an accessory placenta.

Maternal Surface of Placenta

The *cobblestone appearance* of the maternal surface of the placenta is produced by slightly bulging villous areas—the **cotyledons**—which are separated by grooves formerly occupied by **placental septa** (Fig. 8-9A).

Fetal Surface of Placenta

The umbilical cord usually attaches near the center of the fetal surface, and its epithelium is continuous with the amnion adhering to the chorionic plate of the placenta

Figure 8–11 Placental abnormalities. In placenta accreta, there is abnormal adherence of the placenta to the myometrium (muscle layer). In placenta percreta, the placenta has penetrated the full thickness of the myometrium. In placenta previa, the placenta overlies the internal os of the uterus, blocking the cervical canal.

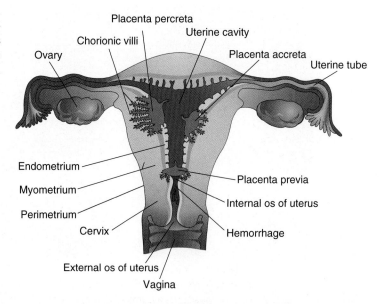

ABSENCE OF AN UMBILICAL ARTERY

In approximately 1 in 200 newborn infants, only one umbilical artery is present (Fig. 8-12), a condition that may be associated with chromosomal and fetal abnormalities. Absence of an umbilical artery is accompanied by a 15% to 20% incidence of cardiovascular anomalies in the fetus. Absence of an artery results from either agenesis or degeneration of this vessel early in development.

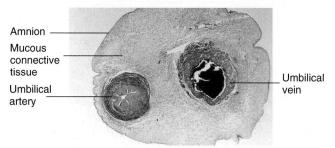

Figure 8–12 Transverse section of the umbilical cord. Note that the cord is covered by a single-layered epithelium derived from the enveloping amnion. It has a core of mucous connective tissue. Observe also that the cord has one umbilical artery and one vein. Usually, there are two arteries. (*Courtesy Professor V. Becker, Pathologisches Institut der Universität, Erlangen, Germany.*)

(Fig. 8-9*B*). The chorionic vessels radiating to and from the umbilical cord are visible through the smooth, transparent amnion. The **umbilical vessels** branch on the fetal surface, forming the **chorionic vessels**, which enter the chorionic villi (Fig. 8-5).

Umbilical Cord

The umbilical cord is usually 1 to 2 cm in diameter and 30 to 90 cm in length (Fig. 8-10). *Doppler ultrasonography* may be used for prenatal diagnosis of the position and structural abnormalities of the umbilical cord. Long cords have a tendency to prolapse through the cervix or to coil around the fetus. Prompt recognition of *prolapse of the cord* is important because, during delivery, it may be compressed between the presenting body part of the fetus and the mother's bony pelvis, causing fetal anoxia. If the deficiency of oxygen persists for more than 5 minutes, the infant's brain may be damaged.

The umbilical cord usually has *two arteries and one vein* surrounded by mucoid connective tissue (*Wharton jelly*). Because the umbilical vessels are longer than the cord, twisting and bending of the cord is common. The cord frequently forms loops, producing *false knots* that are of no significance; however, in approximately 1% of

pregnancies, *true knots* form in the umbilical cord. These may tighten and cause fetal death secondary to fetal anoxia (Fig. 8-13*C*). In most cases, the knots form during labor as a result of the fetus passing through a loop of the cord. Because these knots are usually loose, they have no clinical significance. Simple looping of the cord around the fetus occasionally occurs. In approximately one fifth of all deliveries, the cord is loosely *looped around the neck* without causing increased fetal risk.

AMNION AND AMNIOTIC FLUID

The **amnion** forms a fluid-filled, membranous *amniotic sac* that surrounds the embryo and fetus. As the amnion enlarges, it gradually obliterates the chorionic cavity and forms the epithelial covering of the umbilical cord (Fig. 8-13*A* and *B*). **Amniotic fluid** plays a major role in fetal growth and development. Initially, most amniotic fluid is

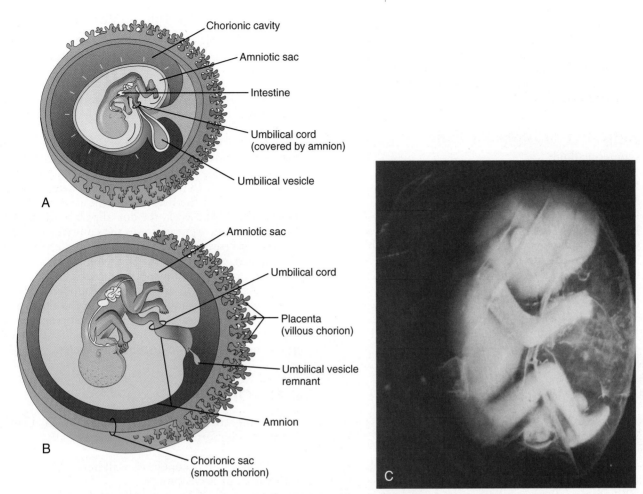

Figure 8–13 Illustrations of how the amnion enlarges, fills the chorionic sac, and envelops the umbilical cord. Observe that part of the umbilical vesicle (yolk sac) is incorporated into the embryo as the primordial gut. Formation of the fetal part of the placenta and degeneration of the chorionic villi are also shown. **A,** At 10 weeks. **B,** At 20 weeks. **C,** A 12-week fetus within its amniotic sac (shown actual size). The fetus and its membranes aborted spontaneously. It was removed from its chorionic sac with the amniotic sac intact.

derived from *maternal tissue fluid* by diffusion across the amniochorionic membrane from the decidua parietalis (see Fig. 8-5). Some fluid is secreted by amniotic cells. Later, there is diffusion of fluid through the chorionic plate from blood in the intervillous space of the placenta. Before keratinization (formation of keratin) of the skin occurs, a major pathway for passage of water and solutes in tissue fluid from the fetus to the amniotic cavity is through the skin. Fluid is also secreted by the fetal respiratory and gastrointestinal tracts and enters the amniotic cavity. Beginning in the 11th week, the fetus contributes to the amniotic fluid by expelling urine into the amniotic cavity.

The water content of amniotic fluid changes every 3 hours. Large amounts of water pass through the amniochorionic membrane into the maternal tissue fluid and into the uterine capillaries. An exchange of fluid with fetal blood also occurs through the umbilical cord and at the site where the amnion adheres to the chorionic plate on the fetal surface of the placenta (see Figs. 8-5 and

8-9B); thus, amniotic fluid is in balance with the fetal circulation.

Amniotic fluid is swallowed by the fetus and absorbed by the fetal respiratory and digestive tracts. It has been estimated that during the final stages of pregnancy, the fetus swallows up to 400 ml of amniotic fluid daily. The fluid is absorbed by the gastrointestinal tract and passes into the fetal bloodstream. The waste products cross the placental membrane and enter the maternal blood in the intervillous space. Excess water in the fetal blood is excreted by the fetal kidneys and returned to the amniotic sac through the fetal urinary tract.

Virtually all of the fluid in the amniotic cavity is water, in which undissolved material (such as desquamated fetal epithelial cells) is suspended. Amniotic fluid contains approximately equal portions of dissolved organic compounds and inorganic salts. Half of the organic constituents are protein; the other half is composed of carbohydrates, fats, enzymes, hormones, and pigments. As pregnancy advances, the composition of the amniotic fluid changes as fetal urine is added. Because fetal urine enters the amniotic fluid, fetal enzyme systems, amino acids, hormones, and other substances can be studied by examining fluid removed by **amniocentesis**. Studies of cells in the amniotic fluid permit the detection of chromosomal abnormalities.

Significance of Amniotic Fluid

The amniotic fluid:

- Permits uniform external growth of the embryo
- Acts as a barrier to infection
- Permits fetal lung development
- Prevents adherence of the amnion to the embryo
- Cushions the embryo against injuries by distributing impacts that the mother may receive
- Helps to control embryonic body temperature by maintaining a relatively constant temperature
- Enables the fetus to move freely, thereby aiding muscular development (e.g., in the limbs)
- Assists in maintaining homeostasis of fluid and electrolytes

UMBILICAL VESICLE

The umbilical vesicle (yolk sac) can be observed sonographically early during the fifth week of gestation. At 32 days, the umbilical vesicle is large (see Fig. 8-1C). By 10 weeks, the umbilical vesicle has shrunk to a pear-shaped remnant approximately 5 mm in diameter (Fig. 8-13A). By 20 weeks, the umbilical vesicle is very small (Fig. 8-13B).

DISORDERS OF AMNIOTIC FLUID VOLUME

A low volume of amniotic fluid—*oligohydramnios*—results, in some cases, from placental insufficiency, with diminished placental blood flow. Preterm rupture of the amniochorionic membrane is the most common cause of oligohydramnios. In the presence of renal agenesis (failure of kidney formation), the lack of fetal urine in the amniotic fluid is the main cause of oligohydramnios. A similar decrease in amniotic fluid occurs with obstructive uropathy (urinary tract obstruction). Complications of oligohydramnios include fetal abnormalities (pulmonary hypoplasia, facial defects, and limb defects) caused by fetal compression by the uterine wall.

A high volume of amniotic fluid is termed *polyhydramnios*. Most cases of polyhydramnios (60%) are idiopathic (of unknown cause); 20% of cases are caused by maternal factors, whereas 20% are fetal in origin. Polyhydramnios may be associated with severe anomalies of the central nervous system, such as meroencephaly (anencephaly) (see Chapter 16). With other anomalies, such as esophageal atresia, amniotic fluid accumulates because it cannot pass to the fetal stomach and the intestines for absorption.

Significance of Umbilical Vesicle

The umbilical vesicle is nonfunctional as far as yolk storage is concerned, but its presence is essential for several reasons:

- It has a role in the *transfer of nutrients* to the embryo during the second and third weeks before the uteroplacental circulation is established.
- *Blood* first develops in the well-vascularized, extraembryonic mesoderm covering the wall of the umbilical vesicle beginning in the third week (see Chapter 5), and it continues to develop there until hematopoietic activity begins in the liver during the sixth week.
- During the fourth week, the dorsal part of the umbilical vesicle is incorporated into the embryo as the *primordial gut* (see Fig. 6-1). Its endoderm, derived from the epiblast, gives rise to the epithelium of the trachea, bronchi, lungs, and alimentary tract.
- *Primordial germ cells* appear in the endodermal lining of the wall of the umbilical vesicle in the third week and subsequently migrate to the developing gonads (see Chapter 13). They differentiate into the spermatogonia in males and the oogonia in females.

ALLANTOIS

Although the allantois is not functional in human embryos, it is important for three reasons:

- Blood formation occurs in its wall during the third to fifth weeks of development.
- Its blood vessels become the umbilical vein and arteries.
- The intraembryonic portion of the allantois runs from the umbilicus to the urinary bladder, with which it is continuous (see Fig. 13-11E). As the bladder enlarges, the allantois involutes to form a thick tube, the **urachus** (see Fig. 13-11G). After birth, the urachus becomes a fibrous cord, the median umbilical ligament, which extends from the apex of the urinary bladder to the umbilicus.

PREMATURE RUPTURE OF FETAL MEMBRANES

Premature rupture of the amniochorionic membrane is the most common event leading to premature labor and delivery and the most common complication resulting in oligohydramnios. Loss of amniotic fluid removes the major protection the fetus has against infection. Rupture of the membrane may cause various fetal anomalies that constitute amniotic band syndrome, or amniotic band disruption complex. These anomalies are associated with a variety of abnormalities, ranging from constriction of digits to major scalp, craniofacial, and visceral defects. The cause of these anomalies is probably related to constriction by encircling amniotic bands (Fig. 8-14).

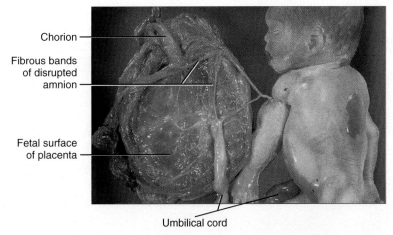

Chorion

Fibrous bands
of disrupted
amnion

Fetal surface
of placenta

Umbilical cord

Figure 8–14 A fetus with amniotic band syndrome, showing amniotic bands constricting the left arm. *(Courtesy Professor V. Becker, Pathologisches Institut der Universität, Erlangen, Germany.)*

FETAL MEMBRANES IN MULTIPLE PREGNANCIES

Multiple gestations are associated with higher risks of fetal morbidity and mortality than single gestations. The risks are progressively greater as the number of fetuses increases. In North America, *twins* naturally occur approximately once in every 85 pregnancies, *triplets* approximately once in every 90^2 pregnancies, *quadruplets* approximately once in every 90^3 pregnancies, and *quintuplets* approximately once in every 90^4 pregnancies.

Twins and Fetal Membranes

Twins that originate from two zygotes are **dizygotic (DZ) twins** (fraternal twins) (Fig. 8-15), whereas twins that originate from one zygote are **monozygotic (MZ) twins** (identical twins) (Fig. 8-16). The fetal membranes and placentas vary according to the origin of the twins. *Approximately two thirds of twins are dizygotic, and the rate of DZ twinning increases with maternal age.*

The study of twins is important in human genetics because it is useful for comparing the effects of genes and environment on development. If an abnormal condition does not show a simple genetic pattern, comparison of its incidence in MZ and DZ twins may show that heredity is involved.

Dizygotic Twins

Because they result from the fertilization of two oocytes by two sperms, DZ twins may be of the same sex or different sexes. For the same reason, they are no more alike genetically than brothers or sisters born at different times. *DZ twins always have two amnions and two chorions* (Fig. 8-15A), but the chorions and placentas may be fused (Fig. 8-15B). DZ twinning shows a hereditary tendency. The recurrence risk in families with one set of DZ twins is approximately triple that of the general population. The incidence of DZ twinning shows considerable racial variation, ranging from 1 in 500 in Asian populations, to 1 in 125 in white populations, to as high as 1 in 20 in some African populations.

Monozygotic Twins

Because they result from the fertilization of one oocyte and develop from one zygote (Fig. 8-16), *MZ twins are of the same sex, are genetically identical, and are similar in physical appearance.* Physical differences between MZ twins are environmentally induced, such as by anastomosis of the placental vessels, resulting in differences in blood supply from the placenta (Fig. 8-17). MZ twinning usually begins in the blastocyst stage, approximately at the end of the first week, and results from division of the embryoblast into two embryonic primordia (Fig. 8-16). Subsequently, two embryos, each in its own amniotic sac, develop within one chorionic sac and share a common placenta, a monochorionic-diamniotic twin placenta. Uncommonly, early separation of the embryonic blastomeres (e.g., during the two- to eight-cell stage) results in MZ twins with two amnions, two chorions, and two placentas that may or may not be fused (Fig. 8-18). In such cases, it is impossible to determine, from the membranes alone, whether the twins are monozygotic or dizygotic.

TWIN TRANSFUSION SYNDROME

Twin transfusion syndrome occurs in 15% to 30% of monochorionic-diamniotic MZ twins. Arterial blood may be preferentially shunted from one twin through arteriovenous anastomoses in the placenta into the venous circulation of the other twin. The donor twin is small, pale, and anemic (see Fig. 8-17), whereas the recipient twin is large and polycythemic (i.e., having a higher than normal red blood cell count). The placenta shows similar abnormalities; the part of the placenta supplying the anemic twin is pale, whereas the part supplying the polycythemic twin is dark red. In lethal cases, death results from anemia in the donor twin and from congestive heart failure in the recipient twin.

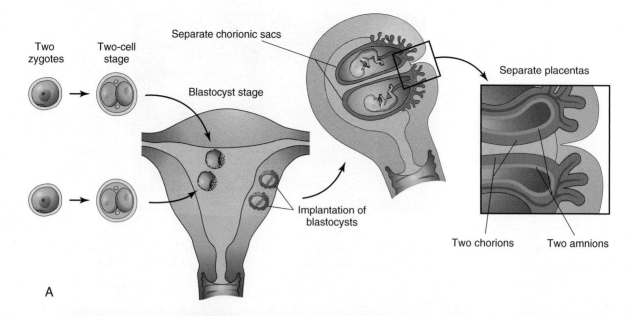

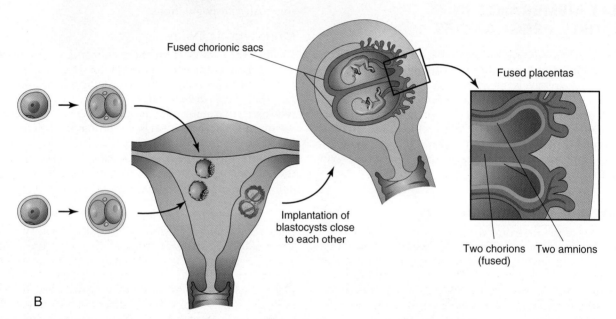

Figure 8–15 Dizygotic twins developing from two zygotes. The relationship of the fetal membranes and placentas are shown for instances in which the blastocysts implant separately **(A)** and the blastocysts implant close together **(B)**. In both cases, there are two amnions and two chorions.

ZYGOSITY OF TWINS

Establishment of the zygosity of twins has become important, particularly because of the introduction of tissue and organ transplantation (e.g., bone marrow transplants). Twin zygosity is now determined by molecular testing. Any two people who are not MZ twins are virtually certain to show differences in some of the large number of DNA markers that can be studied.

Late division of the early embryonic cells (i.e., division of the embryonic disc during the second week) results in MZ twins with one amniotic sac and one chorionic sac. A

monochorionic-monoamniotic twin placenta is associated with a fetal mortality rate approaching 50%. The umbilical cords are frequently so entangled that circulation of the blood through their vessels ceases, and one or both fetuses die. Ultrasonography plays an important role in the diagnosis of twin pregnancies and the management of various conditions that may complicate MZ twinning, such as intrauterine growth restriction, intrauterine fetal distress, and premature labor.

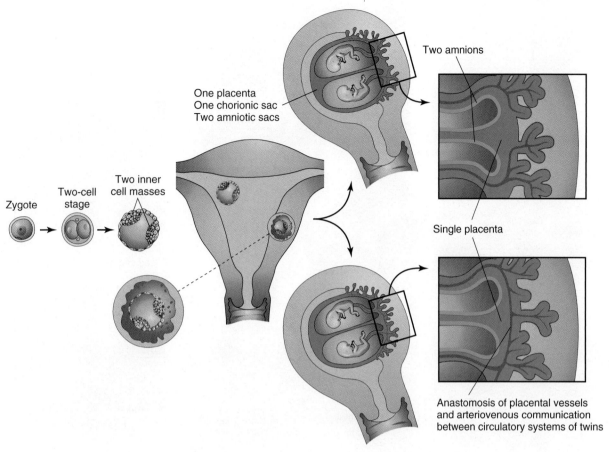

One placenta
One chorionic sac
Two amniotic sacs

Two amnions

Single placenta

Anastomosis of placental vessels and arteriovenous communication between circulatory systems of twins

Zygote   Two-cell stage   Two inner cell masses

Figure 8–16 Illustrations of how approximately 65% of monozygotic twins develop from one zygote by division of the inner cell mass. These twins always have separate amnions, a single chorionic sac, and a common placenta. If there is anastomosis of the placental vessels, one twin may receive most of the nutrition from the placenta (see Fig. 8-17).

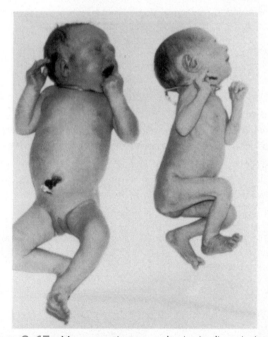

Figure 8–17 Monozygotic, monochorionic-diamniotic twins. Note the wide discrepancy in size resulting from an uncompensated arteriovenous anastomosis of the placental vessels. Blood was shunted from the smaller twin to the larger one, producing the *twin transfusion syndrome.*

CONJOINED TWINS

If the embryonic disc does not divide completely, various types of conjoined (MZ) twins may form. These twins are named according to the regions of the body that are attached; for example, *thoracopagus* indicates anterior union of the thoracic regions. In some cases, the twins are connected to each other by skin only or by cutaneous and other tissues, such as fused livers. Some conjoined twins can be separated successfully by surgery. The incidence of conjoined twins is 1 in 50,000 to 1 in 100,000 births.

Other Types of Multiple Births

Triplets may be derived from:

- One zygote and be identical
- Two zygotes and consist of identical twins and a singleton
- Three zygotes and be of the same sex or of different sexes, in which case the infants are no more similar than infants from three separate pregnancies

Similar combinations occur in quadruplets, quintuplets, sextuplets, and septuplets.

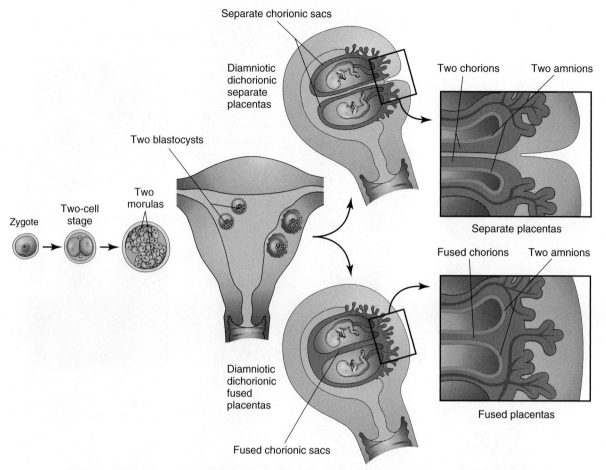

Figure 8–18 Illustrations of how approximately 35% of monozygotic twins develop from one zygote. Separation of the blastomeres may occur at any point from the two-cell stage to the morula stage, producing two identical blastocysts. Each embryo subsequently develops its own amniotic and chorionic sacs. The placentas may be separate or fused. In most cases, there is a single placenta resulting from secondary fusion, whereas in fewer cases, there are two placentas. In the latter cases, examination of the placenta suggests that they are dizygotic twins. This explains why some monozygotic twins are incorrectly classified as dizygotic twins at birth.

CLINICALLY ORIENTED QUESTIONS

1. What is meant by the term *stillbirth*? Do older women have more stillborn infants?

2. An infant was born dead, reportedly because of a "cord accident." What does this mean? Do these accidents always kill the infant? If not, what defects may be present?

3. What is the scientific basis of the home pregnancy tests that are sold in drugstores?

4. What is the proper name for what laypeople sometimes refer to as the *bag of waters*? What is meant by a *dry birth*? Does premature rupture of this "bag" induce the birth of the infant?

5. What does the term *fetal distress* mean? How is the condition recognized? What causes fetal distress?

6. Some say that twins are born more commonly to older mothers. Is this true? Others maintain that twinning is hereditary. Is this correct?

The answers to these questions are at the back of the book.

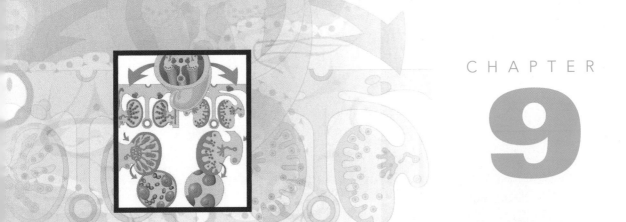

Body Cavities, Mesenteries, and Diaphragm

E arly in the fourth week of development, the **intraembryonic coelom**—the primordium of the body cavities—appears as a horseshoe-shaped cavity (Fig. 9-1*A*). The curve or bend in this cavity at the cranial end of the embryo represents the future *pericardial cavity*, and its limbs indicate the future *pleural and peritoneal cavities*. The distal part of each limb of the intraembryonic coelom is continuous with the **extraembryonic coelom** at the lateral edges of the embryonic disc (Fig. 9-1*B*). This communication is important because most of the midgut normally herniates through this communication into the umbilical cord. The intraembryonic coelom provides room for the abdominal organs to develop and move. During embryonic lateral folding, the limbs of the coelom are brought together on the ventral aspect of the embryo (Fig. 9-2*A* to *F*).

 EMBRYONIC BODY CAVITY

The intraembryonic coelom gives rise to three well-defined body cavities during the fourth week (Figs. 9-2 and 9-4): a *pericardial cavity*, two *pericardioperitoneal canals* connecting the pericardial and the peritoneal cavities, and a large *peritoneal cavity*.

These body cavities are lined by the mesothelium—a parietal wall derived from the somatic mesoderm and a visceral wall derived from the splanchnic mesoderm (Fig. 9-3*E*). The mesothelium forms the major portion of the peritoneum. The **peritoneal cavity** is connected to the extraembryonic coelom at the umbilicus (Fig. 9-4*C* and *D*). The peritoneal cavity loses its connection with the extraembryonic coelom during the 10th week as the intestines return to the abdomen from the umbilical cord (see Chapter 12).

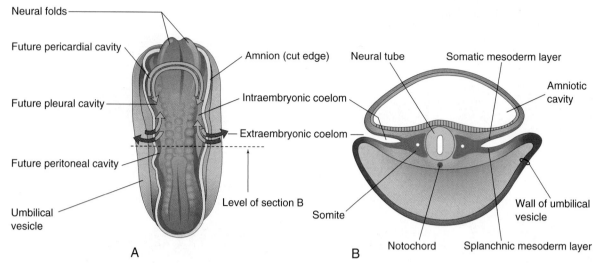

Figure 9–1 **A,** Dorsal view of a 22-day embryo, showing the outline of the horseshoe-shaped intraembryonic coelom. The amnion has been removed and the coelom is shown as if the embryo were translucent. The continuity of the intraembryonic coelom, as well as the communication of its right and left limbs with the extraembryonic coelom, is indicated by *arrows.* **B,** Transverse section through the embryo at the level shown in **A.**

During the formation of the head fold, the heart and **pericardial cavity** move ventrocaudally, anterior to the foregut (Fig. 9-2*A, B, D,* and *E*). As a result, the pericardial cavity opens into the **pericardioperitoneal canals,** which pass dorsal to the foregut (Fig. 9-4*B* and *D*). After embryonic folding, the caudal parts of the foregut, midgut, and hindgut are suspended in the peritoneal cavity from the dorsal abdominal wall by the **dorsal mesentery** (Figs. 9-2*F* and 9-3*B* to *E*).

Mesenteries

A mesentery is a double layer of peritoneum that begins as an extension of the visceral peritoneum that covers an organ. It connects the organ to the body wall and conveys its vessels and nerves. Transiently, the dorsal and ventral mesenteries divide the peritoneal cavity into right and left halves (Fig. 9-3*C*). The ventral mesentery soon disappears (see Fig. 9-3*E*), except where it is attached to the caudal part of the foregut (primordium of stomach and proximal part of the duodenum). The peritoneal cavity then becomes a continuous space (Figs. 9-3*A* and 9-4*D*). The arteries supplying the primordial gut—*celiac arterial trunk* (foregut), the *superior mesenteric artery* (midgut), and the *inferior mesenteric artery* (hindgut)—pass between the layers of the dorsal mesentery (Fig. 9-3*C*).

 ## Division of Embryonic Body Cavity

Each pericardioperitoneal canal lies lateral to the proximal part of the foregut (future esophagus) and dorsal to the **septum transversum**—a thick plate of mesoderm that occupies the space between the thoracic cavity and the omphaloenteric duct (Fig. 9-4*A* and *B*). The septum transversum is the primordium of the **central tendon of the diaphragm.** Partitions form in each

pericardioperitoneal canal, separating the pericardial cavity from the pleural cavities; and the pleural cavities from the peritoneal cavity (Fig. 9-3*A*). Because of the growth of the **bronchial buds** (primordia of bronchi and lungs) into the pericardioperitoneal canals (Fig. 9-5*A*), a pair of membranous ridges is produced in the lateral wall of each canal. The cranial ridges—the *pleuropericardial folds*—are located superior to the developing lungs. The caudal ridges—the *pleuroperitoneal folds*—are located inferior to the lungs.

As the **pleuropericardial folds** enlarge, they form partitions that separate the pericardial cavity from the pleural cavities. These partitions—**pleuropericardial membranes**—contain the **common cardinal veins** (Fig. 9-5*A* and *B*), which drain the venous system into the sinus venosus of the primordial heart (Chapter 14). Subsequently, they grow laterally from the caudal end of the trachea into the pericardioperitoneal canals (future pleural canals). As the **primordial pleural cavities** expand ventrally around the heart, they extend into the body wall, splitting the mesenchyme into two layers: (1) an outer layer that becomes the thoracic wall and (2) an inner layer (pleuropericardial membrane) that becomes the fibrous pericardium, the outer layer of the pericardial sac that encloses the heart (Fig. 9-5*C* and *D*).

The *pleuropericardial membranes* project into the cranial ends of the **pericardioperitoneal canals** (Fig. 9-5*B*). With subsequent growth of the common cardinal veins, positional displacement of the heart, and expansion of the pleural cavities, the pleuropericardial membranes become mesentery-like folds extending from the lateral thoracic wall. By the seventh week, the pleuropericardial membranes fuse with the mesenchyme ventral to the esophagus, separating the pericardial cavity from the pleural cavities (Fig. 9-5*C*). The primordial mediastinum consists of a mass of mesenchyme that extends from the sternum to the vertebral column, separating the

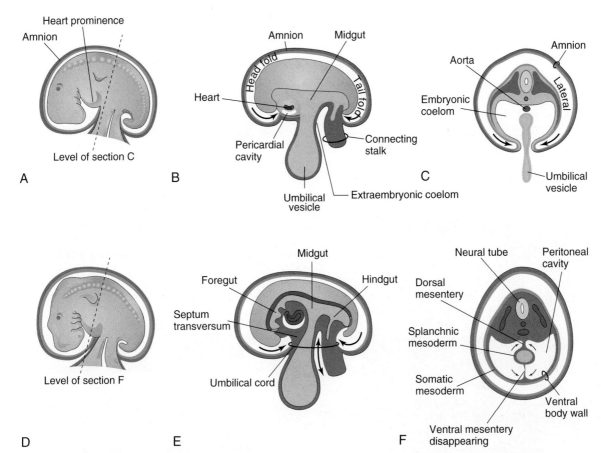

Figure 9–2 Embryonic folding and its effects on the intraembryonic coelom and other structures. **A,** Lateral view of an embryo (approximately 26 days). **B,** Schematic sagittal section of the embryo, showing the head and tail folds. **C,** Transverse section at the level shown in **A,** indicating how fusion of the lateral folds gives the embryo a cylindric form. **D,** Lateral view of an embryo (approximately 28 days). **E,** Schematic sagittal section of the embryo, showing the reduced communication between the intraembryonic and extraembryonic coeloms (*double-headed arrow*). **F,** Transverse section, as indicated in **D,** showing the formation of the ventral body wall and the disappearance of the ventral mesentery. The *arrows* indicate the junction of the somatic and the splanchnic layers of the mesoderm. The somatic mesoderm will become the parietal peritoneum lining the abdominal wall, and the splanchnic mesoderm will become the visceral peritoneum covering the organs (e.g., stomach).

developing lungs (Fig. 9-5D). The right pleuropericardial opening closes slightly earlier than the left one and produces a larger pleuropericardial membrane.

As the **pleuroperitoneal folds** enlarge, they project into the pericardioperitoneal canals. Gradually, the folds become membranous, forming the **pleuroperitoneal membranes** (Fig. 9-6B and C). Eventually, these membranes separate the pleural cavities from the peritoneal cavity. The *pleuroperitoneal membranes* are produced as the developing lungs and pleural cavities expand and invade the body wall. They are attached dorsolaterally to the abdominal wall and their crescentic free edges initially project into the caudal ends of the **pericardioperitoneal canals**. During the sixth week, the pleuroperitoneal membranes extend ventromedially until their free edges fuse with the dorsal mesentery of the esophagus and the septum transversum (see Fig. 9-6C). This membrane separates the pleural cavities from the peritoneal cavity.

Closure of the pleuroperitoneal openings is assisted by the migration of myoblasts (primordial muscle cells) into the pleuroperitoneal membranes. The pleuroperitoneal opening on the right side closes slightly before the left one.

DEVELOPMENT OF DIAPHRAGM

The diaphragm is a dome-shaped, musculotendinous partition that separates the thoracic and abdominal cavities. It is a composite structure that develops from four embryonic components (Fig. 9-6):

- Septum transversum
- Pleuroperitoneal membranes
- Dorsal mesentery of esophagus
- Muscular growth from lateral body walls

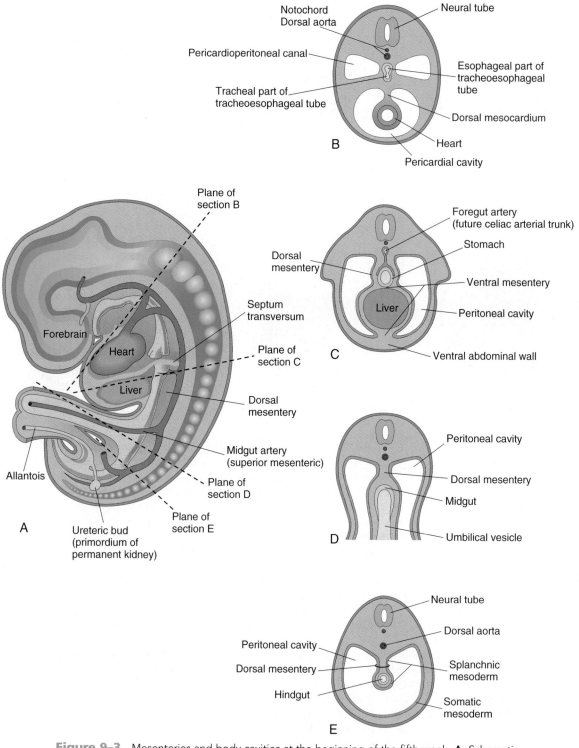

Figure 9–3 Mesenteries and body cavities at the beginning of the fifth week. **A,** Schematic sagittal section. Note that the dorsal mesentery serves as a pathway for the arteries that supply the developing gut. Nerves and lymphatics also pass between the layers of this mesentery. **B to E,** Transverse sections through the embryo at the levels shown in **A.** The ventral mesentery disappears except in the region of the terminal esophagus, stomach, and first part of the duodenum. Note that the right and left parts of the peritoneal cavity, which are separate in **C,** are continuous in **E.**

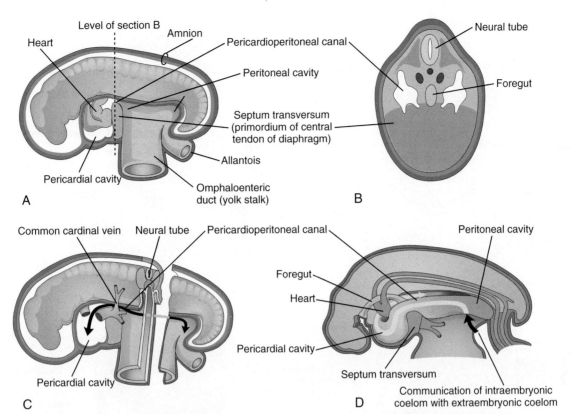

Figure 9–4 Illustration of an embryo (approximately 24 days). **A,** The lateral wall of the pericardial cavity has been removed to show the primordial heart. **B,** Transverse section of the embryo, showing the relationship of the pericardioperitoneal canals to the septum transversum and the foregut. **C,** Lateral view of the embryo, with the heart removed. The embryo has also been sectioned transversely to show the continuity of the intraembryonic and extraembryonic coeloms (*black arrow*). **D,** Illustration of the pericardioperitoneal canals that arise from the dorsal wall of the pericardial cavity and pass on each side of the foregut to join the peritoneal cavity. The *arrow* shows the communication of the extraembryonic coelom with the intraembryonic coelom and the continuity of the intraembryonic coelom at this stage.

Septum Transversum

This transverse septum, which is composed of mesodermal tissue, is the **primordium of the central tendon of the diaphragm** (Fig. 9-6D and E). The septum transversum grows dorsally from the ventrolateral body wall and forms a semicircular shelf that separates the heart from the liver. After the head folds ventrally during the fourth week, the septum transversum forms a thick incomplete partition between the pericardial and abdominal cavities (Fig. 9-4). The septum transversum expands and fuses with the mesenchyme ventral to the esophagus and the pleuroperitoneal membranes (Fig. 9-6C).

Pleuroperitoneal Membranes

The pleuroperitoneal membranes fuse with the dorsal mesentery of the esophagus and the septum transversum (Fig. 9-6C). This fusion completes the partition between the thoracic and abdominal cavities and forms the **primordial diaphragm**. The pleuroperitoneal membranes represent relatively small parts of the diaphragm in a neonate (Fig. 9-6E).

Dorsal Mesentery of Esophagus

The septum transversum and the pleuroperitoneal membranes fuse with the dorsal mesentery of the esophagus. This mesentery becomes the median portion of the diaphragm. The **crura of the diaphragm**—a pair of diverging muscle bundles that cross in the median plane anterior to the aorta (Fig. 9-6E)—develop from myoblasts (primordial muscle cells) that grow into the dorsal mesentery of the esophagus.

Muscular Growth from Lateral Body Walls

During the 9th to 12th weeks, the lungs and pleural cavities enlarge, "burrowing" into the lateral body walls (Fig. 9-5). During this process, the tissue of the body wall is split into two layers:

- An external layer that becomes part of the definitive thoracic and abdominal wall
- An internal layer that contributes muscle to the peripheral portions of the diaphragm, external to the parts derived from the pleuroperitoneal membranes (Fig. 9-6D and E)

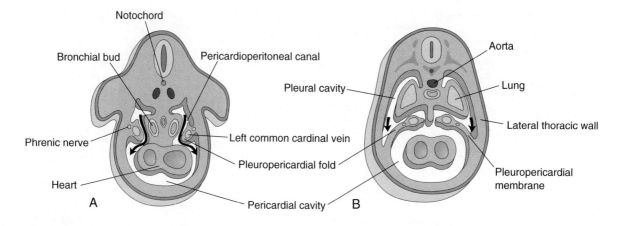

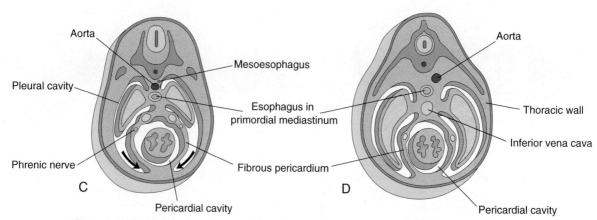

Figure 9–5 Transverse sections through an embryo cranial to the septum transversum, showing successive stages in the separation of the pleural cavities from the pericardial cavity. Growth and development of the lungs, expansion of the pleural cavities, and formation of the fibrous pericardium are also shown. **A,** At 5 weeks. The *arrows* indicate the communications between the pericardioperitoneal canals and the pericardial cavity. **B,** At 6 weeks. The *arrows* indicate the development of the pleural cavities as they expand into the body wall. **C,** At 7 weeks. Expansion of the pleural cavities ventrally (*arrows*) around the heart is evident. The pleuropericardial membranes are now fused in the median plane with each other and with the mesoderm ventral to the esophagus. **D,** At 8 weeks. Continued expansion of the lungs and the pleural cavities and formation of the fibrous pericardium and the thoracic wall are shown.

Further extension of the developing pleural cavities into the lateral body walls forms the right and left **costo-diaphragmatic recesses** (Fig. 9-7), establishing the characteristic dome-shaped configuration of the diaphragm.

Positional Changes and Innervation of the Diaphragm

During the fourth week of development, the septum transversum lies opposite the third to fifth cervical somites. During the fifth week, myoblasts from these somites migrate into the developing diaphragm, bringing their nerve fibers with them. Consequently, the **phrenic nerves** that supply motor innervation to the diaphragm arise from the ventral primary rami of the third, fourth, and fifth cervical spinal nerves, which join together on each side to form a phrenic nerve. The phrenic nerves also

supply sensory fibers to the superior and inferior surfaces of the right and left domes of the diaphragm.

Rapid growth of the dorsal part of the embryo's body results in an *apparent descent of the diaphragm*. By the sixth week, the developing diaphragm is at the level of the thoracic somites. The phrenic nerves now have a descending course. By the beginning of the eighth week, the dorsal part of the diaphragm lies at the level of the first lumbar vertebra. The phrenic nerves in the embryo enter the diaphragm by passing through the pleuropericardial membranes. For this reason, the phrenic nerves subsequently lie on the fibrous pericardium of the heart, which is derived from the pleuropericardial membranes (Fig. 9-5C and D).

The costal border of the diaphragm receives sensory fibers from the lower intercostal nerves because of the origin of the peripheral part of the diaphragm from the lateral body walls (Fig. 9-6D and E).

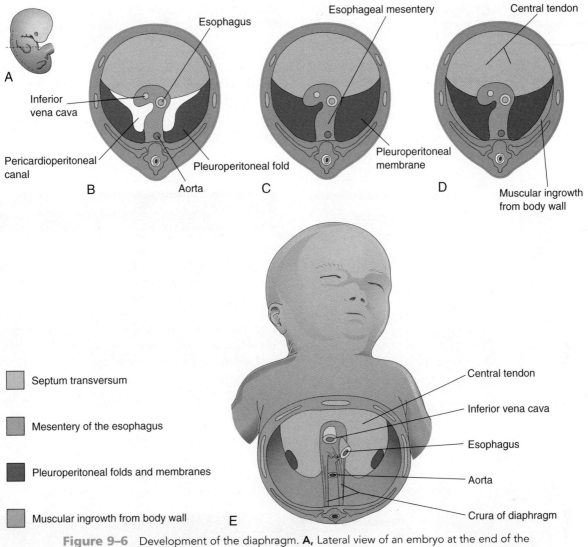

Figure 9–6 Development of the diaphragm. **A,** Lateral view of an embryo at the end of the fifth week (actual size), indicating the level of **B** to **D** sections. **B** to **E** show the developing diaphragm as viewed inferiorly. **B,** Transverse section, showing the unfused pleuroperitoneal membranes. **C,** Similar section at the end of the sixth week, after fusion of the pleuroperitoneal membranes with the other two diaphragmatic components. **D,** Transverse section of a 12-week embryo, after ingrowth of the fourth diaphragmatic component from the body wall. **E,** View of the diaphragm of a newborn infant, indicating the embryologic origin of its components.

CONGENITAL DIAPHRAGMATIC HERNIA

A posterolateral defect of the diaphragm is the only relatively common congenital anomaly involving the diaphragm (Fig. 9-8*A*). This diaphragmatic defect occurs in approximately 1 in 2200 newborn infants and is associated with **congenital diaphragmatic hernia** (CDH) (herniation of abdominal contents into the thoracic cavity).

The *most common cause of pulmonary hypoplasia*, CDH can lead to life-threatening respiratory difficulties. If severe lung hypoplasia is present, some primordial alveoli may rupture, causing air to enter the pleural cavity (*pneumothorax*). Usually unilateral, CDH results from defective formation or fusion of the pleuroperitoneal membrane with the other three parts of the diaphragm (Fig. 9-6*B*). This defect produces a large opening in the posterolateral region of the diaphragm. If a pleuroperitoneal canal is still open when the intestines return to the abdomen from the umbilical cord in the 10th week, some intestine and other viscera may pass into the thorax and compress the lungs. Often the stomach, spleen, and most of the intestines herniate (Figs. 9-8*B* and 9-8*C*). The defect usually occurs on the left side, and it is likely related to the earlier closure of the right pleuroperitoneal opening. Ultrasonographic and magnetic resonance imaging can provide a *prenatal diagnosis* of CDH.

EVENTRATION OF DIAPHRAGM

In the uncommon condition of **diaphragmatic eventration**, part of the diaphragm has defective musculature, causing it to balloon into the thoracic cavity as an aponeurotic (membranous) sheet, forming a large diaphragmatic pouch. Consequently, the abdominal viscera are displaced superiorly into the pocket-like outpouching of the diaphragm. This congenital anomaly results mainly from failure of the muscular tissue from the body wall to extend into the pleuroperitoneal membrane on the affected side.

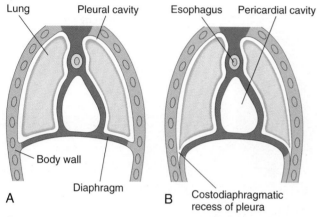

Figure 9–7 Extension of the pleural cavities into the body walls to form the peripheral parts of the diaphragm, the costodiaphragmatic recesses, and the characteristic dome-shaped configuration of the diaphragm.

RETROSTERNAL (PARASTERNAL) HERNIA

Herniations may occur through the sternocostal hiatus, the opening for the superior epigastric vessels in the retrosternal area. This hiatus is located between the sternal and the costal parts of the diaphragm. Herniation of the intestine into the pericardial sac may occur or, conversely, part of the heart may descend into the peritoneal cavity in the epigastric region. Large defects are commonly associated with body wall defects in the umbilical region (e.g., omphalocele; see Chapter 12).

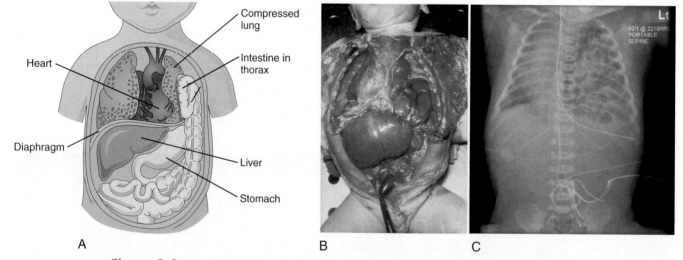

Figure 9–8 **A,** This "window view" overlooking the thorax and the abdomen shows the herniation of the intestine into the thorax through a posterolateral defect in the left side of the diaphragm. Note that the left lung is compressed and hypoplastic. **B,** Diaphragmatic hernia. Note the herniation of the stomach and the small intestine into the thorax through a posterolateral defect in the left side of the diaphragm, similar to that shown in Figure 9-8A. Note that the heart is pushed to the right side of the thorax. **C,** Radiograph showing a diaphragmatic hernia on the left side. Note the loops of small intestine in the thoracic cavity and the displacement of the heart into the right thoracic cavity. (**B,** *Courtesy of Dr. Nathan E. Wiseman, Professor of Surgery, Children's Hospital, University of Manitoba, Winnipeg, Manitoba, Canada.* **C,** *From Dr. Frank Gaillard, Radiopaedia.org, with permission.*)

CLINICALLY ORIENTED QUESTIONS

1. There have been reports of an infant who was born with its stomach and liver in its chest. Is this possible?

2. Can an infant with most of its abdominal viscera in the chest survive? Some say that diaphragmatic defects can be operated on before birth. Is this true?

3. Do the lungs develop normally in infants who are born with a congenital diaphragmatic hernia?

4. A man underwent routine chest radiography approximately 1 year ago and was told that a small part of his small intestine was in his chest. Is it possible for him to have a congenital diaphragmatic hernia without being aware of it? Would his lung on the affected side be normal?

The answers to these questions are at the back of the book.

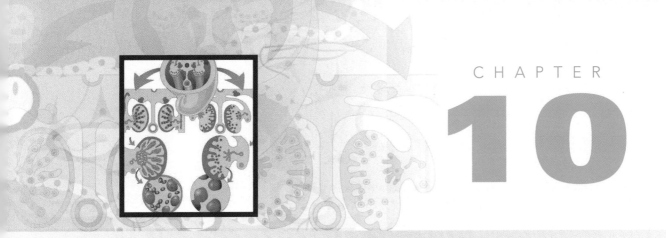

Pharyngeal Apparatus

T he **pharyngeal apparatus** (Fig. 10-1) consists of the following: *pharyngeal arches, pharyngeal pouches, pharyngeal grooves,* and *pharyngeal membranes.* These embryonic structures contribute to the formation of the face and neck.

 PHARYNGEAL ARCHES

The pharyngeal arches begin to develop early in the fourth week as **neural crest cells** migrate from the hindbrain into the mesenchyme of the future head and neck regions. Initially, each pharyngeal arch consists of a core of mesenchyme (embryonic connective tissue) and is covered externally by ectoderm and internally by endoderm (Fig. 10-1*D* and *E*). The first pair of arches, the primordia of the jaws, appears as surface elevations lateral to the developing pharynx (Fig. 10-1). Other arches soon appear as obliquely disposed, rounded ridges on each side of the future head and neck regions. By the end of the fourth week, four well-defined pairs of arches are visible (Fig. 10-1*A*).

The pharyngeal arches support the lateral walls of the primordial pharynx, which is derived from the cranial part of the foregut. The **stomodeum** (primordial mouth) initially appears as a slight depression of the surface ectoderm (Fig. 10-1*A*). It is separated from the cavity of the primordial pharynx by a bilaminar membrane—the **oropharyngeal membrane**—composed of fused ectoderm and endoderm. The oropharyngeal membrane ruptures at

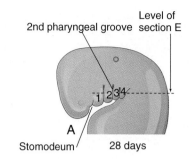

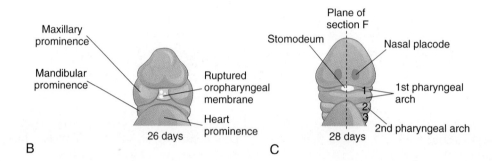

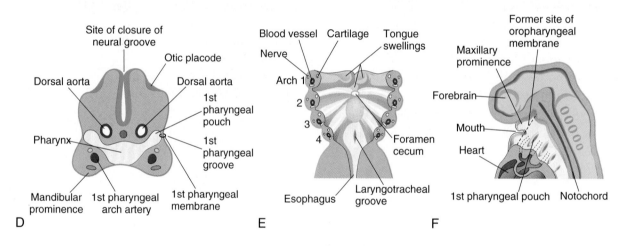

Germ Layer Derivatives

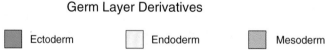

Figure 10–1 Illustrations of the human pharyngeal apparatus. **A,** Lateral view showing the development of four pharyngeal arches. **B** and **C,** Ventral (facial) views showing the relationship of the pharyngeal arches to the stomodeum. **D,** Frontal section through the cranial region of an embryo. **E,** Horizontal section showing the arch components and the floor of the primordial pharynx. **F,** Sagittal section of the cranial region of an embryo, showing the openings of the pharyngeal pouches in the lateral wall of the primordial pharynx.

approximately 26 days (Fig. 10-1C), bringing the primordial pharynx and foregut into communication with the amniotic cavity. The pharyngeal arches contribute extensively to the formation of the face, nasal cavities, mouth, larynx, pharynx, and neck (Figs. 10-2 to 10-4).

The **first pharyngeal arch** develops two prominences (Figs. 10-1B and 10-2): the smaller maxillary prominence and the larger mandibular prominence. The **second pharyngeal arch** makes a major contribution to the formation of the hyoid bone (see Fig. 10-5B).

Pharyngeal Arch Components

A typical pharyngeal arch has the following components (Fig. 10-3A and B):

- A pharyngeal arch artery (aortic arch artery) that arises from the truncus arteriosus of the primordial heart and courses around the primordial pharynx to enter the dorsal aorta
- A cartilaginous rod that forms the skeleton of the arch

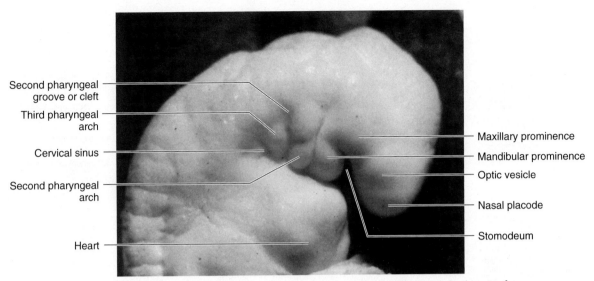

Figure 10–2   A Carnegie stage 13, 4½-week human embryo. *(Courtesy the late Professor Emeritus Dr. K.V. Hinrichsen, Medizinische Fakultät, Institut für Anatomie, Ruhr-Universität Bochum, Bochum, Germany.)*

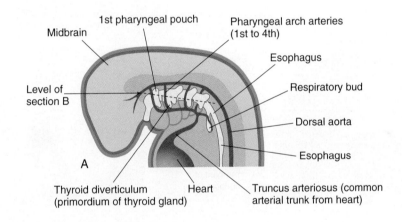

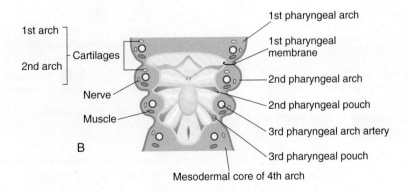

Germ Layer Derivatives

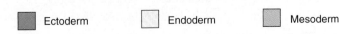

Ectoderm   Endoderm   Mesoderm

Figure 10–3   **A,** Illustration of the pharyngeal pouches and pharyngeal arch arteries. **B,** Horizontal section through the embryo showing the floor of the primordial pharynx and illustrating the germ layer origin of the pharyngeal arch components.

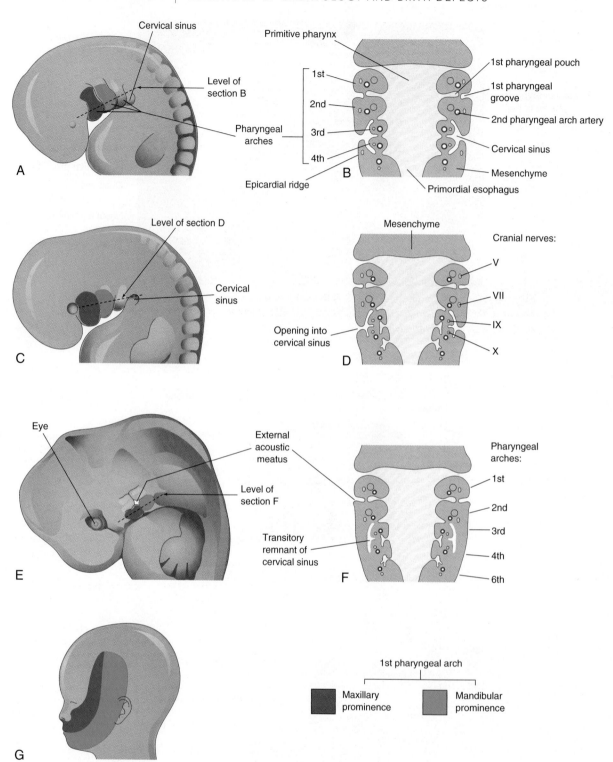

Figure 10–4 **A,** Lateral view of the head, neck, and thoracic regions of an embryo (approximately 32 days), showing the pharyngeal arches and the cervical sinus. **B,** Diagrammatic section through the embryo at the level seen in **A,** showing growth of the second arch over the third and fourth arches. **C,** An embryo of approximately 33 days. **D,** Section of the embryo at the level seen in **C,** showing early closure of the cervical sinus. **E,** An embryo of approximately 41 days. **F,** Section of the embryo at the level seen in **E,** showing the transitory cystic remnant of the cervical sinus. **G,** Illustration of a 20-week fetus, showing the area of the face derived from the first pair of pharyngeal arches.

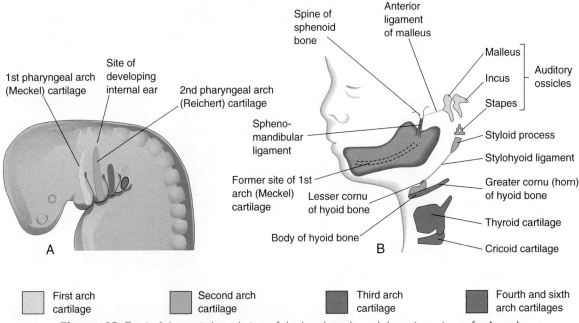

Figure 10–5 **A,** Schematic lateral view of the head, neck, and thoracic regions of a 4-week embryo, showing the location of the cartilages in the pharyngeal arches. **B,** Similar view of a 24-week fetus, showing the adult derivatives of the arch cartilages. Note that the mandible is formed by intramembranous ossification of the mesenchymal tissue surrounding the first arch cartilage.

First arch cartilage

Second arch cartilage

Third arch cartilage

Fourth and sixth arch cartilages

- A muscular component that is the primordium of the muscles in the head and neck
- A nerve that supplies the mucosa and muscles derived from each arch

Derivatives of Pharyngeal Arch Arteries

The transformation of the pharyngeal arch arteries into the adult arterial pattern of the head and neck is described in the section on the pharyngeal arch artery derivatives in Chapter 14.

Derivatives of Pharyngeal Arch Cartilages

The dorsal end of the **first pharyngeal arch cartilage** becomes ossified to form two middle ear bones, the **malleus** and **incus** (Fig. 10-5 and Table 10-1). The middle section of the cartilage regresses, but its *perichondrium* forms the **anterior ligament of the malleus** and the **sphenomandibular ligament**. Ventral parts of the first arch cartilage form the primordium of the mandible. Each half of the mandible forms lateral to and in close association with its cartilage. The cartilage disappears as the mandible develops around it by *intramembranous ossification*.

The dorsal end of the **second pharyngeal arch cartilage** ossifies to form the **stapes** of the middle ear and the styloid process of the temporal bone. The part of the cartilage between the **styloid process** and the hyoid bone regresses; its perichondrium forms the **stylohyoid ligament**. The ventral end of the second arch cartilage ossifies to form the lesser cornu and the superior part of the body of the **hyoid bone**.

The **third pharyngeal arch cartilage** ossifies to form the greater cornu and the inferior part of the body of the hyoid bone. The **fourth and sixth pharyngeal arch**

cartilages fuse to form the laryngeal cartilages, except for the epiglottis. The epiglottic and thyroid cartilages appear to develop from neural crest cells (see Fig. 10-22A to C). The cricoid cartilage develops from mesoderm.

Derivatives of Pharyngeal Arch Muscles

The muscular components of the arches form various muscles in the head and neck; for example, the musculature of the first pharyngeal arch forms the **muscles of mastication** and others (Fig. 10-6A and B and Table 10-1).

Derivatives of Pharyngeal Arch Nerves

Each arch is supplied by its own cranial nerve (CN). The *special visceral efferent (branchial) components* of the cranial nerves supply muscles derived from the pharyngeal arches (Fig. 10-7A and Table 10-1). Because the mesenchyme from the pharyngeal arches contributes to the dermis and the mucous membranes of the head and neck, these areas are supplied with the *special visceral afferent nerves*. The facial skin is supplied by the fifth cranial nerve (CN V, or **trigeminal nerve**); however, only the caudal two branches (*maxillary* and *mandibular*) supply derivatives of the first pharyngeal arch (Fig. 10-7B). CN V is the principal sensory nerve of the head and neck and is the motor nerve for the muscles of mastication. Its sensory branches innervate the face, teeth, and mucous membranes of the nasal cavities, palate, mouth, and tongue (Fig. 10-7C). The seventh cranial nerve (CN VII, or **facial nerve**), the ninth cranial nerve (CN IX, or **glossopharyngeal nerve**), and the 10th cranial nerve (CN X, or **vagus nerve**) supply the second, third, and caudal (fourth to sixth) arches, respectively. The fourth arch is supplied by the superior laryngeal branch

Table 10–1 Structures Derived from Pharyngeal Arch Components*

ARCH	NERVE	MUSCLES	SKELETAL STRUCTURES	LIGAMENTS
First (mandibular)	Trigeminal† (CN V)	Muscles of mastication‡ Mylohyoid and anterior belly of digastric Tensor tympani Tensor veli palatini	Malleus Incus	Anterior ligament of malleus Sphenomandibular ligament
Second (hyoid)	Facial (CN VII)	Muscles of facial expression§ Stapedius Stylohyoid Posterior belly of digastric	Stapes Styloid process Lesser cornu of hyoid bone Upper part of body of hyoid bone	Stylohyoid ligament
Third	Glossopharyngeal (CN IX)	Stylopharyngeus	Greater cornu of hyoid bone Lower part of body of hyoid bone	
Fourth and sixth‖	Superior laryngeal branch of vagus (CN X) Recurrent laryngeal branch of vagus (CN X)	Cricothyroid Levator veli palatini Constrictors of pharynx Intrinsic muscles of larynx Striated muscles of esophagus	Thyroid cartilage Cricoid cartilage Arytenoid cartilage Corniculate cartilage Cuneiform cartilage	

*The derivatives of the pharyngeal arch arteries are described in Chapter 14.
†The ophthalmic division of the fifth cranial nerve (CN V) does not supply any pharyngeal arch components.
‡Temporalis, masseter, medial, and lateral pterygoids.
§Buccinator, auricularis, frontalis, platysma, and orbicularis oris and oculi.
‖The fifth pharyngeal arch regresses. The cartilaginous components of the fourth and sixth arches fuse to form the cartilages of the larynx.

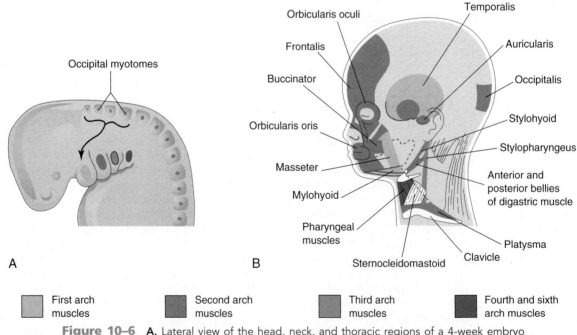

Figure 10–6 **A,** Lateral view of the head, neck, and thoracic regions of a 4-week embryo showing the muscles derived from the pharyngeal arches. The *arrow* shows the pathway taken by myoblasts from the occipital myotomes to form the tongue musculature. **B,** The head and neck regions of a 20-week fetus, showing the muscles derived from the pharyngeal arches. Parts of the platysma and sternocleidomastoid muscles have been removed to show the deeper muscles. Note that myoblasts from the second arch migrate from the neck to the head, where they give rise to the muscles of facial expression. These muscles are supplied by the facial nerve (cranial nerve VII), the nerve of the second pharyngeal arch.

PHARYNGEAL POUCHES

The primordial pharynx widens cranially where it joins the *stomodeum*, and narrows caudally, where it joins the *esophagus* (Figs. 10-3A and 10-4B). The endoderm of the pharynx lines the internal aspects of the pharyngeal arches and passes into the **pharyngeal pouches** (Figs. 10-1D and E and 10-8A). These pairs of pouches develop in a craniocaudal sequence between the arches. The first pair of pouches, for example, lies between the first and second pharyngeal arches. Four pairs of pharyngeal pouches are well defined; the fifth pair is absent or rudimentary. The endoderm of the pouches contacts the ectoderm of the pharyngeal grooves, and together they form the double-layered **pharyngeal membranes** (Fig. 10-3B).

Derivatives of Pharyngeal Pouches

The **first pharyngeal pouch** gives rise to the **tubotympanic recess** (Fig. 10-8B). The first pharyngeal membrane contributes to the formation of the **tympanic membrane** (eardrum) (Fig. 10-8C). The cavity of the tubotympanic recess gives rise to the **tympanic cavity** and the **mastoid antrum**. The connection of the tubotympanic recess with the pharynx forms the **pharyngotympanic tube** (auditory tube).

The **second pharyngeal pouch** is largely obliterated as the **palatine tonsil** develops (Figs. 10-8C and 10-9). A part of this pouch remains as the **tonsillar sinus (fossa)**. The endoderm of the second pouch proliferates and grows into the underlying mesenchyme. The central parts of these buds break down, forming **tonsillar crypts**. The pouch endoderm forms the surface epithelium and the lining of the crypts. The mesenchyme around the crypts differentiates into lymphoid tissue, which soon organizes into the lymphatic nodules of the palatine tonsil.

The **third pharyngeal pouch** expands and develops a solid, bulbar, dorsal part and a hollow, elongate ventral part (Fig. 10-8B). The connection between the pouch and the pharynx is reduced to a narrow duct that soon degenerates. By the sixth week of development, the epithelium of each bulbar dorsal part begins to differentiate into an **inferior parathyroid gland**. The epithelium of the elongated ventral parts of the third pair of pouches proliferates, obliterating their cavities. These parts come together in the median plane to form the **thymus**. The primordia of the thymus and parathyroid glands lose their connections with the pharynx. Later, the inferior parathyroid glands separate from the thymus and lie on the dorsal surface of the thyroid gland, whereas the thymus descends into the superior mediastinum (Figs. 10-8C and 10-9). The mesenchyme surrounding the thymic primordium is derived from *neural crest cells*.

The dorsal part of each **fourth pharyngeal pouch** develops into a **superior parathyroid gland**, which lies on the dorsal surface of the thyroid gland (Fig. 10-8B). The parathyroid glands derived from the third pouches descend with the thymus and are carried to a more inferior position than the parathyroid glands that are derived from the fourth pouches (Fig. 10-9). The elongated ventral part of each fourth pouch develops into the

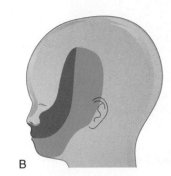

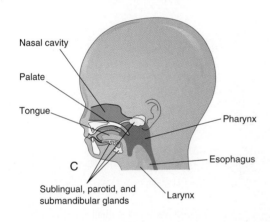

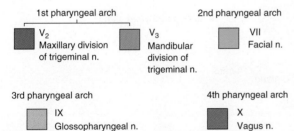

Figure 10–7 **A,** Lateral view of the head, neck, and thoracic regions of a 4-week embryo, showing the cranial nerves that supply the pharyngeal arches. **B,** The head and neck regions of a 20-week fetus, showing the superficial distribution of the two caudal branches of the first arch nerve (cranial nerve V). **C,** Sagittal section of the fetal head and neck, showing the deep distribution of the sensory fibers of the nerves to the teeth and mucosa of the tongue, pharynx, nasal cavity, palate, and larynx.

of the vagus nerve, whereas the sixth arch is supplied by its recurrent laryngeal branch. The nerves of the second to sixth pharyngeal arches (Fig. 10-7B) innervate the mucous membranes of the tongue, pharynx, and larynx (Fig. 10-7C).

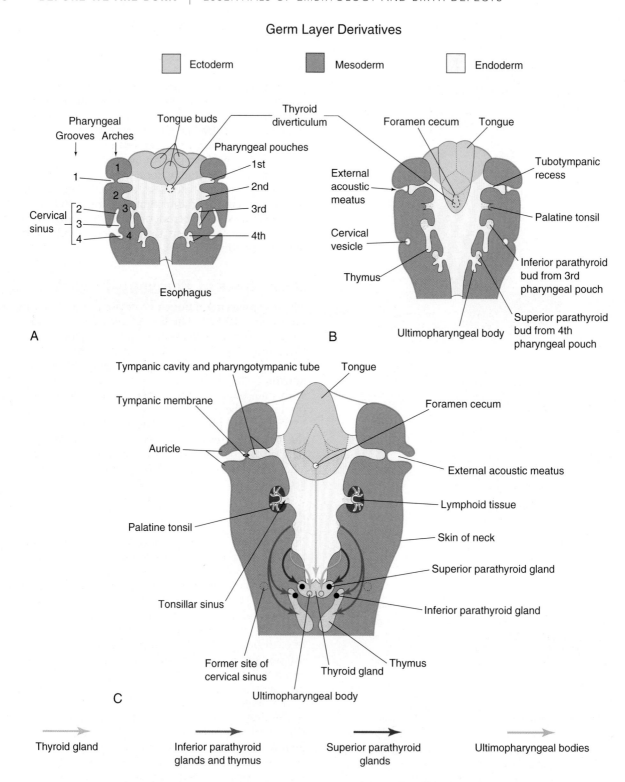

Figure 10–8   Schematic horizontal sections at the level shown in Figure 10-4*A*, showing the adult derivatives of the pharyngeal pouches. **A,** At 5 weeks. Note that the second pharyngeal arch grows over the third and fourth arches, burying the second to fourth pharyngeal grooves in the cervical sinus. **B,** At 6 weeks. **C,** At 7 weeks. Note the migration of the developing thymus, parathyroid, and thyroid glands into the neck.

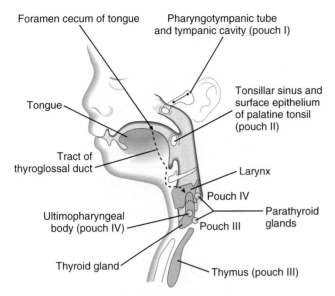

Figure 10–9   A sagittal section of the head, neck, and upper thoracic regions of a 20-week fetus, showing the adult derivatives of the pharyngeal pouches and the descent of the thyroid gland into the neck.

CONGENITAL AURICULAR SINUSES AND CYSTS

Small auricular sinuses and cysts are usually located in a triangular area of skin anterior to the auricle of the external ear (Fig. 10-10*D*); however, they may occur in other sites around the auricle or in its lobule (earlobe). Although some sinuses and cysts are remnants of the first pharyngeal groove, others represent ectodermal folds sequestered during formation of the auricle from the auricular hillocks (swellings that contribute to the auricle).

CERVICAL (BRANCHIAL) SINUSES

Cervical sinuses are uncommon, and almost all that open externally on the side of the neck result from failure of the second pharyngeal groove and the cervical sinus to obliterate (Figs. 10-10*B* and 10-11*A*). The sinus typically opens along the anterior border of the sternocleidomastoid muscle in the inferior third of the neck. Anomalies of the other pharyngeal grooves occur in approximately 5% of cases.

External cervical sinuses are commonly detected during infancy because of the discharge of mucous material from their orifices in the neck. These *lateral cervical sinuses* are bilateral in approximately 10% of cases and are commonly associated with auricular sinuses.

Internal cervical sinuses open into the pharynx and are very rare. Almost all of these sinuses result from persistence of the proximal part of the second pharyngeal pouch, so they usually open into the tonsillar sinus or near the palatopharyngeal arch (Fig. 10-10*B* and *D*). Normally, this pouch disappears as the palatine tonsil develops; its normal remnant is the tonsillar sinus.

ultimopharyngeal body, which fuses with the thyroid gland, giving rise to the **parafollicular cells (C cells)** of the thyroid gland. These cells produce calcitonin, a hormone involved in the regulation of calcium. C cells differentiate from **neural crest cells** that migrate from the pharyngeal arches into the fourth pair of pharyngeal pouches.

If the **fifth pharyngeal pouch** develops, it is rudimentary and becomes part of the fourth pharyngeal pouch.

PHARYNGEAL GROOVES

The head and neck regions of the embryo exhibit four pharyngeal grooves on each side during the fourth and fifth weeks (Fig. 10-1*A*). These grooves separate the pharyngeal arches externally. Only one pair of grooves contributes to the adult structures; the first pair persists as the **external acoustic meatus** (ear canal) (Fig. 10-8*C*). The other grooves lie in a slit-like depression—the **cervical sinus**—and are usually obliterated with it as the neck develops (Fig. 10-4*B* to *F*).

BRANCHIAL FISTULA

An abnormal canal that opens internally into the tonsillar sinus and externally on the side of the neck is a *branchial fistula*. This rare anomaly results from persistence of parts of the second pharyngeal groove and the second pharyngeal pouch (Figs. 10-10*C* and *D* and 10-11*B*). The fistula ascends from its opening in the neck, through the subcutaneous tissue and the platysma muscle, to reach the tonsillar sinus.

CERVICAL CYSTS

The third and fourth pharyngeal arches are buried in the cervical sinus (Fig. 10-8*A*). Remnants of parts of the cervical sinus, the second pharyngeal groove, or both may persist and form a spherical or elongated cyst (Fig. 10-10*D*). Cervical cysts often do not become apparent until late childhood or early adulthood, when they produce a slowly enlarging, painless swelling in the neck (Fig. 10-12). The cysts enlarge because of the accumulation of fluid and cellular debris derived from desquamation of their epithelial linings (Fig. 10-13).

CERVICAL VESTIGES

Normally the pharyngeal cartilages disappear, except for the parts that form ligaments or bones; however, in unusual cases, cartilaginous or bony remnants of the pharyngeal arch cartilages appear under the skin on the side of the neck. These are usually found anterior to the inferior third of the sternocleidomastoid muscle (Fig. 10-10*D*).

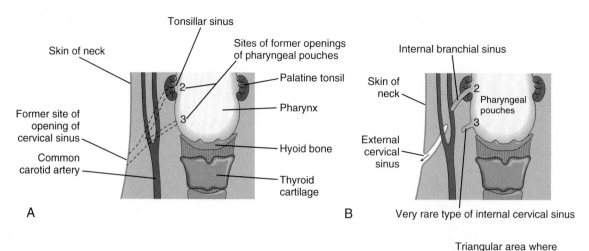

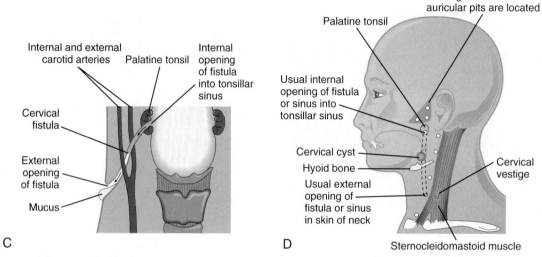

Figure 10–10 **A,** The adult pharyngeal and neck regions, indicating the former sites of openings of the cervical sinus and the pharyngeal pouches (2 and 3). The *broken lines* indicate possible courses of cervical fistulas. **B,** The embryologic basis for various types of cervical sinus. **C,** Illustration of a cervical fistula resulting from the persistence of parts of the second pharyngeal groove and the second pharyngeal pouch. **D,** Possible sites of cervical cysts and openings of the cervical sinuses and fistulas. A cervical vestige is also shown.

FIRST ARCH SYNDROME

Abnormal development of the first pharyngeal arch results in various congenital anomalies of the eyes, ears, mandible, and palate that together constitute *first pharyngeal arch syndrome* (Fig. 10-14). This syndrome is believed to result from insufficient migration of neural crest cells into the first arch during the fourth week. There are two main clinical manifestations of first arch syndrome:

* **Treacher Collins syndrome** (mandibulofacial dysostosis), is most often caused by an autosomal dominant gene defect (TCOF1), and results in underdevelopment of the zygomatic bones of the face—malar hypoplasia. Characteristic features of the syndrome include down-slanting palpebral fissures, defects of the lower eyelids, deformed external ears, and sometimes abnormalities of the middle and internal ears.

* **Pierre Robin sequence** consists of hypoplasia of the mandible, cleft palate, and defects of the eye and ear. Many cases of this syndrome are sporadic; however, some appear to have a genetic basis. In *Robin morphogenetic complex,* the initiating defect is a small mandible (micrognathia), which results in posterior displacement of the tongue and obstruction to full closure of the palatine processes, resulting in bilateral cleft palate.

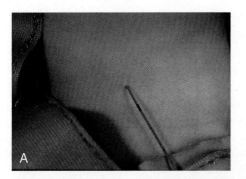

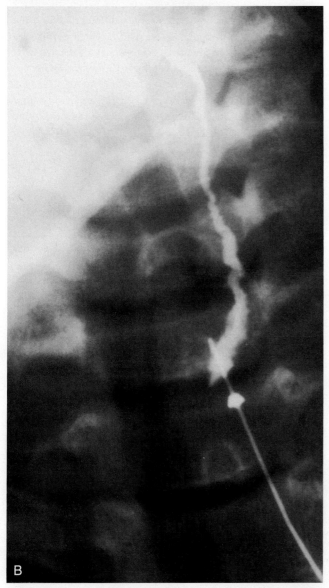

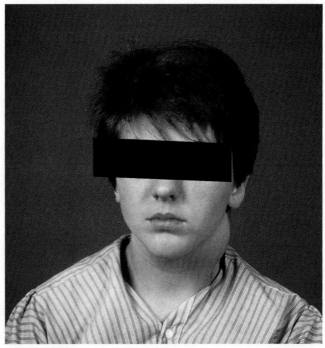

Figure 10–12 A boy with swelling in the neck produced by a cervical cyst. Cervical cysts often lie free in the neck, just inferior to the angle of the mandible, or they may be found anywhere along the anterior border of the sternocleidomastoid muscle. (*Courtesy Dr. Pierre Soucy, Division of Paediatric Surgery, Children's Hospital of Eastern Ontario, Ottawa, Ontario, Canada.*)

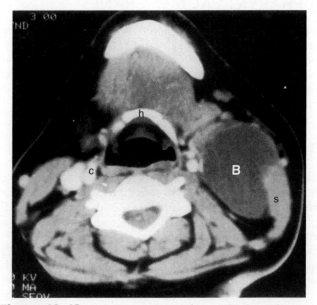

Figure 10–11 **A,** A child's neck, showing a catheter inserted into the external opening of a cervical sinus. The catheter allows definition of the length of the tract, which facilitates surgical excision. **B,** A fistulogram of a complete cervical fistula. The radiograph was taken after injection of a contrast medium to show the course of the fistula through the neck. (*Courtesy Dr. Pierre Soucy, Division of Paediatric Surgery, Children's Hospital of Eastern Ontario, Ottawa, Ontario, Canada.*)

Figure 10–13 A large cervical (cleft) cyst (*B*) shown by computed tomography of the neck region of a woman who had a "lump" in the neck, similar to that shown in Figure 10-12. The low-density cyst is anterior to the right sternocleidomastoid muscle (*s*) at the level of the hyoid bone (*h*). The normal appearance of the left carotid sheath (*c*) is shown for comparison with the compressed sheath on the right side. (*From McNab T, McLennan MK, Margolis M: Radiology rounds. Can Fam Physician 41:1673, 1995.*)

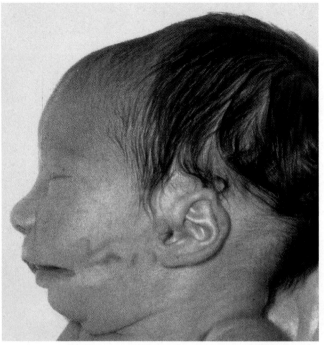

Figure 10–14 An infant with first arch syndrome, a pattern of anomalies resulting from insufficient migration of the neural crest cells into the first pharyngeal arch. Note the following characteristics: deformed auricle of the external ear, preauricular appendage, defect in the cheek between the auricle and the mouth, hypoplasia of the mandible, and macrostomia (large mouth).

 ## PHARYNGEAL MEMBRANES

These membranes form where the epithelia of a groove and a pouch approach each other. The pharyngeal membranes appear in the floors of the pharyngeal grooves during the fourth week (Fig. 10-1*B* and *D*). Only the first pair contributes to the formation of adult structures, the **tympanic membrane** (Fig. 10-8*C*).

 ## DEVELOPMENT OF THYROID GLAND

The thyroid gland is the first endocrine gland to develop. It begins to form at approximately 24 days from a median endodermal thickening in the floor of the primordial pharynx (Fig. 10-15*A*). This thickening soon forms a small outpouching known as the **thyroid primordium**. As the embryo and tongue grow, the developing thyroid gland descends in the neck, passing ventral to the developing hyoid bone and the laryngeal cartilages. For a short time, it is connected to the tongue by the **thyroglossal duct** (Fig. 10-15*B* and *C*). As a result of rapid cell proliferation, the lumen of the thyroid diverticulum soon obliterates, and then it divides into right and left lobes that are connected by the **thyroid isthmus**.

By 7 weeks, the thyroid gland has assumed its definitive shape and has usually reached its final site in the neck (Fig. 10-15*D*). By this time, the thyroglossal duct has usually degenerated. The proximal opening of the thyroglossal duct persists as a small, blind pit—the **foramen**

DiGEORGE SYNDROME

Infants with DiGeorge (*velocardiofacial*) syndrome are born without a thymus and parathyroid glands. The disease is characterized by *congenital hypoparathyroidism* (hypocalcemia); increased susceptibility to infections (from immune deficiency—specifically, defective T-cell function); palate abnormalities, micrognathia (airway obstruction due to retropositioned tongue); low-set, notched ears; nasal clefts; and cardiac abnormalities (defects of the arch of the aorta and the heart). *DiGeorge syndrome occurs when the third and fourth pharyngeal pouches do not differentiate into the thymus and parathyroid glands.* The facial abnormalities result primarily from abnormal development of the first arch components during formation of the face and ears. *DiGeorge syndrome commonly involves a microdeletion (22q11.2 region), mutation of the* HIRA *and* UFDIL *genes, and neural crest cell defects.* The incidence of DiGeorge syndrome is one in 2,000 to 4,000 births.

ECTOPIC PARATHYROID GLANDS

The parathyroids are highly variable in number and location. They may be found anywhere near or within the thyroid gland or the thymus (Fig. 10-16). The superior glands are more constant in position than the inferior ones. Occasionally, an inferior parathyroid gland does not descend and remains near the bifurcation of the common carotid artery. In other cases, it may accompany the thymus into the thorax.

ABNORMAL NUMBER OF PARATHYROID GLANDS

In unusual cases, there may be more than four parathyroid glands. Supernumerary parathyroid glands probably result from division of the primordia of the original glands. Absence of a parathyroid gland results from failure of one of the primordia to differentiate or from atrophy of a gland early in development.

cecum in the dorsum of the tongue (Fig. 10-8*C*). A **pyramidal thyroid lobe** extends superiorly from the isthmus in approximately 50% of individuals. This lobe may be attached to the hyoid bone by fibrous tissue, smooth muscle, or both.

At 11 weeks, colloid begins to appear in the **thyroid follicles**; thereafter, iodine concentration and the synthesis of thyroid hormones can be demonstrated.

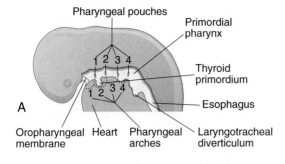

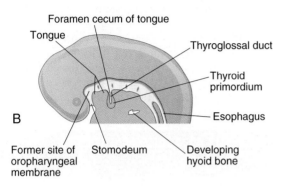

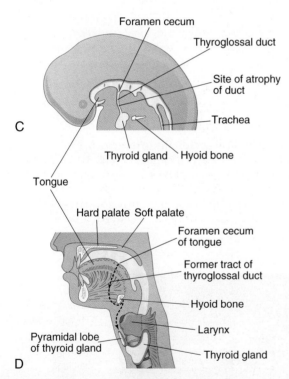

Figure 10–15 Development of the thyroid gland. **A to C,** Schematic sagittal sections of the head and neck regions of 4-week, 5-week, and 6-week embryos, showing successive stages in the development of the thyroid gland. **D,** Similar section of an adult head and neck, showing the path taken by the thyroid gland during its embryonic descent (indicated by the former tract of the thyroglossal duct).

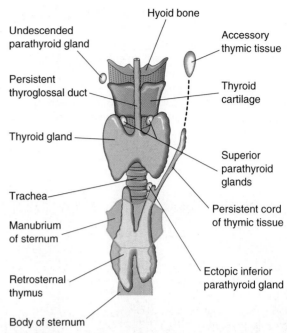

Figure 10–16 Anterior view of the thyroid gland, thymus, and parathyroid glands, showing various possible congenital anomalies.

THYROGLOSSAL DUCT CYSTS AND SINUSES

A remnant of the thyroglossal duct may persist and form a cyst in the tongue or in the anterior part of the neck, usually just inferior to the hyoid bone (Fig. 10-17). The swelling produced by a *thyroglossal duct cyst* usually develops as a painless, progressively enlarging, movable median mass (Fig. 10-18). The cyst may contain some thyroid tissue. After infection of a cyst, perforation of the skin occurs in some cases, forming a **thyroglossal duct sinus** that usually opens in the median plane of the neck, anterior to the laryngeal cartilages (Fig. 10-19A).

ECTOPIC THYROID GLAND

Infrequently, an ectopic thyroid gland is located along the normal route of its descent from the tongue (Fig. 10-15C). **Lingual thyroid glandular tissue** is the most common type. Incomplete descent of the thyroid gland results in a **sublingual thyroid gland** that appears high in the neck, at or just inferior to the hyoid bone (Figs. 10-20 and 10-21). As a rule, an ectopic sublingual thyroid gland is the only thyroid tissue present. It is clinically important to differentiate an ectopic thyroid gland from a thyroglossal duct cyst or from accessory thyroid tissue to prevent *inadvertent surgical removal of the thyroid gland* because this may be the only thyroid tissue present. Failure to recognize the thyroid gland may leave the person permanently dependent on thyroid medication.

DEVELOPMENT OF TONGUE

Near the end of the fourth week, a median triangular elevation appears in the floor of the primordial pharynx, just rostral to the foramen cecum (Fig. 10-22A). This swelling—the **median lingual swelling**—is the first indication of tongue development. Two oval **lateral lingual swellings** soon develop on each side of the median swelling. The swellings result from the proliferation of mesenchyme in the ventromedial parts of the first pair of pharyngeal arches. The lateral swellings rapidly increase in size, merge, and overgrow the median tongue swelling.

The merged lateral swellings form the anterior two thirds, or the oral part, of the tongue (Fig. 10-22C). The plane of fusion of the lateral swellings is indicated superficially by the midline groove of the tongue and internally by the fibrous lingual septum. The median lingual swelling forms no recognizable part of the adult tongue.

Formation of the posterior third, or the pharyngeal part, of the tongue is indicated by two elevations that develop caudal to the foramen cecum (Fig. 10-22A):

- The **copula** forms by fusion of the ventromedial parts of the second pair of pharyngeal arches.
- The **hypopharyngeal eminence** develops caudal to the copula from mesenchyme in the ventromedial parts of the third and fourth pairs of pharyngeal arches.

CONGENITAL LINGUAL CYSTS AND FISTULAS

Cysts in the tongue may be derived from remnants of the thyroglossal duct (Fig. 10-15B). They may enlarge and produce pharyngeal pain, dysphagia (difficulty in swallowing), or both. Fistulas may also arise as a result of persistence of the lingual parts of the thyroglossal duct; such fistulas open through the *foramen cecum* into the oral cavity.

The copula is gradually overgrown by the hypopharyngeal eminence and disappears (Fig. 10-22B and C). As a result, the pharyngeal part of the tongue develops from the rostral part of the hypopharyngeal eminence. The line of fusion of the anterior and posterior parts of the tongue is roughly indicated by a V-shaped groove called the

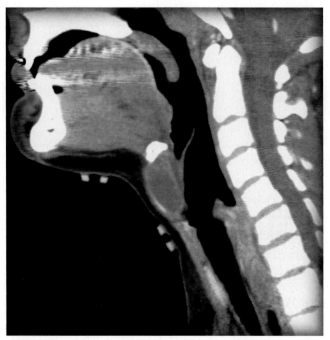

Figure 10–17 CT-Scan of a thyroglossal duct cyst in a child. The cyst is located in the neck anterior to the thyroid cartilage. *(From Dr. Frank Gaillard, Radiopaedia.org, with permission.)*

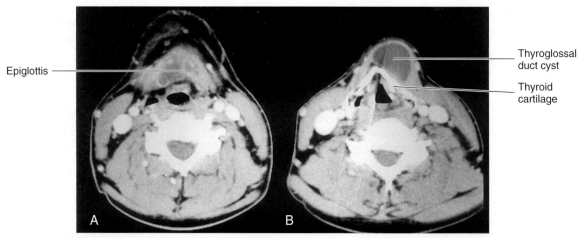

Figure 10–18 Computed tomography scans. **A,** The level of the thyrohyoid membrane and the base of the epiglottis. **B,** The level of the thyroid cartilage, which is calcified. The thyroglossal duct cyst extends cranially to the margin of the hyoid bone. *(Courtesy of Dr. Gerald S. Smyser, Altru Health System, Grand Forks, ND.)*

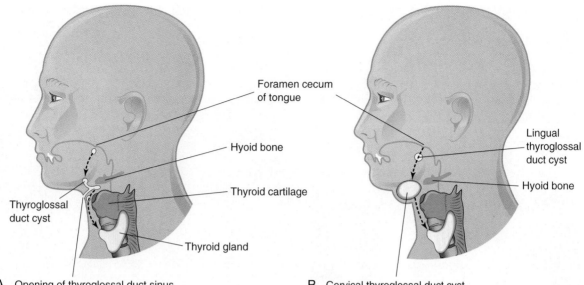

A Opening of thyroglossal duct sinus

B Cervical thyroglossal duct cyst

Figure 10–19 **A,** The head and neck, showing the possible locations of thyroglossal duct cysts. A thyroglossal duct sinus is also shown. The *broken line* indicates the course taken by the thyroglossal duct during the descent of the developing thyroid gland from the foramen cecum to its final position in the anterior part of the neck. **B,** Similar sketch showing lingual and cervical thyroglossal duct cysts. Most thyroglossal duct cysts are located just inferior to the hyoid bone.

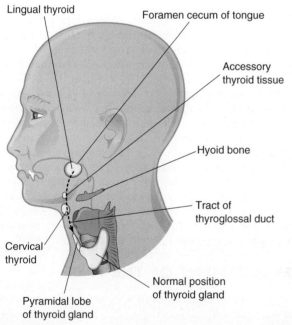

Figure 10–20 The head and neck, showing the usual sites of ectopic thyroid tissue. The *broken line* indicates the path followed by the thyroid gland during its descent, as well as the former tract of the thyroglossal duct.

terminal sulcus (Fig. 10-22C). The pharyngeal arch mesenchyme forms the connective tissue and vasculature of the tongue. The intrinsic tongue muscles are derived from myoblasts that migrate from the occipital somites (see Fig. 10-6A). The hypoglossal nerve (CN XII) accompanies the myoblasts during their migration and innervates the tongue muscles as they develop.

ANKYLOGLOSSIA

The lingual frenulum normally connects the inferior surface of the tongue to the floor of the mouth (Fig. 10-23). Ankyloglossia (tongue-tie) occurs in approximately 1 in 300 North American infants, but it is usually of no functional significance. A short frenulum usually stretches with time, making surgical correction of the anomaly unnecessary.

Papillae and Taste Buds of Tongue

The **lingual papillae** appear by the end of the eighth week. The vallate and foliate papillae appear first, close to the terminal branches of the glossopharyngeal nerve. The fungiform papillae appear later, near the terminations of the chorda tympani branch of the facial nerve. Filiform papillae, the most common papillae, develop during the early fetal period (10–11 weeks). They contain afferent nerve endings that are sensitive to touch.

Taste buds develop during weeks 11 to 13 by inductive interaction between the epithelial cells of the tongue and invading gustatory nerve cells from the chorda tympani, glossopharyngeal, and vagus nerves. Facial responses in the fetus can be induced by bitter-tasting substances at 26 to 28 weeks, indicating that reflex pathways between taste buds and facial muscles are established by this stage.

Nerve Supply of Tongue

The sensory supply to the mucosa of almost the entire anterior tongue (oral part) is from the lingual branch of the mandibular division of the trigeminal nerve (CN V), the nerve of the first pharyngeal arch (Fig. 10-22C).

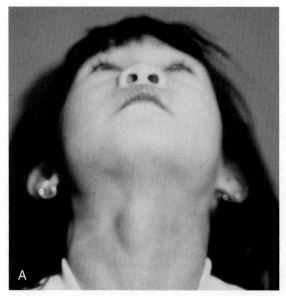
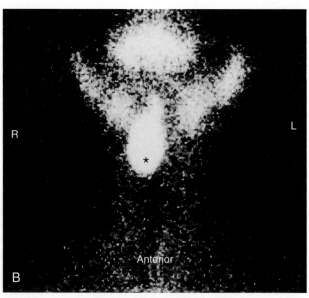

Figure 10–21 **A,** A sublingual thyroid mass in a 5-year-old girl. **B,** Technetium 99m pertech-netate scan showing an ectopic sublingual thyroid gland (*) without evidence of functioning thyroid tissue in the lower neck. *(From Leung AKC, Wong AL, Robson WLLM: Ectopic thyroid gland simulating a thyroglossal duct cyst: A case report. Can J Surg 38:87, 1995.)*

Although the facial nerve is the nerve of the second pharyngeal arch, its chorda tympani branch supplies the taste buds in the anterior tongue, except for the vallate papillae. Because the second arch component, the copula, is overgrown by the third arch component (hypopharyngeal eminence), the facial nerve does not supply any of the tongue mucosa, except for the taste buds. The vallate papillae in the anterior tongue are innervated by the glossopharyngeal nerve of the third pharyngeal arch (Fig. 10-22C). The posterior tongue (pharyngeal part) is innervated mainly by the glossopharyngeal nerve (CN IX). The superior laryngeal branch of the vagus nerve of the fourth arch supplies a small area of the tongue anterior to the epiglottis (Fig. 10-22C). All muscles of the tongue are supplied by the hypoglossal nerve (CN XII), except for the palatoglossus, which is supplied from the pharyngeal plexus by fibers arising from the vagus nerve.

DEVELOPMENT OF SALIVARY GLANDS

During the sixth and seventh weeks, the salivary glands begin as solid epithelial buds from the endoderm of the primordial oral cavity (Fig. 10-7C). The ends of the buds grow into the underlying mesenchyme. The connective tissue in the glands is derived from neural crest cells. All secretory (parenchymal) tissue arises by proliferation of the oral epithelium.

The **parotid glands** are the first to appear (early in the sixth week). They develop early in the sixth week from the oral ectodermal lining near the angles of the stomodeum. The buds grow toward the ears and branch to form solid cords with rounded ends. Later, the cords canalize and become ducts by approximately 10 weeks. The rounded ends of the cords differentiate into acini, which begin to secrete at 18 weeks. The capsule and

the connective tissue develop from the surrounding mesenchyme.

The **submandibular glands** appear late in the sixth week. They develop from endodermal buds in the floor of the stomodeum. Solid cellular processes grow posteriorly, lateral to the developing tongue. Later they branch and differentiate. Acini begin to form at 12 weeks and secretory activity begins at 16 weeks. Growth of the submandibular glands continues after birth, with the formation of mucous acini. Lateral to the developing tongue, a linear groove forms that soon closes over to form the *submandibular duct.*

The **sublingual glands** appear in the eighth week, approximately 2 weeks later than the other salivary glands (Fig. 10-7). They develop from multiple endodermal epithelial buds in the **paralingual sulcus.** These buds branch and canalize to form 10 to 12 ducts that open independently into the floor of the mouth.

DEVELOPMENT OF THE FACE

The facial primordia begin to appear around the **primordial stomodeum** early in the fourth week (Fig. 10-24A). Facial development depends on the inductive influence of organizing centers. The **prosencephalic organizing center,** derived from the prechordal mesoderm that migrates from the primitive streak, is located rostral to the notochord and ventral to the prosencephalon, or forebrain (see Chapter 6). The **rhombencephalic organizing center** is ventral to the rhombencephalon (hindbrain).

The **five facial primordia,** which appear around the *stomodeum,* are:

- The single frontonasal prominence
- The paired maxillary prominences
- The paired mandibular prominences

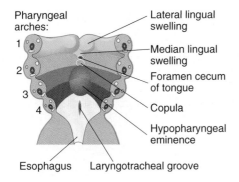

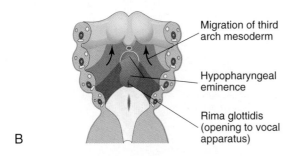

Pharyngeal arches:
1
2
3
4

Lateral lingual swelling
Median lingual swelling
Foramen cecum of tongue
Copula
Hypopharyngeal eminence

A   Esophagus   Laryngotracheal groove

Migration of third arch mesoderm
Hypopharyngeal eminence
Rima glottidis (opening to vocal apparatus)

B

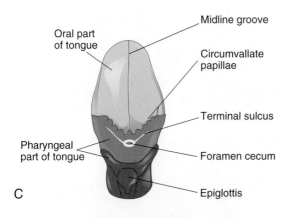

Oral part of tongue
Pharyngeal part of tongue

Midline groove
Circumvallate papillae
Terminal sulcus
Foramen cecum
Epiglottis

C

Arch Derivatives of Tongue

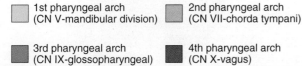

☐ 1st pharyngeal arch (CN V-mandibular division)
☐ 2nd pharyngeal arch (CN VII-chorda tympani)
■ 3rd pharyngeal arch (CN IX-glossopharyngeal)
■ 4th pharyngeal arch (CN X-vagus)

Figure 10–22 **A** and **B**, Schematic horizontal sections through the pharynx at the level shown in Figure 10-4A, showing successive stages in the development of the tongue during the fourth and fifth weeks. **C**, The adult tongue, showing the pharyngeal arch derivation of the nerve supply of its mucosa.

Both paired prominences are derivatives of the first pair of pharyngeal arches. The prominences are produced by mesenchyme derived from **neural crest cells** that migrate into the arches during the fourth week of development. These cells are the major source of connective

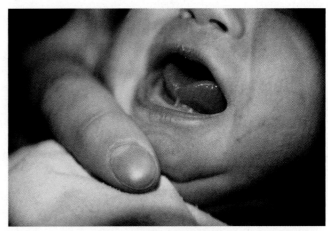

Figure 10–23 An infant with ankyloglossia, or tongue-tie. Note the short frenulum, which extends to the tip of the tongue. Tongue-tie interferes with protrusion of the tongue and may make breast-feeding difficult. (*Courtesy Dr. Evelyn Jain, Lakeview Breastfeeding Clinic, Calgary, Alberta, Canada.*)

tissue components, including cartilage, bone, and ligaments in the facial and oral regions.

The **frontonasal prominence** surrounds the ventrolateral part of the forebrain, which gives rise to the optic vesicles that form the eyes (Figs. 10-24A and 10-25). The frontal part of the frontonasal prominence forms the forehead; the nasal part of the frontonasal prominence forms the rostral boundary of the stomodeum and the nose.

The **maxillary prominences** form the lateral boundaries of the stomodeum, whereas the **mandibular prominences** constitute the caudal boundary of the primordial mouth (Figs. 10-24A and 10-25). The lower jaw and the lower lip are the first parts of the face to form. They result from merging of the medial ends of the mandibular prominences.

By the end of the fourth week, bilateral oval thickenings of the surface ectoderm—**nasal placodes**—have developed on the inferolateral parts of the frontonasal prominence (Figs. 10-25 and 10-26A and B). Initially, these placodes are convex, but later, they are stretched to produce a flat depression in each placode. The mesenchyme in the margins of the placodes proliferates, producing horseshoe-shaped elevations—the medial and lateral **nasal prominences** (Figs. 10-24B and 10-26D and E). As a result, the nasal placodes lie in depressions, called **nasal pits** (Figs. 10-24B and 10-26C and D). These pits are the primordia of the anterior nares (nostrils) and nasal cavities (Fig. 10-26E). Proliferation of mesenchyme in the maxillary prominences causes them to enlarge and grow medially toward each other and the nasal prominences (Figs. 10-24B and C and 10-25). The medial migration of the maxillary prominences moves the medial nasal prominences toward the median plane and each other. Each lateral nasal prominence is separated from the maxillary prominence by a cleft called the **nasolacrimal groove** (Fig. 10-24B).

By the end of the fifth week, **six auricular hillocks**—*primordia of the auricle*—(mesenchymal swellings) form

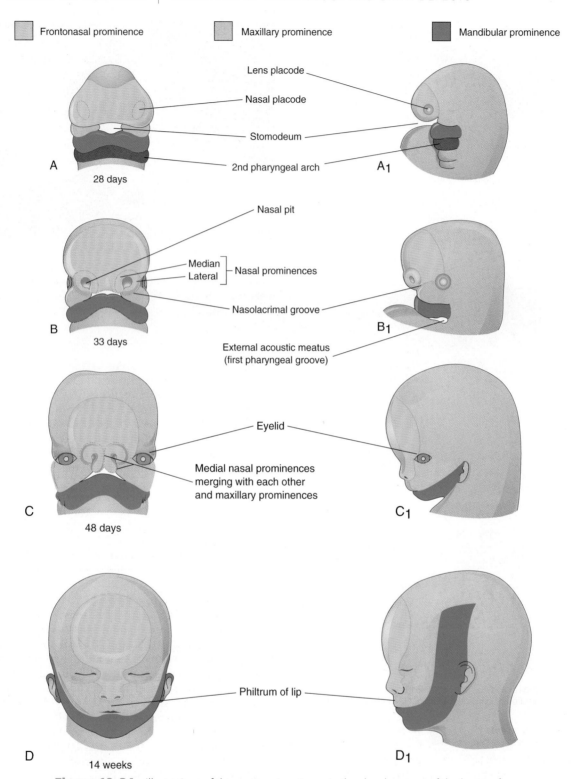

Figure 10–24 Illustrations of the progressive stages in the development of the human face.

around the first pharyngeal groove (three on each side), the primordium of the external acoustic meatus (canal). Initially, the external ears are positioned in the neck region; however, as the mandible develops, they ascend to the side of the head at the level of the eyes (Fig. 10-24B and C). By the end of the sixth week, each maxillary prominence has begun to merge with the lateral nasal prominence along the line of the nasolacrimal groove

(Fig. 10-27A and B). This establishes continuity between the side of the nose, formed by the lateral nasal prominence, and the cheek region, formed by the maxillary prominence.

The **nasolacrimal duct** develops from a rod-like thickening of ectoderm in the floor of the *nasolacrimal groove*. This thickening gives rise to a solid epithelial cord that separates from the ectoderm and sinks into

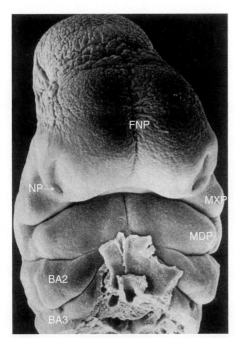

Figure 10–25 Scanning electron micrograph showing a ventral view of a human embryo at approximately 33 days (stage 15; crown–rump length [CRL], 8 mm). Observe the prominent frontonasal prominence *(FNP)* surrounding the telencephalon (forebrain). Also observe the nasal pits *(NP)* located in the ventrolateral regions of the frontonasal prominence. Medial and lateral nasal prominences surround these pits. The wedge-shaped maxillary prominences *(MXP)* form the lateral boundaries of the stomodeum. The fusing mandibular prominences *(MDP)* are located just caudal to the stomodeum. The second pharyngeal arch *(BA2)* is clearly visible and shows overhanging margins (opercula). The third pharyngeal (branchial) arch *(BA3)* is also clearly visible. *(From Hinrichsen K: The early development of morphology and patterns of the face in the human embryo. Adv Anat Embryol Cell Biol 98:1, 1985.)*

the mesenchyme. Later, as a result of apoptosis (programmed cell death), the cord canalizes to form the nasolacrimal duct. The cranial end of this duct expands to form the *lacrimal sac*. In the late fetal period, the nasolacrimal duct drains into the inferior meatus in the lateral wall of the nasal cavity. The duct usually becomes completely patent only after birth.

Between weeks 7 and 10, the medial nasal prominences merge with each other and with the maxillary and lateral nasal prominences (Fig. 10-24C), resulting in disintegration of their contacting surface epithelia. This causes intermingling of the underlying mesenchyme. Merging of the medial nasal and maxillary prominences results in continuity of the upper jaw and lip and separation of the nasal pits from the stomodeum. As the medial nasal prominences merge, they form an intermaxillary segment (Figs. 10-27C to F). The intermaxillary segment gives rise to the following:

- The deep median part of the upper lip
- The premaxillary part of the maxilla and its associated gingiva (gum)
- The primary palate

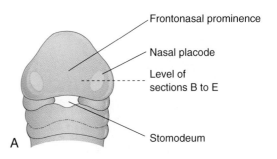
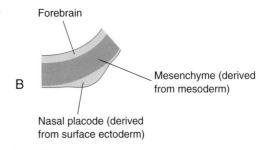
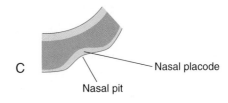
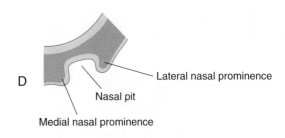
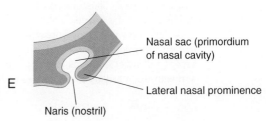

Figure 10–26 Progressive stages in the development of a human nasal sac (primordial nasal cavity). **A,** Ventral view of an embryo at approximately 28 days. **B** to **E,** Transverse sections through the left side of the developing nasal sac.

The lateral parts of the upper lip, most of the maxilla, and the secondary palate form from the maxillary prominences (Fig. 10-24D). These prominences merge laterally with the mandibular prominences. Recent studies show that the lower part of the medial nasal

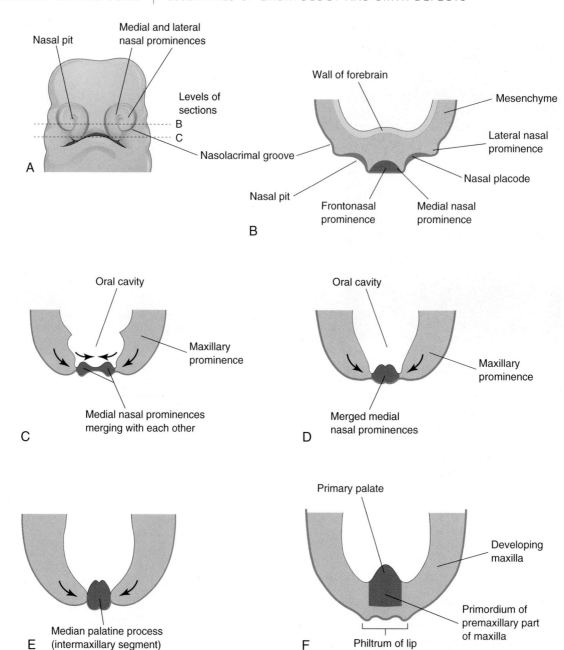

Figure 10–27 Illustrations of the early development of the maxilla, palate, and upper lip. **A,** Facial view of a 5-week embryo. **B** and **C,** Sketches of horizontal sections at the levels shown in **A.** The *arrows* indicate subsequent growth of the maxillary and medial nasal prominences toward the median plane and merging of the prominences with each other. **D** to **F,** Similar sections of older embryos showing merging of the medial nasal prominences with each other and with the maxillary prominences to form the upper lip.

prominences becomes deeply positioned and are covered by medial extensions of the maxillary prominences to form the **philtrum.** The primordial lips and cheeks are invaded by myoblasts from the second pair of pharyngeal arches, which differentiate into the facial muscles (see Fig. 10-6 and Table 10-1). The myoblasts from the first pair of arches differentiate into the muscles of mastication.

DEVELOPMENT OF NASAL CAVITIES

As the face develops, the **nasal placodes** become depressed, forming **nasal pits** (Figs. 10-25 and 10-26). Proliferation of the surrounding mesenchyme forms the medial and lateral **nasal prominences** and results in deepening of the nasal pits and formation of primordial **nasal sacs.** Each nasal sac grows dorsally, ventral to

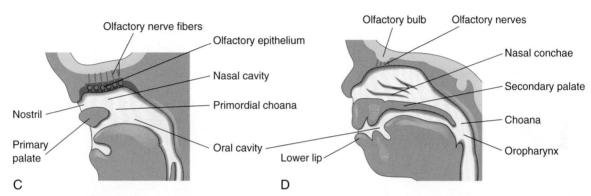

Figure 10–28 Sagittal sections of the head, showing development of the nasal cavities. The nasal septum has been removed. **A,** At 5 weeks. **B,** At 6 weeks, showing breakdown of the oronasal membrane. **C,** At 7 weeks, showing the nasal cavity communicating with the oral cavity and the development of the olfactory epithelium. **D,** At 12 weeks. The palate and the lateral wall of the nasal cavity are evident.

the developing forebrain (Fig. 10-28A). At first, the nasal sacs are separated from the oral cavity by the **oronasal membrane**. This membrane ruptures by the end of the sixth week of development, bringing the nasal and oral cavities into communication (Fig. 10-28B and C). The regions of continuity between the nasal and oral cavities are the **primordial choanae**, which lie posterior to the primary palate. After the *secondary palate* develops, the choanae are located at the junction of the nasal cavity and pharynx (Fig. 10-28D). While these changes are occurring, the superior, middle, and inferior **conchae** develop as elevations of the lateral walls of the nasal cavities (see Fig. 10-30D). Concurrently, the ectodermal epithelium in the roof of each nasal cavity becomes specialized to form the **olfactory epithelium**. Some epithelial cells differentiate into olfactory receptor cells. The axons of these cells constitute the **olfactory nerves**, which grow into the olfactory bulbs of the brain (Fig. 10-28C and D).

Paranasal Sinuses

Some paranasal sinuses, in particular, the **maxillary sinuses**, begin to develop during late fetal life; the remainder of them develop after birth. They form from outgrowths (diverticula) of the walls of the nasal

PARANASAL SINUSES IN NEONATAL AND POSTNATAL DEVELOPMENT

Most of the paranasal sinuses are rudimentary or absent in newborns. The *maxillary sinuses* are small at birth. They grow slowly until puberty and are not fully developed until all of the permanent teeth have erupted in early adulthood. No frontal or sphenoid sinuses are present at birth. The ethmoid cells (sinuses) are small before 2 years, and they do not begin to grow rapidly until 6 to 8 years. At approximately 2 years, the two most anterior ethmoid cells grow into the frontal bone, forming a frontal sinus on each side. Usually, the frontal sinuses are visible on radiographs by 7 years. The two most posterior ethmoid cells grow into the sphenoid bone at approximately 2 years, forming two sphenoid sinuses. Growth of the paranasal sinuses is important in altering the size and shape of the face during infancy and childhood and in adding resonance to the voice during adolescence.

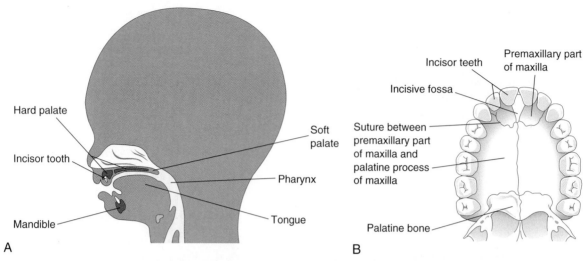

Figure 10–29 **A,** Sagittal section of the head of a 20-week fetus, showing the location of the palate. **B,** The bony palate and the alveolar arch of a young adult. The suture between the premaxillary part of the maxilla and the fused palatal processes of the maxillae is usually visible in the crania of young persons.

cavities, becoming pneumatic (air-filled) extensions of the nasal cavities in the adjacent bones. The original openings of the diverticula persist as the orifices of the adult sinuses.

 DEVELOPMENT OF PALATE

The palate develops from two primordia: the primary palate and the secondary palate.

Palatogenesis begins in the sixth week but is not completed until the 12th week. The critical period of development of the palate is from the end of the sixth week until the beginning of the ninth week.

Primary Palate

Early in the sixth week, the primary palate (**median palatine process**) begins to develop from the deep part of the intermaxillary segment of the maxilla (Figs. 10-27F and 10-28). Initially, this segment is a wedge-shaped mass of mesenchyme between the internal surfaces of the maxillary prominences of the developing maxillae. The primary palate forms the **premaxillary part of the maxilla** (Fig. 10-29B). It represents only a small part of the adult hard palate (the part anterior to the incisive fossa).

Secondary Palate

The secondary palate is the primordium of the hard and soft parts of the palate (Figs. 10-28D and 10-29A and B). The secondary palate begins to develop early in the sixth week from two mesenchymal projections that extend from the internal aspects of the maxillary prominences. Initially, these structures—**lateral palatine processes** (palatal shelves)—project inferomedially on each side of the tongue (Figs. 10-30A to C). As the jaws develop, the tongue becomes relatively smaller and moves inferiorly. During the seventh and eighth weeks, the lateral palatine processes elongate and ascend to a horizontal position superior to the tongue. Gradually, the processes approach each other and fuse in the median plane (Fig. 10-30D to H). They also fuse with the nasal septum and the posterior part of the primary palate. Elevation of the palatine processes to the horizontal position is believed to be caused by an intrinsic force that is generated by the hydration of hyaluronic acid in the mesenchymal cells within the palatine processes. The medial epithelial seam at the edges of the palatine shelves breaks down, allowing for the fusion of the palatine shelves.

The **nasal septum** develops in a downward growth pattern from internal parts of the merged medial nasal prominences (Fig. 10-30C, E, and G). The fusion between the nasal septum and the palatine processes begins anteriorly during the ninth week and is completed posteriorly by the 12th week, superior to the primordium of the hard palate (Fig. 10-30D and F). Bone gradually develops by intramembranous ossification (see Chapter 15) in the primary palate, forming the premaxillary part of the maxilla, which lodges the incisor teeth (Fig. 10-29B). Concurrently, bone extends from the maxillae and palatine bones into the lateral palatine processes to form the **hard palate** (Fig. 10-30E and G). The posterior parts of these processes do not become ossified; they extend posteriorly beyond the nasal septum and fuse to form the **soft palate**,

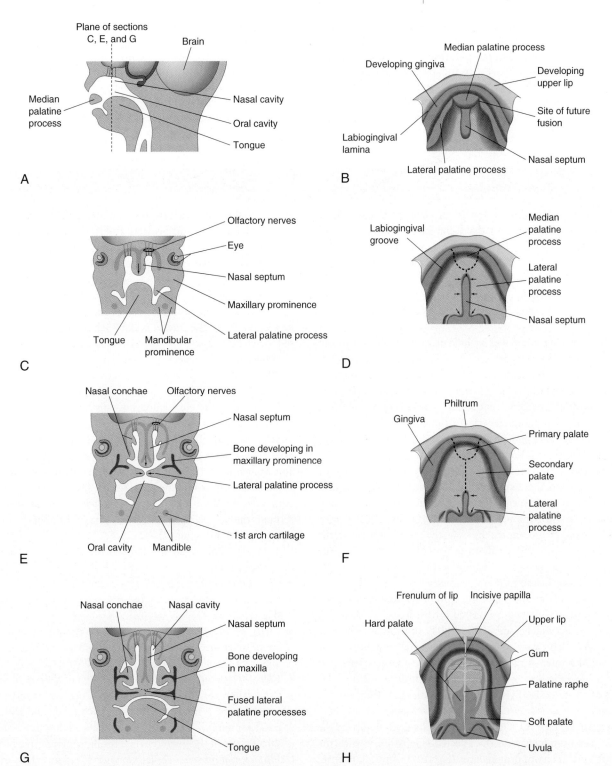

Figure 10–30 **A,** Sagittal section of the embryonic head at the end of the sixth week, showing the median palatine process, or primary palate. **B, D, F,** and **H,** The roof of the mouth from the sixth to 12th weeks, showing the development of the palate. The *broken lines* indicate the sites of fusion of the palatine processes. The *arrows* indicate medial and posterior growth of the lateral palatine processes. **C, E,** and **G,** Frontal sections of the head, showing fusion of the lateral palatine processes with each other and with the nasal septum, and separation of the nasal and oral cavities.

including its conical projection, the **uvula** (Fig. 10-30D, F, and H). The **median palatine raphe** indicates the line of fusion of the lateral palatine processes. A small *nasopalatine canal* persists in the median plane of the palate, between the premaxillary part of the maxilla and the palatine processes of the maxillae. This canal is represented in the adult hard palate by the **incisive fossa** (Fig. 10-29B). An irregular suture runs from the incisive fossa to the alveolar process of the maxilla, between the lateral incisor and the canine teeth on each side, indicating where the embryonic primary and secondary palates fused.

CLEFT LIP AND CLEFT PALATE

Clefts of the upper lip and palate are common. The defects are classified according to developmental criteria, with the incisive fossa and papilla used as reference landmarks (Fig. 10-29B and see Fig. 10-34A). Cleft and cleft palate are especially conspicuous because they result in an abnormal facial appearance and defective speech (Fig. 10-31). Two major groups of cleft lip and cleft palate are recognized (Figs. 10-32 to 10-34):

Anterior cleft anomalies include cleft lip, with or without cleft of the alveolar part of the maxilla. A complete cleft anomaly is one in which the cleft extends through the lip and the alveolar part of the maxilla to the incisive fossa, separating the anterior and posterior parts of the palate (Fig. 10-34E and F). Anterior cleft anomalies result from a deficiency of mesenchyme in the maxillary prominences and the median palatine process (Fig. 10-27D and E).

Posterior cleft anomalies include clefts of the secondary, or posterior, palate that extend through the soft and hard regions of the palate to the incisive fossa, separating the anterior and posterior parts of the palate (Fig. 10-34G and H). Posterior cleft anomalies are caused by defective development of the secondary palate and result from growth distortions in the lateral palatine processes that, in turn, prevent the medial migration and fusion of these processes.

Clefts involving the upper lip, with or without cleft palate, occur in approximately 1 in 1000 births; however, their frequency varies widely, and 60% to 80% of those affected are boys. The clefts vary in severity from small notches in the vermilion border of the lip (Fig. 10-33G) to larger clefts that extend into the floor of the nostril and through the alveolar part of the maxilla (Figs. 10-32A and 10-34E). *Cleft lip can be unilateral or bilateral.*

Unilateral cleft lip (Fig. 10-32A) results from failure of the maxillary prominence on the affected side to unite with the merged medial nasal prominences (Fig. 10-33A to H), in turn, causing a persistent labial groove. The tissues in the floor of the persistent groove break down. As a result, the lip is divided into medial and lateral parts. Sometimes, a bridge of tissue, called a *Simonart band*, joins the parts of the incomplete cleft lip.

Bilateral cleft lip (Figs. 10-32B and 10-34F) results from failure of the mesenchymal masses in the maxillary prominences to meet and unite with the merged medial nasal prominences. When there is a complete bilateral cleft of the lip and the alveolar part of the maxilla, the intermaxillary segment hangs free and projects anteriorly. These defects are especially deforming because of the loss of continuity of the *orbicularis oris muscle*, which closes the mouth and purses the lips.

Median cleft lip is an extremely rare defect. It results from partial or complete failure of the medial nasal prominences to merge and form the intermaxillary segment. Median cleft of the lower lip is also very rare and is caused by failure of the mandibular prominences to merge completely.

The landmark for distinguishing anterior from posterior cleft anomalies is the incisive fossa. Anterior and posterior cleft anomalies are embryologically distinct.

Cleft palate, with or without cleft lip, occurs in approximately 1 in 2500 births and is more common in girls than in boys. The cleft may involve only the uvula, giving it a fish-tail appearance (Fig. 10-34B), or it may extend through the soft and hard regions of the palate (Fig. 10-34C and D). In severe cases associated with cleft lip, the cleft in the palate extends through the alveolar part of the maxilla and the lips on both sides (Fig. 10-34G and H).

Unilateral and bilateral clefts in the palate are classified into three groups:

* *Clefts of the anterior palate* result from failure of the lateral palatine processes to meet and fuse with the primary palate (Fig. 10-34F).
* *Clefts of the posterior palate* result from failure of the lateral palatine processes to meet and fuse with each other and with the nasal septum (Fig. 10-30E).
* *Clefts of the anterior and posterior parts of the palate* result from failure of the lateral palatine processes to meet and fuse with the primary palate, with each other, and with the nasal septum.

Most clefts of the lip and palate result from multiple factors (*multifactorial inheritance*; see Chapter 19). Some clefts of the lip, palate, or both appear as part of syndromes determined by single mutant genes. Other clefts are features of chromosomal syndromes, especially *trisomy 13*. A few cases of cleft lip or cleft palate appear to be caused by teratogenic agents (e.g., anticonvulsant drugs). A sibling of a child with a cleft palate has an elevated risk of having a cleft palate, but no increased risk of cleft lip. A cleft of the lip and the alveolar process of the maxilla that continues through the palate is usually transmitted through a male sex-linked gene.

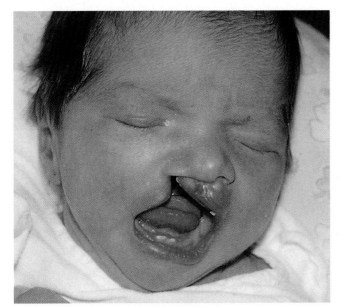

Figure 10–31 Infant with unilateral cleft lip and cleft palate. Clefts of the lip, with or without a cleft palate, occur in approximately 1 in 1000 births; most affected individuals are boys. *(Courtesy of A.E. Chudley, M.D., professor of pediatrics and child health, Children's Hospital and University of Manitoba, Winnipeg, Manitoba, Canada.)*

FACIAL CLEFTS

Various types of facial cleft occur but they are extremely rare. Severe clefts are usually associated with gross anomalies of the head. *Oblique facial clefts* (orbitofacial fissures) are often bilateral and extend from the upper lip to the medial margin of the orbit. When this occurs, the nasolacrimal ducts are open grooves (persistent nasolacrimal grooves). Oblique facial clefts associated with cleft lip result from failure of the maxillary prominences to merge with the lateral and medial nasal prominences. Lateral, or transverse, facial clefts run from the mouth toward the ear. Bilateral clefts result in a very large mouth, a condition called *macrostomia*. In severe cases, the clefts in the cheeks extend almost to the ears.

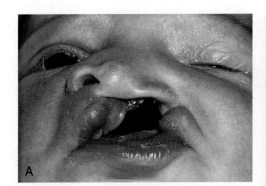
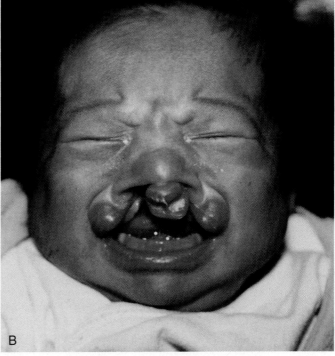

Figure 10–32 Congenital anomalies of the lip and palate. **A,** Infant with a left unilateral cleft lip and a cleft palate. **B,** Infant with a bilateral cleft lip and a cleft palate. *(Courtesy of Dr. Barry H. Grayson and Dr. Bruno L. Vendittelli, New York University Medical Center, Institute of Reconstructive Plastic Surgery, New York, NY.)*

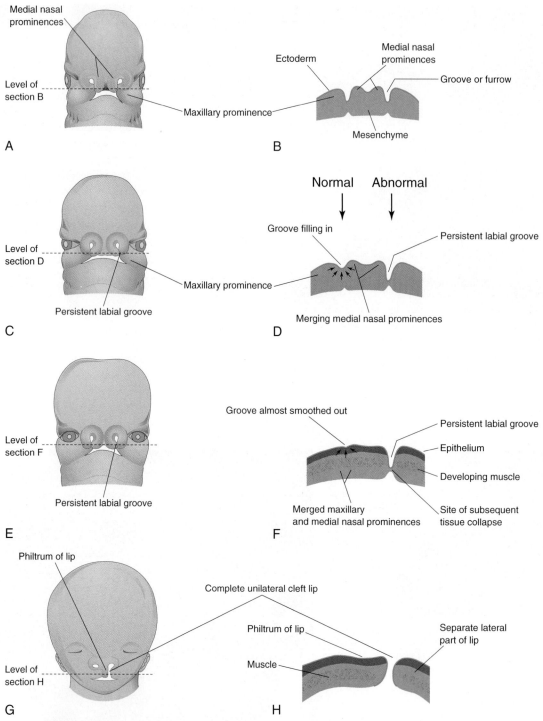

Figure 10–33 Illustrations of the embryologic basis for a complete unilateral cleft lip. **A,** A 5-week embryo. **B,** Horizontal section through the head, showing the grooves between the maxillary prominences and the merging medial nasal prominences. **C,** A 6-week embryo, showing a persistent labial groove on the left side. **D,** Horizontal section through the head, showing the groove gradually filling in on the right side after proliferation of the mesenchyme (*arrows*). **E,** A 7-week embryo. **F,** Horizontal section through the head, showing that the epithelium on the right has almost been pushed out of the groove between the maxillary and medial nasal prominences. **G,** A 10-week fetus with a complete unilateral cleft lip. **H,** Horizontal section through the head after stretching of the epithelium and breakdown of the tissues in the floor of the persistent labial groove on the left side, resulting in the formation of a complete unilateral cleft lip.

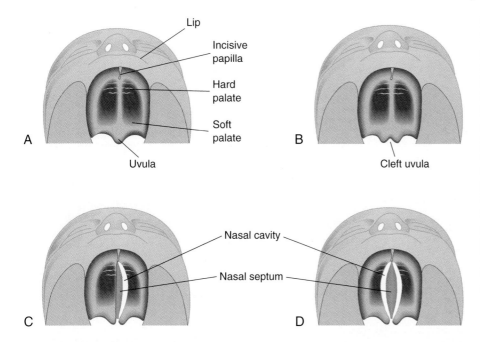

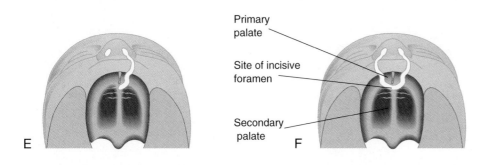

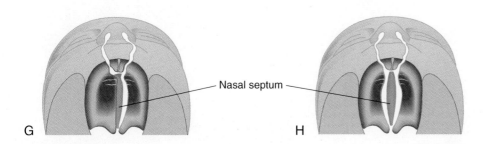

Figure 10–34 Various types of cleft lip and cleft palate. **A,** Normal lip and palate. **B,** Cleft uvula. **C,** Unilateral cleft of the posterior, or secondary, palate. **D,** Bilateral cleft of the posterior palate. **E,** Complete unilateral cleft of the lip and the alveolar process of the maxilla, with a unilateral cleft of the anterior, or primary, palate. **F,** Complete bilateral cleft of the lip and the alveolar processes of the maxillae, with bilateral cleft of the anterior palate. **G,** Complete bilateral cleft of the lip and the alveolar processes of the maxillae, with bilateral cleft of the anterior palate and unilateral cleft of the posterior palate. **H,** Complete bilateral cleft of the lip and the alveolar processes of the maxillae, with complete bilateral cleft of the anterior and posterior palate.

CLINICALLY ORIENTED QUESTIONS

1. What kind of lip defect is a "harelip"? What is the clinical name for this birth defect?

2. Some say that embryos have cleft lips and that this common facial anomaly represents a persistence of this embryonic condition. Are these statements accurate?

3. Neither Clare nor her husband has a cleft lip or a cleft palate, and no one in either one of their families is known to have or to have had these anomalies. What are their chances of having a child with a cleft lip, with or without a cleft palate?

4. Mary's son has a cleft lip and a cleft palate. Her brother has a similar defect involving his lip and palate. Although Mary does not plan to have any more children, her husband says that Mary is entirely to blame for their son's birth defects. Was the defect likely inherited only from Mary's side of the family?

5. A patient's son has minor anomalies involving his external ears, but he does not have hearing problems or a facial malformation. Would his ear abnormalities be considered pharyngeal (branchial) defects?

The answers to these questions are at the back of the book.

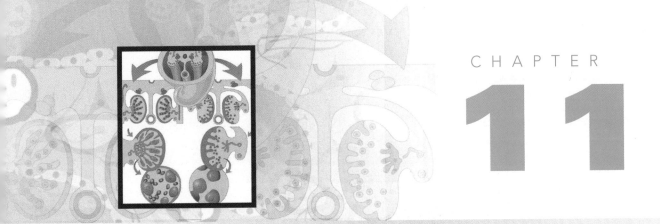

Respiratory System

T he **lower respiratory organs** (larynx, trachea, bronchi, and lungs) begin to form during the fourth week. The primordium of the lower respiratory system—the **laryngotracheal groove**—develops caudal to the fourth pair of pharyngeal pouches (Fig. 11-1*A* and *B*). The endodermal lining of the laryngotracheal groove gives rise to the epithelium and glands of the larynx, trachea, bronchi, and pulmonary epithelium. The connective tissue, cartilage, and smooth muscle in these structures develop from the splanchnic mesoderm surrounding the foregut (see Fig. 11-4*A*). By the end of the fourth week, a pouchlike **laryngotracheal diverticulum** has formed at the largyngotracheal groove (Figs. 11-1*A* and 11-2*A*) and is located ventral to the caudal part of the foregut.

As the diverticulum elongates, its distal end enlarges to form a globular **respiratory bud** (Fig. 11-2*B*). The laryngotracheal diverticulum soon separates from the **primordial pharynx,** but it maintains communication with it through the **primordial laryngeal inlet** (Fig. 11-2*A* and *C*). As the diverticulum elongates, it is invested with splanchnic mesoderm (Fig. 11-2*B*). Longitudinal tracheoesophageal folds develop in the laryngotracheal diverticulum, approach each other, and fuse to form a partition—the **tracheoesophageal septum** (Fig. 11-2*D* and *E*).

This septum divides the cranial part of the foregut into a *ventral part,* the **laryngotracheal tube** (primordium of the larynx, trachea, bronchi, and lungs), and a *dorsal part* (primordium of the oropharynx and esophagus) (Fig. 11-2*F*). The opening of the laryngotracheal tube into the pharynx becomes the **primordial laryngeal inlet** (Figs. 11-2*F* and 11-3*C*).

Figure 11–1 **A,** Sagittal section of the cranial half of the embryo. Lateral view, 4 weeks old. **B,** Horizontal section of the embryo, showing the floor of the primordial pharynx and the location of the laryngotracheal groove.

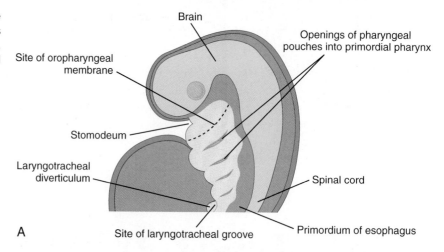

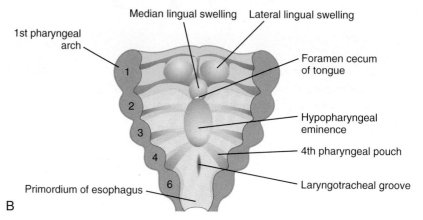

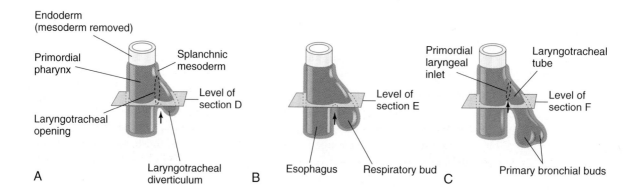

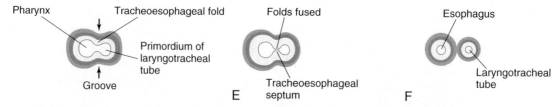

Figure 11–2 Successive stages in the development of the tracheoesophageal septum during the fourth and fifth weeks of development. **A** to **C,** Lateral views of the caudal part of the primordial pharynx, showing the laryngotracheal diverticulum and partitioning of the foregut into the esophagus and the laryngotracheal tube. **D** to **F,** Transverse sections, showing the formation of the tracheoesophageal septum and how it separates the foregut into the laryngotracheal tube and the esophagus. The *arrows* represent cellular changes resulting from growth.

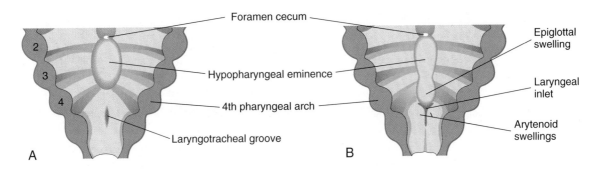

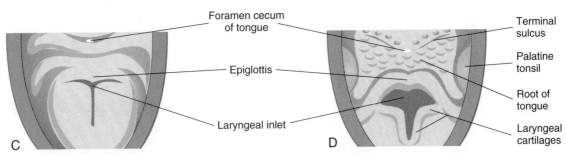

Figure 11–3 Successive stages in the development of the larynx. **A,** At 4 weeks. **B,** At 5 weeks. **C,** At 6 weeks. **D,** At 10 weeks. The epithelium lining the larynx is of endodermal origin. The cartilages and muscles of the larynx arise from the mesenchyme in the fourth and sixth pairs of pharyngeal arches. Note that the laryngeal inlet changes in shape from a slitlike opening to a T-shaped inlet as the mesenchyme surrounding the developing larynx proliferates.

 ## DEVELOPMENT OF LARYNX

The epithelial lining of the larynx develops from the endoderm of the cranial end of the laryngotracheal tube. The cartilages of the larynx develop from cell populations in the fourth and sixth pairs of pharyngeal arches (see Chapter 10). The **laryngeal cartilages** develop from mesenchyme that is derived from *neural crest cells*. The mesenchyme at the cranial end of the laryngotracheal tube proliferates rapidly, producing paired **arytenoid swellings** (Fig. 11-3*B*). These swellings grow toward the tongue, converting **the primordial glottis** into a T-shaped **laryngeal inlet** (Fig. 11-3*C* and *D*). The laryngeal epithelium proliferates rapidly, resulting in *temporary occlusion of the laryngeal lumen*. Recanalization of the larynx occurs by the 10th week. The laryngeal ventricles form during this recanalization process. These recesses are bound by folds of mucous membrane that evolve into the *vocal folds* (cords) and the *vestibular folds*.

The **epiglottis** develops from the caudal part of the *hypopharyngeal eminence*, produced by the proliferation of the mesenchyme in the ventral ends of the third and fourth pharyngeal arches (see Figs. 10-20 and 11-3*B* to *D*). The rostral part of this eminence forms the posterior third or pharyngeal part of the tongue (see Fig. 10-20).

Because the **laryngeal muscles** develop from myoblasts in the fourth and sixth pairs of pharyngeal arches, they are innervated by the laryngeal branches of the vagus nerves (CN X) that supply these arches (see Table 10-1). Growth of the larynx and epiglottis is rapid during the first 3 years after birth, following which the epiglottis has reached its adult form. There is gradual descent of both structures during early childhood.

LARYNGEAL ATRESIA

Laryngeal atresia (obstruction) is a rare anomaly that results in obstruction of the upper fetal airway; it is also known as **congenital high airway obstruction syndrome**. Distal to the atresia or stenosis (narrowing), the airways become dilated, the lungs are enlarged and echogenic (capable of producing echoes during ultrasonography because they are filled with liquid), the diaphragm is either flattened or inverted, and fetal ascites, hydrops, or both (accumulation of serous fluid) is present. Prenatal ultrasonography permits diagnosis of these anomalies.

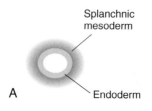

Splanchnic mesoderm

A — Endoderm

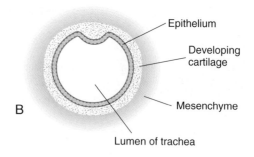

Epithelium

Developing cartilage

Mesenchyme

B

Lumen of trachea

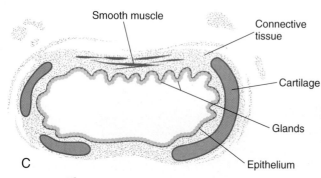

Smooth muscle

Connective tissue

Cartilage

Glands

C — Epithelium

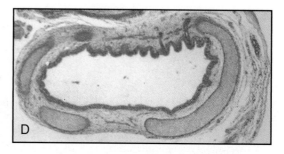

D

Figure 11–4 Transverse sections through the laryngotracheal tube, showing progressive stages in the development of the trachea. **A,** At 4 weeks. **B,** At 10 weeks. **C,** At 11 weeks. Note that the endoderm of the tube gives rise to the epithelium and the glands of the trachea and that the mesenchyme surrounding the tube forms the connective tissue, muscle, and cartilage (drawing of the micrograph shown in **D**). **D,** Photomicrograph of a transverse section of the developing trachea at 12 weeks. *(From Moore KL, Persaud TVN, Shiota K: Color Atlas of Clinical Embryology, 2nd ed. Philadelphia, WB Saunders, 2000.)*

DEVELOPMENT OF TRACHEA

The endodermal lining of the laryngotracheal tube distal to the larynx differentiates into the epithelium and the glands of the trachea and the pulmonary epithelium. The cartilage, connective tissue, and muscles of the trachea are derived from the splanchnic mesoderm surrounding the laryngotracheal tube (Fig. 11-4).

DEVELOPMENT OF BRONCHI AND LUNGS

The **respiratory bud** (lung bud) that developed at the caudal end of the laryngotracheal diverticulum during the fourth week (Fig. 11-2*B*) soon divides into two outpouchings called **primary bronchial buds** (Figs. 11-2*C* and 11-7*A*). Later, **secondary and tertiary bronchial buds**

TRACHEOESOPHAGEAL FISTULA

A **tracheoesophageal fistula** (TEF) is an abnormal passage between the trachea and the esophagus (Figs. 11-5 and 11-6*A*). It occurs at a rate of approximately 1 in 3000 to 1 in 4500 live births and predominantly affects males. In most cases, the fistula is associated with **esophageal atresia**. TEF results from incomplete division of the cranial part of the foregut into respiratory and esophageal parts during the fourth week. Incomplete fusion of the tracheoesophageal folds results in a **defective tracheoesophageal septum** and communication between the trachea and esophagus.

TEF *is the most common anomaly of the lower respiratory tract.* Four main varieties of TEF may develop. The usual anomaly is a blind ending of the superior part of the esophagus (*esophageal atresia*) and a joining of the inferior part to the trachea near its bifurcation (Figs. 11-5*A* and 11-6*B*).

Infants with this type of TEF and esophageal atresia cough and choke when swallowing because of the accumulation of excessive amounts of liquid in the mouth and upper respiratory tract. When the infant attempts to swallow milk, it rapidly fills the esophageal pouch and is regurgitated. Gastric contents may also reflux from the stomach through the fistula into the trachea and lungs which may result in pneumonia or pneumonitis (inflammation of the lungs). Other varieties of TEF are shown in Fig. 11-5*B* to *D*. **Polyhydramnios** (see Chapter 8) is often associated with esophageal atresia and TEF. Excess amniotic fluid accumulates because fluid cannot pass to the stomach and intestines for absorption and subsequent transfer through the placenta to the maternal blood for disposal.

TRACHEAL STENOSIS AND ATRESIA

Narrowing (stenosis) and obstruction (atresia) of the trachea are uncommon anomalies that are usually associated with one of the varieties of TEF. Stenoses and atresias probably result from unequal partitioning of the foregut into the esophagus and the trachea. In some cases, a web of tissue obstructs airflow (*incomplete tracheal atresia*).

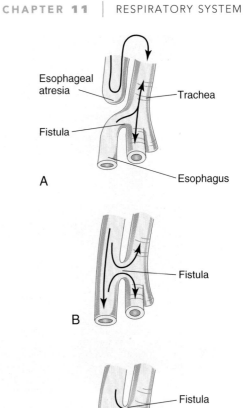

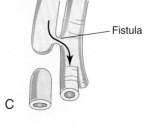

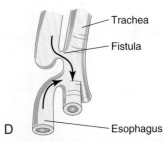

Figure 11–5 The main varieties of tracheoesophageal fistula, shown in order of frequency. Possible directions of the flow of the contents are indicated by *arrows*. **A,** Esophageal atresia is associated with tracheoesophageal fistula in more than 85% of cases. **B,** Fistula between the trachea and the esophagus; this type of anomaly accounts for approximately 4% of cases. **C,** Atresia of the proximal esophagus ending in a tracheal esophageal fistula with the distal esophagus having a blind pouch. Air cannot enter the distal esophagus and the stomach. **D,** Atresia of the proximal segment of the esophagus, with fistulas between the trachea and both the proximal and the distal segments of the esophagus. All infants born with tracheoesophageal fistula have esophageal dysmotility, and most have reflux.

form and grow laterally into the *pericardioperitoneal canals* (Fig. 11-7A). Together with the surrounding splanchnic mesoderm, the bronchial buds differentiate into the bronchi and their ramifications in the lungs (Fig. 11-7B). Early in the fifth week, the connection of each bronchial bud with the trachea enlarges to form the primordia of main bronchi (Fig. 11-8).

The embryonic right main bronchus is slightly larger than the left one and is oriented more vertically. This embryonic relationship persists in adults; consequently, a foreign body is more liable to enter the right main bronchus than the left one. The main bronchi subdivide into **secondary bronchi that form lobar, segmental, and intrasegmental branches** (Fig. 11-8). On the right, the superior secondary bronchus supplies the upper (superior) lobe of the lung, whereas the inferior secondary bronchus subdivides into two bronchi, one connecting to the middle lobe of the right lung and the other connecting to the lower (inferior) lobe. On the left, the two secondary bronchi supply the upper and lower lobes of the lung. Each secondary bronchus undergoes progressive branching.

The **segmental bronchi**—10 in the right lung and 8 or 9 in the left lung—begin to form by the seventh week. As this development occurs, the surrounding mesenchyme also divides. Each segmental bronchus, with its surrounding mass of mesenchyme, is the primordium of a **bronchopulmonary segment.** By 24 weeks, approximately 17 orders of branching have occurred and **respiratory bronchioles** have developed (Fig. 11-9B). An additional seven orders of airways develop after birth.

As the bronchi develop, cartilaginous plates are formed from the surrounding splanchnic mesenchyme. The bronchial smooth muscle and connective tissue and the pulmonary connective tissue and capillaries are also derived from this mesenchyme. As the lungs develop, they acquire a layer of **visceral pleura** from the splanchnic mesoderm (Fig. 11-7). With expansion, the lungs and pleural cavities grow caudally into the mesenchyme of the body wall and soon lie close to the heart. The thoracic body wall becomes lined by a layer of **parietal pleura**, derived from the somatic mesoderm (Fig. 11-7B).

Maturation of Lungs

Maturation of the lungs is divided into four stages: pseudoglandular, canalicular, terminal saccular, and alveolar.

Pseudoglandular Period (6–16 Weeks)

The developing lungs resemble, on a histologic basis, an exocrine gland during the early part of this period (Fig. 11-9A). By 16 weeks, all of the major elements of the lung have formed, except those involved with gas

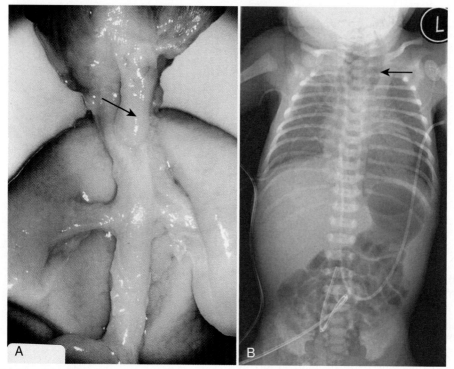

Figure 11–6 **A,** Tracheoesophageal fistula in a 17-week fetus. The upper esophageal segment ends blindly (*pointer*). **B,** Radiograph of an infant with esophageal atresia. Air in the distal gastrointestinal tract indicates the presence of a tracheoesophageal fistula (*arrow,* blind proximal esophageal sac). (**A,** *From Kalousek DK, Fitch N, Paradice BA: Pathology of the Human Embryo and Previable Fetus. New York, Springer Verlag, 1990.* **B,** *Courtesy of Dr. J. Been, Dr. M. Shuurman, and Dr. S. Robben, Maastricht University Medical Centre, Maastricht, Netherlands.*)

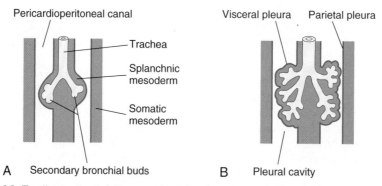

Figure 11–7 Illustrations of the growth of the developing lungs into the splanchnic mesoderm adjacent to the medial walls of the pericardioperitoneal canals (primordial pleural cavities). Development of the layers of the pleura is also shown. **A,** At 5 weeks. **B,** At 6 weeks.

exchange. Respiration is not possible; hence, *fetuses born during this period are unable to survive.*

Canalicular Period (16–26 Weeks)

The canalicular period overlaps the pseudoglandular period because cranial segments of the lungs mature faster than caudal segments. During the canalicular period, the lumina of the bronchi and the terminal bronchioles become larger and the lung tissue becomes highly vascular (Fig. 11-9B). By 24 weeks, each terminal bronchiole has given rise to two or more **respiratory bronchioles,** each of which then divides into three to six tubular passages called the primordial **alveolar ducts.** Respiration is possible toward the end of the canalicular stage because some thin-walled **terminal sacs** (primordial alveoli) have developed at the ends of the respiratory bronchioles and the lung tissue is well vascularized. Although a fetus born at 24 to 26 weeks may survive if given intensive care, it often dies because its respiratory and other systems are relatively immature.

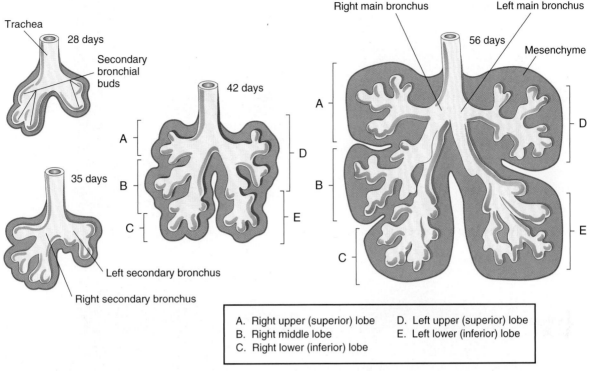

A. Right upper (superior) lobe   **D.** Left upper (superior) lobe
B. Right middle lobe   **E.** Left lower (inferior) lobe
C. Right lower (inferior) lobe

Figure 11–8 Successive stages in the development of the bronchial buds, the bronchi, and the lungs.

Terminal Sac Stage (26 Weeks to Birth)

During this period, many more terminal sacs develop, their epithelium becomes very thin, and capillaries begin to bulge into these sacs (see Fig. 11-9C). The intimate contact between epithelial and endothelial cells establishes the **blood-air barrier**, permitting adequate gas exchange for survival. By 26 weeks, the terminal sacs are lined mainly by squamous epithelial cells of endodermal origin—**type I pneumocytes**—across which gas exchange occurs. The capillary network proliferates rapidly in the mesenchyme around the developing alveoli, and there is concurrent active development of lymphatic capillaries. Scattered among the squamous epithelial cells are rounded secretory epithelial cells—**type II pneumocytes**—*which secrete pulmonary surfactant*, a complex mixture of phospholipids and proteins. Surfactant forms as a monomolecular film over the interior walls of the alveolar sacs and counteracts surface tension forces at the air-alveolar interface. This facilitates expansion of the terminal sacs (primordial alveoli).

The maturation of alveolar type II cells and the production of surfactant vary widely in fetuses of different ages. *Surfactant production begins by 20 weeks*, but surfactant is present in only small amounts in premature infants. It does not reach adequate levels until the late fetal period. Both increased surfactant production induced by antenatal corticosteroids and postnatal surfactant replacement therapy have increased the rates of survival of these infants.

Alveolar Period (32 Weeks to 8 Years)

Exactly when the terminal saccular period ends and the alveolar period begins depends on the definition of the term **alveolus** (Fig. 11-9D). At the beginning of the alveolar period, each respiratory bronchiole terminates in a cluster of thin-walled terminal sacs that are separated from one another by loose connective tissue. These terminal sacs represent future alveolar ducts. The **alveolocapillary membrane** (pulmonary diffusion barrier, or respiratory membrane) is sufficiently thin to allow gas exchange. The transition from dependence on the placenta for gas exchange to autonomous gas exchange after birth requires the following adaptive changes in the lungs:

● Production of surfactant in the alveolar sacs
● Transformation of the lungs into gas-exchanging organs
● Establishment of parallel pulmonary and systemic circulations

Approximately 95% of characteristic **mature alveoli** develop postnatally. Before birth, the primordial alveoli appear as small bulges on the walls of the respiratory bronchioles and terminal sacs (future alveolar ducts). After birth, the primordial alveoli enlarge as the lungs expand; however, most of the increase in the size of the lungs results from a continued increase in the number of respiratory bronchioles and primordial alveoli rather than from an increase in the size of the alveoli. Alveolar

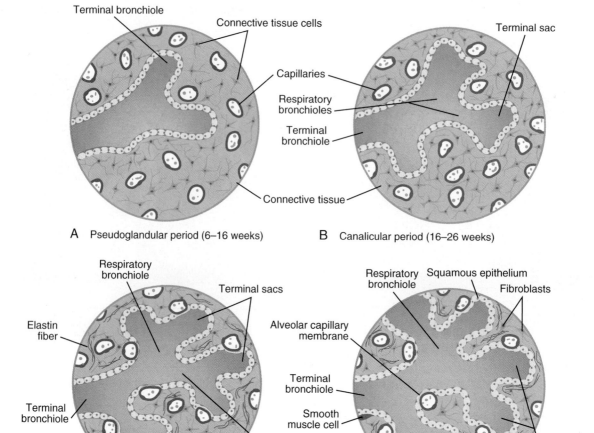

Figure 11–9   Diagram of histologic sections, showing progressive stages of lung development. **A** and **B**, Early stages of lung development. In **C** and **D**, note that the alveolocapillary membrane is thin and that some capillaries bulge into the terminal saccules.

development is largely complete by 3 years of age, but new alveoli may be added until approximately 8 years of age. Unlike mature alveoli, immature alveoli have the potential for forming additional primordial alveoli.

Approximately 150 million primordial alveoli, one half the number in adults, are present in the lungs of a full-term newborn infant. On chest radiographs, therefore, the lungs of newborn infants appear denser than adult lungs. Between the third and the eighth year, the adult complement of 300 million alveoli is achieved.

Three factors that are essential for normal lung development are:

● Adequate thoracic space for lung growth
● Adequate amniotic fluid volume
● Fetal breathing movements

Fetal breathing movements occur before birth, exerting sufficient force to cause aspiration of some amniotic fluid into the lungs. These fetal breathing movements

occur approximately 50% of the time and only during rapid eye movement sleep. These movements stimulate lung development, possibly by creating a pressure gradient between the lungs and the amniotic fluid. By birth, the fetus has had the advantage of several months of breathing exercise. Fetal breathing movements increase as the time of delivery approaches.

At birth, the lungs are approximately half-filled with fluid derived from the amniotic cavity, the lungs, and the tracheal glands. Aeration of the lungs at birth occurs not so much by the inflation of empty collapsed organs as by the rapid replacement of intra-alveolar fluid by air. The fluid in the lungs is cleared at birth by three routes:

● Through the mouth and nose by pressure on the thorax during vaginal delivery
● Into the pulmonary capillaries and pulmonary arteries and veins
● Into the lymphatics

OLIGOHYDRAMNIOS AND LUNG DEVELOPMENT

When oligohydramnios (an insufficient amount of amniotic fluid) is severe and chronic (e.g., because of amniotic fluid leakage), lung development is retarded because restriction of the fetal thorax by the uterine walls impedes lung growth. Pulmonary hypoplasia occurs as a result and may be severe.

RESPIRATORY DISTRESS SYNDROME

Respiratory distress syndrome (RDS) affects approximately 2% of live newborn infants, and those born prematurely are the most susceptible. RDS is also known as *hyaline membrane disease*. Affected infants have rapid, labored breathing shortly after birth. An estimated 30% of all neonatal disease results from RDS or its complications. *Surfactant deficiency is a major cause of RDS*. The lungs are underinflated and the alveoli contain fluid with a high protein content—*hyaline membrane*. This membrane is believed to be derived from a combination of substances in the circulation and from the injured pulmonary epithelium. Prolonged intrauterine asphyxia may produce irreversible changes in type II alveolar cells, making them incapable of producing surfactant. Not all of the growth factors and hormones that control surfactant production have been identified, but *corticosteroids* and *thyroxine* are potent stimulators of surfactant production.

LUNGS OF NEWBORN INFANTS

Fresh, healthy neonatal lungs always contain some air; consequently, pulmonary tissue samples float in water. By contrast, a diseased lung that is partially filled with fluid may not float. Of medicolegal significance is the fact that the lungs of a stillborn infant are firm and sink when placed in water because they contain fluid, not air.

LUNG HYPOPLASIA

In infants with a congenital diaphragmatic hernia (see Chapter 9), the lung is unable to develop normally because it is compressed by the abnormally positioned abdominal viscera. Lung hypoplasia is characterized by markedly reduced lung volume. Many infants with a congenital diaphragmatic hernia die of pulmonary insufficiency, despite optimal postnatal care, because their lungs are too hypoplastic to support extrauterine life.

CLINICALLY ORIENTED QUESTIONS

1. What stimulates the infant to start breathing at birth? Is "slapping the buttocks" necessary?

2. An infant reportedly died approximately 72 hours after birth from the effects of respiratory distress syndrome. What is respiratory distress syndrome? By what other name is this condition known? Is its cause genetic or environmental?

3. Can an infant born 22 weeks after fertilization survive?

The answers to these questions are at the back of the book.

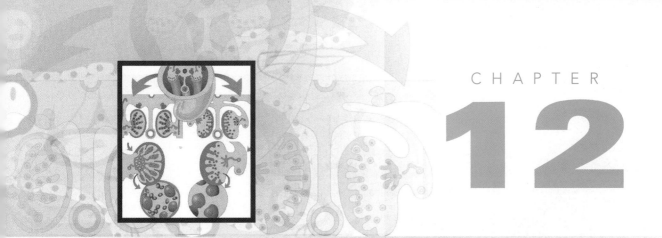

Alimentary System

T he alimentary system is the digestive tract from the mouth to the anus with all its associative glands and organs. At the beginning of the fourth week, the **primordial gut** is closed at its cranial end by the **oropharyngeal membrane** (Fig. 12-1*B*) and at its caudal end by the **cloacal membrane** (Fig. 12-1). The endoderm of the primordial gut gives rise to most of the epithelium and glands of the alimentary system. The epithelium at the cranial and caudal ends of the tract is derived from the ectoderm of the **stomodeum** and the **proctodeum** (anal pit), respectively (see Fig. 12-1).

The muscular and connective tissue and other layers of the wall of the digestive tract are derived from the splanchnic mesenchyme surrounding the primordial gut. The gut is divided into three parts: foregut, midgut, and hindgut. *The regional differentiation of the primordial gut is established by sonic and Indian hedgehog genes (Shh and Ihh) that are expressed in the endoderm and the surrounding mesoderm.* The endodermal signaling provides temporal and positional information for the development of the gut.

FOREGUT

The derivatives of the foregut are as follows:

- The primordial pharynx and its derivatives
- The lower respiratory system
- The esophagus and stomach
- The duodenum, just distal to the opening of the bile duct
- The liver, biliary apparatus (hepatic ducts, gallbladder, and bile duct), and pancreas

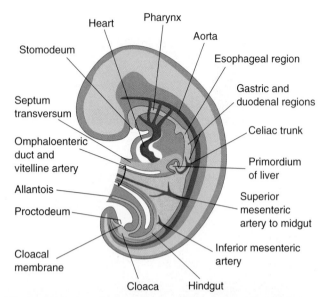

Figure 12–1 Median section of a 4-week embryo, showing the early alimentary system and its blood supply.

All of the foregut derivatives except the pharynx, the respiratory tract, and most of the esophagus are supplied by the **celiac trunk**, the artery of the foregut (Figs. 12-1 and 12-2*A*).

Development of Esophagus

The esophagus elongates rapidly and reaches its final relative length by the seventh week. Its epithelium and glands are derived from the endoderm. The epithelium proliferates and partly or completely obliterates the esophageal lumen; however, recanalization normally occurs by the end of the eighth week. The striated muscle of the esophagus is derived from the mesenchyme in the fourth and sixth pharyngeal arches. The smooth muscle, mainly in the inferior third of the esophagus, develops from the surrounding splanchnic mesenchyme.

ESOPHAGEAL ATRESIA

Blockage of the esophagus occurs in approximately 1 in 3000 to 1 in 4500 live births. Approximately one third of affected infants are born prematurely. Esophageal atresia is frequently associated with **tracheoesophageal fistula** (see Figs. 11-5 and 11-6). Esophageal atresia results from deviation of the *tracheoesophageal septum* in a posterior direction (see Figs. 11-2 and 11-6); as a result, separation of the esophagus from the laryngotracheal tube is incomplete. In some cases, the atresia results from *failure of esophageal recanalization* during the eighth week of development. A fetus with esophageal atresia is unable to swallow amniotic fluid, resulting in polyhydramnios.

ESOPHAGEAL STENOSIS

Narrowing of the lumen of the esophagus (stenosis) can occur anywhere along the esophagus, but it usually occurs in the distal one third, either as a web or as a long segment of esophagus with a threadlike lumen. The stenosis usually results from incomplete recanalization of the esophagus during the eighth week.

Development of Stomach

During the fourth week, a slight dilation of the tubelike foregut indicates the site of the primordial stomach. It first appears as a fusiform enlargement that is oriented in the median plane (Fig. 12-2). The primordial stomach enlarges and broadens ventrodorsally. Its dorsal border grows more quickly than its ventral border. This site of rapid growth demarcates the **greater curvature of the stomach** (Fig. 12-2*D*).

Rotation of Stomach

As the stomach enlarges, it rotates 90 degrees in a clockwise direction around its longitudinal axis. The effects of rotation on the stomach are as follows (Figs. 12-2 and 12-3):

- The ventral border (lesser curvature) moves to the right, and the dorsal border (greater curvature) moves to the left (Fig. 12-2*C* to *F*).
- Before rotation, the cranial and caudal ends of the stomach are in the median plane (Fig. 12-2*B*).
- During rotation and growth of the stomach, its cranial region moves to the left and slightly inferiorly, and its caudal region moves to the right and superiorly (Fig. 12-2*C* to *E*).
- After rotation, the stomach assumes its final position, with its long axis almost transverse to the long axis of the body (Fig. 12-2*E*). This rotation and growth explains why the left vagus nerve supplies the anterior wall of the adult stomach and the right vagus nerve innervates its posterior wall.

CONGENITAL HYPERTROPHIC PYLORIC STENOSIS

Anomalies of the stomach are uncommon, except for hypertrophic pyloric stenosis, which affects 1 in 150 male infants and 1 in 750 female infants. Infants with this anomaly have marked **muscular thickening of the pylorus** of the stomach, the distal sphincteric region of the stomach. The muscles in the pyloric region are hypertrophied, which results in *severe stenosis (narrowing) of the pyloric canal* and obstruction to the passage of food. As a result, the stomach becomes markedly distended and its contents are expelled with considerable force (**projectile vomiting**). Surgical relief of the pyloric obstruction is the usual treatment.

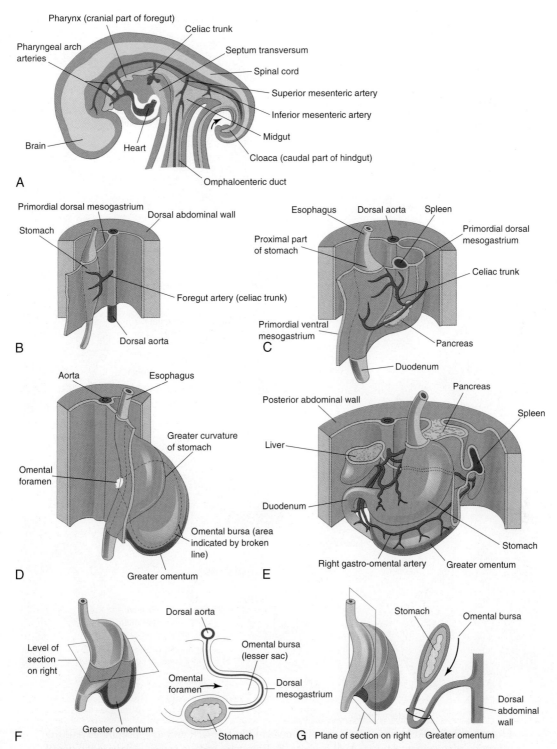

Figure 12–2 Illustrations of the development and rotation of the stomach and the formation of the omental bursa and greater omentum. **A,** Median section of a 28-day embryo. **B,** Antero-lateral view of a 28-day embryo. **C,** Embryo at approximately 35 days. **D,** Embryo at approximately 40 days. **E,** Embryo at approximately 48 days. **F,** Lateral view of the stomach and greater omentum of an embryo at approximately 52 days. **G,** Sagittal section, showing the omental bursa and greater omentum. The *arrow* in **F** and **G** indicates the site of the omental foramen.

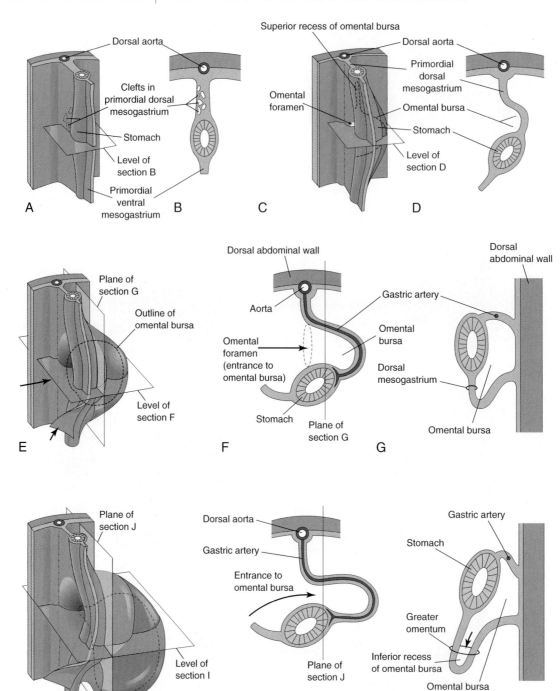

Figure 12–3 Illustrations of the development of the stomach and its mesenteries and the formation of the omental bursa. **A,** At 5 weeks. **B,** Transverse section showing clefts in the dorsal mesogastrium. **C,** Later stage, after coalescence of the clefts to form the omental bursa. **D,** Transverse section showing the initial appearance of the omental bursa. **E,** The dorsal mesentery has elongated and the omental bursa has enlarged. **F** and **G,** Transverse and sagittal sections, respectively, showing elongation of the dorsal mesogastrium and expansion of the omental bursa. **H,** At 6 weeks, showing the greater omentum and expansion of the omental bursa. **I** and **J,** Transverse and sagittal sections, respectively, showing the inferior recess of the omental bursa and the omental foramen. The *arrows* in **E, F,** and **I,** indicate the site of the omental foramen. In **J,** the *arrow* indicates the recess of the omental bursa.

Mesenteries of Stomach

The stomach is suspended from the **dorsal** wall of the abdominal cavity by the primordial **dorsal mesogastrium** (Figs. 12-2B and C and 12-3A to D). This mesentery, originally located in the median plane, is carried to the left during rotation of the stomach. The **primordial ventral mesogastrium**—attaches the stomach and duodenum to the liver and the ventral abdominal wall (Figs. 12-2C and 12-3A and B).

Omental Bursa

Isolated clefts develop in the mesenchyme that forms the dorsal mesogastrium (see Fig. 12-3A and B). The clefts soon coalesce to form a single cavity—the **omental bursa** (*lesser peritoneal sac*), a large recess of the peritoneal cavity (Figs. 12-2F and G and 12-3C and D). Rotation of the stomach pulls the dorsal mesogastrium to the left, thereby enlarging the bursa.

The omental bursa lies between the stomach and the posterior abdominal wall. As the stomach enlarges, the omental bursa expands and hangs over the developing intestines. This part of the omental bursa is called the **greater omentum** (Fig. 12-3G to J and see Fig. 12-13A). The two layers of the greater omentum eventually fuse (see Fig. 12-13F). The omental bursa communicates with the main part of the peritoneal cavity through a small opening—the **omental foramen** (Figs. 12-2D and F and 12-3C and F).

Development of Duodenum

Early in the fourth week, the duodenum develops from the caudal part of the foregut and the cranial part of the midgut (Fig. 12-4A). The developing duodenum elongates, forming a C-shaped loop that projects ventrally (Fig. 12-4B to D). As the stomach rotates, the duodenal

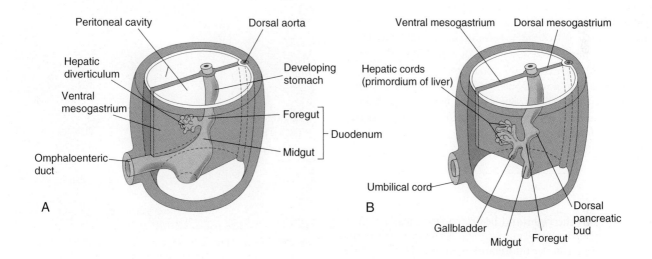

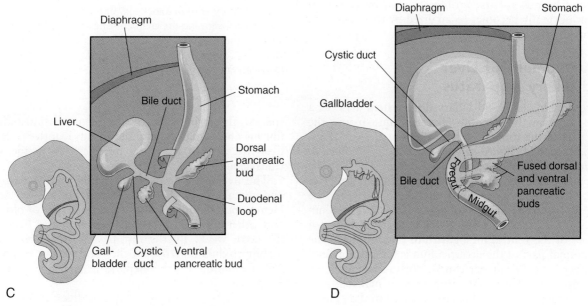

Figure 12–4 Illustrations of progressive stages in the development of the duodenum, liver, pancreas, and extrahepatic biliary apparatus. **A,** At 4 weeks. **B** and **C,** At 5 weeks. **D,** At 6 weeks.

DUODENAL STENOSIS

Partial occlusion of the duodenal lumen—**duodenal stenosis**—is usually caused by incomplete recanalization of the duodenum. Most stenoses involve the horizontal (third) part or the ascending (fourth) part of the duodenum, or both. Because of the occlusion, the stomach contents are often vomited.

DUODENAL ATRESIA

Complete occlusion of the duodenum—**duodenal atresia**—results from failure of reformation of the lumen (Fig. 12-5B). Most atresias involve the descending and horizontal parts of the duodenum and are located distal to the opening of the bile duct. In infants with duodenal atresia, vomiting begins within a few hours of birth. The vomitus almost always contains bile. **Polyhydramnios** also occurs because duodenal atresia prevents normal absorption of amniotic fluid by the intestines. A diagnosis of duodenal atresia is suggested by the presence of a "double-bubble sign" on plain radiographs or ultrasound scans. This sign is caused by a distended, gas-filled stomach and the proximal duodenum. Between 20% and 30% of affected infants have Down syndrome, and an additional 20% are premature.

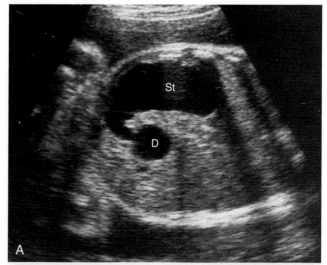

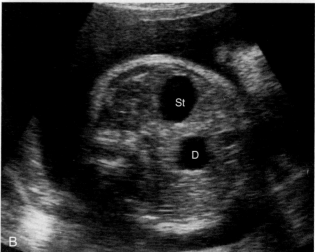

Figure 12-5 Ultrasound scans of a fetus at 33 weeks gestation (31 weeks after fertilization), showing duodenal atresia. **A,** An oblique scan shows the dilated, fluid-filled stomach (St) entering the proximal duodenum (D), which is also enlarged because of the atresia (blockage) distal to it. **B,** Transverse ultrasound scan, showing the characteristic "double-bubble" appearance of the stomach and duodenum when there is duodenal atresia. (Courtesy of Dr. Lyndon M. Hill, Magee-Women's Hospital, Pittsburgh, PA.)

loop rotates to the right and lies retroperitoneally (external to peritoneum). Because of its derivation from the foregut and midgut, the duodenum is supplied by branches of both the celiac and the superior mesenteric arteries (Fig. 12-1). The lumen of the duodenum is temporarily obliterated because of the proliferation of its epithelial cells, but normally becomes recanalized by the end of the embryonic period.

Development of Liver and Biliary Apparatus

The liver, gallbladder, and biliary duct system arise as a ventral outgrowth—**hepatic diverticulum**—from the caudal part of the foregut early in the fourth week (Figs. 12-4A and 12-6A). *Wnt/β-catenin signaling is involved in the induction of the hepatic diverticulum.* The hepatic diverticulum extends into the septum transversum (Fig. 12-6B), a mass of splanchnic mesoderm between the developing heart and the midgut. The diverticulum enlarges and divides into two parts as it grows between the layers of the **ventral mesogastrium** (Fig. 12-4A). The larger, cranial part of the diverticulum is the **primordium of the liver,** and the smaller caudal portion becomes the biliary apparatus. The proliferating endodermal cells give rise to interlacing cords of hepatocytes and to the epithelial lining of the intrahepatic part of the biliary apparatus. The **hepatic cords** anastomose around endothelium-lined

spaces, the primordia of the **hepatic sinusoids.** The fibrous and hematopoietic tissue and Kupffer cells of the liver are derived from the mesenchyme in the septum transversum.

The liver grows rapidly and fills a large part of the abdominal cavity (Figs. 12-4 and Fig. 12-6C and D). **Hematopoiesis** (formation of various types of blood cells and other formed elements) begins in the liver during the sixth week. By the ninth week, the liver accounts for approximately 10% of the total weight of the fetus. **Bile formation** by the hepatic cells begins during the 12th week.

The caudal portion of the hepatic diverticulum becomes the **gallbladder;** the stalk forms the **cystic duct** (Fig. 12-4B and C). Initially, the *extrahepatic biliary apparatus* is

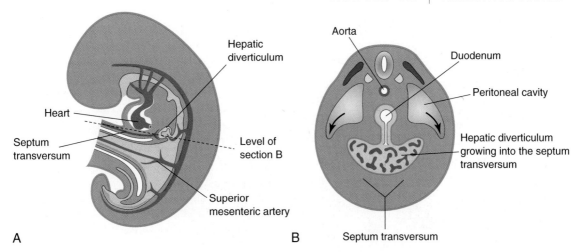

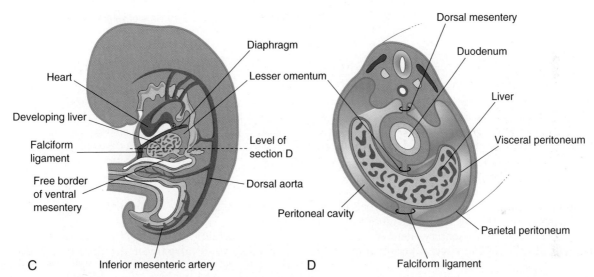

Figure 12–6 Illustrations of how the caudal part of the septum transversum becomes stretched and membranous as it forms the ventral mesentery. **A,** Median section of a 4-week embryo. **B,** Transverse section of the embryo, showing expansion of the peritoneal cavity (*arrows*). **C,** Sagittal section of a 5-week embryo. **D,** Transverse section of the embryo after formation of the dorsal and ventral mesenteries.

ANOMALIES OF LIVER AND BILIARY DUCTS

Minor variations of liver lobulation are common, as are variations of the hepatic ducts, bile duct, and cystic duct. For example, **accessory hepatic ducts** may be present, and an awareness of their possible presence is important from a surgical perspective. Congenital anomalies of the liver are rare.

EXTRAHEPATIC BILIARY ATRESIA

Extrahepatic biliary atresia, the most serious anomaly involving the extrahepatic biliary system, is uncommon. Failure of the bile ducts to canalize often results from persistence of the solid stage of duct development. Jaundice occurs soon after birth.

Ventral Mesentery

The *double-layered ventral mesentery* (Figs. 12-6C and D and 12-7) gives rise to two structures:

- The lesser omentum, which passes from the liver to the lesser curvature of the stomach (hepatogastric ligament) and from the liver to the duodenum (*hepatoduodenal ligament*)
- The falciform ligament, which extends from the liver to the ventral abdominal wall

occluded with epithelial cells. The stalk connecting the hepatic and cystic ducts to the duodenum becomes the **bile duct**, which attaches to the ventral aspect of the duodenal loop. As the duodenum grows and rotates, the entrance of the bile duct is carried to the dorsal aspect of the duodenum (Fig. 12-4C and D).

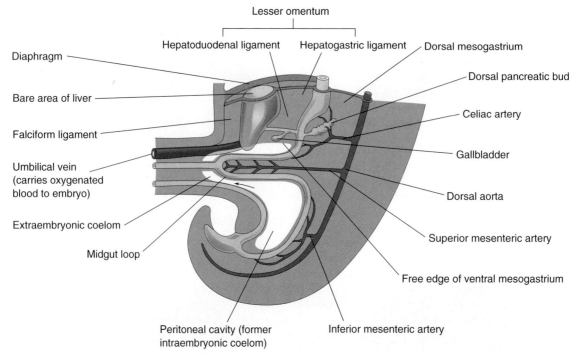

Figure 12–7 Median section of the caudal half of an embryo at the end of the fifth week, showing the liver and its associated ligaments. The *arrow* indicates the communication of the peritoneal cavity with the extraembryonic coelom. Because of the rapid growth of the liver and the midgut loop, the abdominal cavity temporarily becomes too small to contain the developing intestines; consequently, they enter the extraembryonic coelom in the proximal part of the umbilical cord (see Fig. 12-11*B*).

The **umbilical vein** passes in the free border of the falciform ligament on its way from the umbilical cord to the liver. The ventral mesentery, derived from the mesogastrium, also forms the **visceral peritoneum of the liver.**

Development of Pancreas

The pancreas develops between the layers of both mesenteries from the dorsal and ventral **pancreatic buds,** which arise from the caudal part of the foregut (Fig. 12-8*A*). Most of the pancreas is derived from the **dorsal pancreatic bud,** which appears first. It grows rapidly between the layers of the dorsal mesentery. *Formation of the dorsal pancreatic bud depends on signals from the notochord (activin and fibroblast growth factor 2) that block the expression of sonic hedgehog (Shh) in the endoderm. Expression of pancreatic and duodenal homeobox factors (PDX-1 and MafA) is critical for the development of the pancreas.*

The **ventral pancreatic bud** develops near the entry of the bile duct into the duodenum (Fig. 12-8*A* and *B*). As the duodenum rotates to the right and becomes C-shaped, the ventral pancreatic bud is carried dorsally with the bile duct (Fig. 12-8*C* to *F*). It soon lies posterior to the dorsal pancreatic bud and later fuses with it (Fig. 12-8*G*). As the pancreatic buds fuse, their ducts anastomose.

The ventral pancreatic bud forms the *uncinate process* and part of the *head of the pancreas.* As the stomach, duodenum, and ventral mesentery rotate, the pancreas

comes to lie along the dorsal abdominal wall (Fig. 12-8*D* and *G*).

The **pancreatic duct** forms from the duct of the ventral bud and the distal part of the duct of the dorsal bud (Fig. 12-8*G*). In approximately 9% of people, the proximal part of the duct of the dorsal bud persists as an **accessory pancreatic duct** that opens into the *minor duodenal papilla.* The connective tissue sheath and the interlobular septa of the pancreas develop from the surrounding splanchnic mesenchyme. **Insulin secretion** begins at approximately 10 weeks. The glucagon- and somatostatin-containing cells develop before differentiation of the insulin-secreting cells occurs. With increasing fetal age, total pancreatic insulin and glucagon content also increases.

ANNULAR PANCREAS

Annular pancreas is an uncommon anomaly and probably results from the growth of a bifid ventral pancreatic bud around the duodenum (Fig. 12-9*A* to *C*). The parts of the bifid ventral bud then fuse with the dorsal bud, forming a pancreatic ring. The ringlike, annular part of the pancreas consists of a thin, flat band of pancreatic tissue surrounding the descending, or second, part of the duodenum. An annular pancreas may cause obstruction of the duodenum shortly after birth, but many cases are not diagnosed until adulthood. Males are affected much more frequently than females.

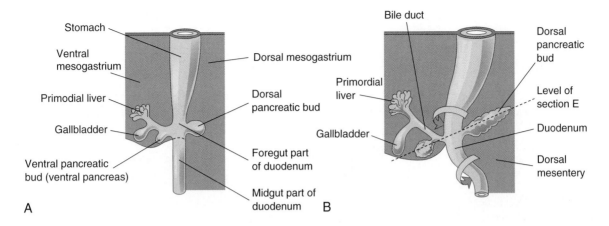

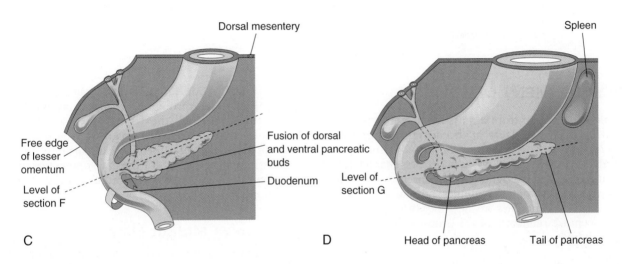

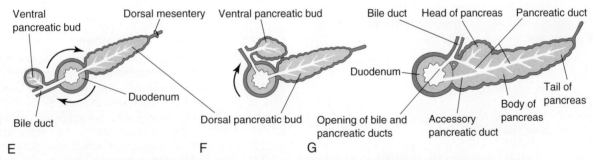

Figure 12–8 **A** to **D,** Illustrations of successive stages in the development of the pancreas from the fifth to the eighth weeks. **E** to **G,** Transverse sections through the duodenum and the developing pancreas. Growth and rotation (*arrows*) of the duodenum bring the ventral pancreatic bud toward the dorsal bud; the two buds subsequently fuse. Note that the bile duct initially attaches to the ventral aspect of the duodenum and is carried around to the dorsal aspect as the duodenum rotates. The pancreatic duct is formed by the union of the distal part of the dorsal pancreatic duct and the entire ventral pancreatic duct. The proximal part of the dorsal pancreatic duct usually obliterates, but it may persist as an accessory pancreatic duct.

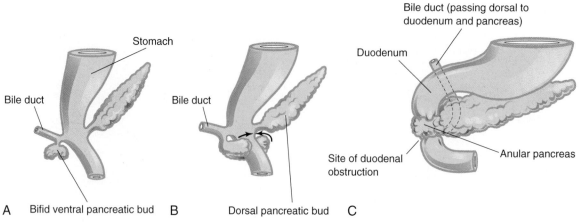

Figure 12–9   **A** and **B**, Illustrations of the probable embryologic basis of an annular pancreas. **C**, An annular pancreas encircling the duodenum. This anomaly sometimes produces obstruction of the duodenum.

 # DEVELOPMENT OF SPLEEN

The spleen is derived from a mass of mesenchymal cells located between the layers of the dorsal mesogastrium (Fig. 12-10A and B). The spleen begins to develop during the fifth week, but does not acquire its characteristic shape until early in the fetal period. The spleen is lobulated in the fetus, but the lobules normally disappear before birth. The notches in the superior border of the adult spleen are remnants of the grooves that separated the fetal lobules.

ACCESSORY SPLEENS

One or more small splenic masses (polysplenia) may develop (10% of the population), commonly near the hilum of the spleen or adjacent to the tail of the pancreas.

MIDGUT

The derivatives of the midgut are:

● The small intestine, including the duodenum distal to the opening of the bile duct
● The cecum, appendix, ascending colon, and right half to two thirds of the transverse colon

All of these derivatives are supplied by the **superior mesenteric artery** (Fig. 12-7). The **midgut loop** is suspended from the dorsal abdominal wall by an elongated mesentery. The midgut elongates and forms a ventral, U-shaped loop that projects into the proximal part of the umbilical cord. This projection of the intestine, occurring at the beginning of the sixth week, is called a **physiologic umbilical herniation** (Figs. 12-11 and 12-12). Umbilical herniation occurs because there is not enough room in the abdomen for the rapidly growing midgut.

The midgut loop communicates with the umbilical vesicle (yolk sac) through the narrow **omphaloenteric duct** (yolk stalk) until the 10th week (Fig. 12-11A and C). The cranial limb of the loop grows rapidly and forms most of the small intestine. The caudal limb undergoes very little change, except for the development of the **cecal diverticulum**, which is the primordium of the cecum and appendix (Fig. 12-11C to E).

Rotation of Midgut Loop

While in the umbilical cord, the midgut loop rotates 90 degrees counterclockwise around the axis of the **superior mesenteric artery** (see Fig. 12-11B). This rotation brings the cranial limb (small intestine) of the midgut loop to the right and the caudal limb (large intestine) to the left.

Return of Midgut to Abdomen

During the 10th week, with enlargement of the abdominal cavity, the intestines return to the abdomen (*reduction of the physiologic midgut hernia*) (Fig. 12-11C and D). The small intestine returns first, passing posterior to the superior mesenteric artery, and occupies the central part of the abdomen. As the large intestine returns, it undergoes a further 180-degree counterclockwise rotation (Fig. 12-11C_1 and D_1). Later, it comes to occupy the right side of the abdomen. The ascending colon becomes recognizable as the posterior abdominal wall progressively elongates (Figs. 12-11E and 12-13A).

Fixation of Intestines

Rotation of the stomach and duodenum causes the duodenum and pancreas to fall to the right, where they are pressed against the posterior abdominal wall by the colon. The adjacent layers of peritoneum fuse and subsequently disappear (see Fig. 12-13C and F); consequently, most of the duodenum and the head of the pancreas become retroperitoneal (posterior to peritoneum). The mesentery of the ascending colon fuses with the parietal peritoneum on the posterior abdominal wall.

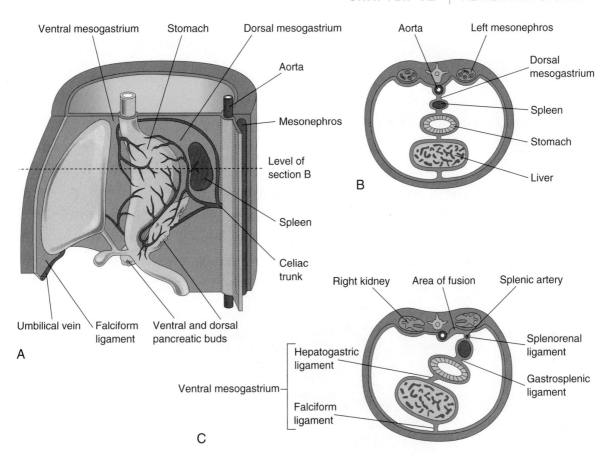

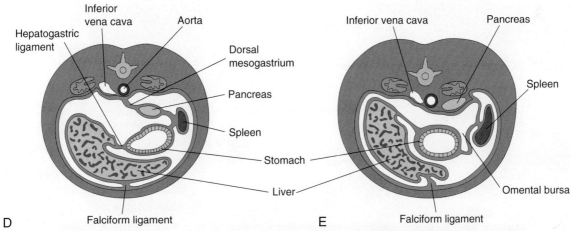

Figure 12–10 **A,** The left side of the stomach and associated structures at the end of the fifth week. Note that the pancreas, spleen, and celiac trunk are located between the layers of the dorsal mesogastrium. **B,** Transverse section of the liver, stomach, and spleen at the level shown in **A,** showing their relationship to the dorsal and ventral mesenteries. **C,** Transverse section of a fetus, showing fusion of the dorsal mesogastrium with the peritoneum on the posterior abdominal wall. **D** and **E,** Similar sections, showing movement of the liver to the right and rotation of the stomach. Observe the fusion of the dorsal mesogastrium to the dorsal abdominal wall, which results in the pancreas becoming retroperitoneal.

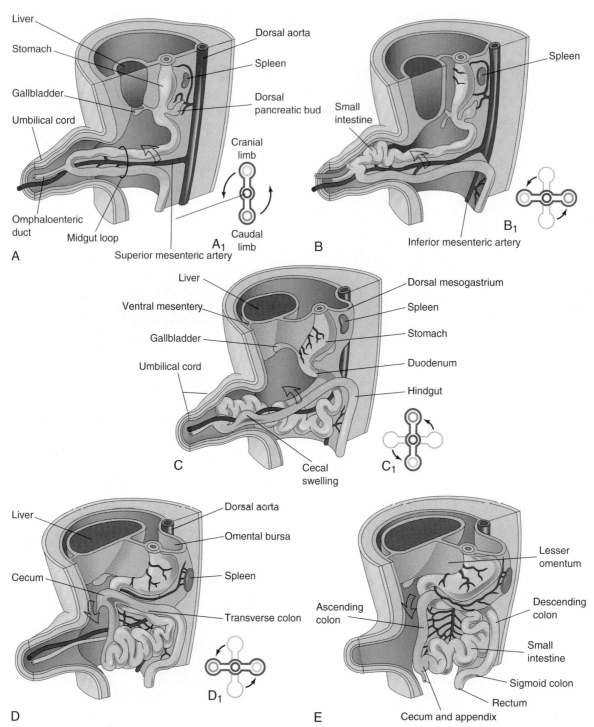

Figure 12–11 Illustrations of the rotation of the midgut, as seen from the left. **A,** During the sixth week, the midgut loop is situated in the proximal part of the umbilical cord. **A₁,** Transverse section through the midgut loop, showing the initial relationship of the limbs of the midgut loop to the superior mesenteric artery. **B,** A later stage, showing the beginning of midgut rotation. **B₁,** Illustration of the 90-degree counterclockwise rotation that carries the cranial limb of the midgut to the right. **C,** At approximately 10 weeks, the intestines return to the abdomen. **C₁,** Illustration of a further rotation of 90 degrees. **D,** By approximately 11 weeks, all of the intestines return to the abdomen. **D₁,** A further 90-degree rotation of the gut, for a total of 270 degrees. **E,** The later fetal period, showing the cecum rotating to its normal position in the lower right quadrant of the abdomen.

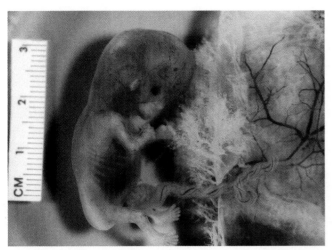

Figure 12–12 Physiologic hernia in a 58-day embryo attached to its chorionic sac. Note the herniated intestine derived from the midgut loop in the proximal part of the umbilical cord. *(Courtesy of Dr. D.K. Kalousek, Department of Pathology, University of British Columbia, Children's Hospital, Vancouver, British Columbia, Canada.)*

The mesentery of the ascending colon becomes retroperitoneal (see Fig. 12-13*B* and *E*). The other derivatives of the midgut loop retain their mesenteries.

Cecum and Appendix

The *primordium of the cecum and the appendix* appears in the sixth week as a swelling on the antimesenteric border of the caudal limb of the midgut loop (Figs. 12-11*C* to *E* and 12-14*A*). Initially, the appendix is a small diverticulum of the cecum. It subsequently increases rapidly in length so that at birth it is a relatively long tube arising from the distal end of the cecum (Fig. 12-14*D*). After birth, the unequal growth of the walls of the cecum results in the appendix entering its medial side (see Fig. 12-14*E*). *The appendix is subject to considerable variation in position.* As the ascending colon elongates, the appendix may pass posterior to the cecum (*retrocecal appendix*) or the colon (*retrocolic appendix*).

CONGENITAL OMPHALOCELE

Congenital omphalocele results in persistence of the herniation of the abdominal contents into the proximal part of the umbilical cord (Figs. 12-15 and 12-16). This is caused by failure of the body walls to fuse at the umbilical ring because of defective growth of mesenchyme. Herniation of the intestines occurs in approximately 1 in 5000 births; herniation of the liver and intestines occurs less frequently (1 in 10,000 births). The size of the hernia depends on its contents. The abdominal cavity is proportionately small when an omphalocele is present because the impetus for it to grow is absent.

UMBILICAL HERNIA

When the intestines herniate through an imperfectly closed umbilicus, an umbilical hernia forms. This common type of hernia differs from an omphalocele. In umbilical hernias, the protruding mass (usually consisting of part of the greater omentum and small intestine) is covered by subcutaneous tissue and skin. The hernia protrudes during crying, straining, or coughing.

HINDGUT

The derivatives of the hindgut are:

- The left third to half of the transverse colon, the descending colon and sigmoid colon, the rectum, and the superior part of the anal canal
- The epithelium of the urinary bladder and most of the urethra

All of these derivatives are supplied by the **inferior mesenteric artery** (Fig. 12-7). The descending colon becomes retroperitoneal as its mesentery fuses with the peritoneum on the left posterior abdominal wall (Fig. 12-13*B* and *E*). The mesentery of the sigmoid colon is retained.

GASTROSCHISIS AND CONGENITAL EPIGASTRIC HERNIA

Gastroschisis results from a defect near the median plane of the abdominal wall (Fig. 12-17). The viscera protrude into the amniotic cavity and are bathed by amniotic fluid. The term *gastroschisis*, which literally means "split stomach," is a misnomer because it is the anterior abdominal wall, not the stomach, that is split. The defect usually occurs on the right side, lateral to the median plane, and is more common in boys than in girls. The anomaly results from incomplete closure of the lateral folds during the fourth week of development (see Chapter 6).

NONROTATION OF MIDGUT

Nonrotation of the midgut (*left-sided colon*) is a relatively common condition (Fig. 12-18*A* and *B*) resulting in the caudal limb of the midgut loop returning to the abdomen first. The small intestine then lies on the right side of the abdomen, and the entire large intestine lies on the left. Although patients are generally asymptomatic, if **volvulus** (twisting) occurs, the superior mesenteric artery may be obstructed, resulting in infarction and gangrene of the associated intestine.

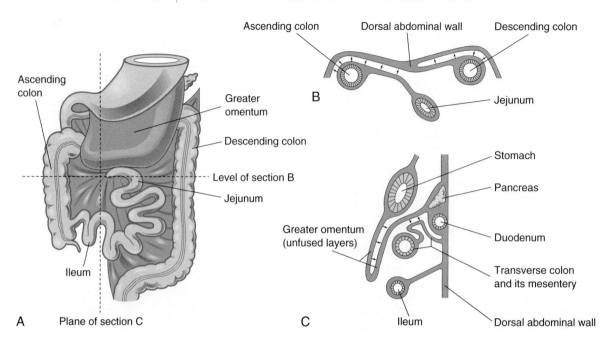

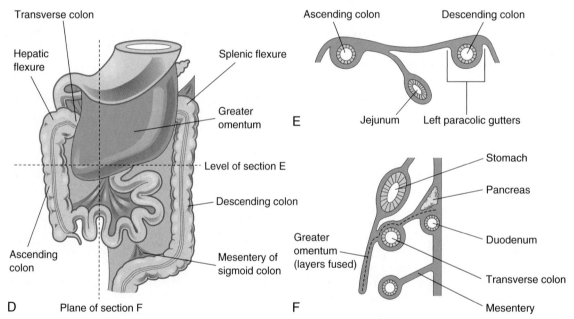

Figure 12–13 Fixation of the intestines. **A,** Ventral view of the intestines before their fixation. **B,** Transverse section at the level shown in **A.** The *arrows* indicate areas of subsequent fusion. **C,** Sagittal section at the plane shown in **A,** illustrating the greater omentum overhanging the transverse colon. The *arrows* indicate areas of subsequent fusion. **D,** Ventral view of the intestines after their fixation. **E,** Transverse section at the level shown in **D** after disappearance of the mesentery of the ascending and descending colon. **F,** Sagittal section at the plane shown in **D,** illustrating fusion of the greater omentum with the mesentery of the transverse colon and fusion of the layers of the greater omentum.

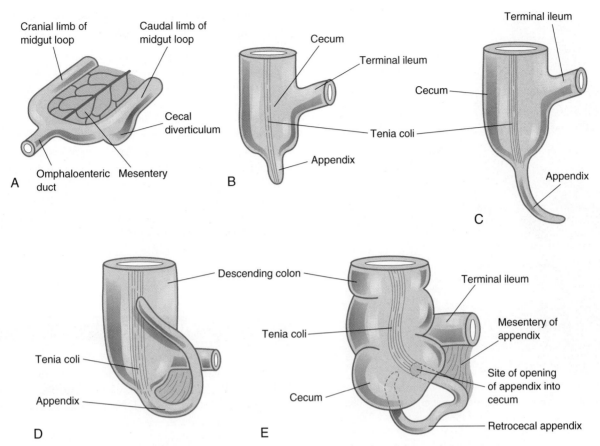

Figure 12–14 Successive stages in the development of the cecum and appendix. **A,** At 6 weeks. **B,** At 8 weeks. **C,** At 12 weeks. **D,** At birth. Note that the appendix is relatively long and is continuous with the apex of the cecum. **E,** Adult. Note that the appendix is now relatively short and is located posterior to the cecum.

MIXED ROTATION AND VOLVULUS

With mixed rotation and volvulus, the cecum lies just inferior to the pylorus of the stomach and is fixed to the posterior abdominal wall by peritoneal bands that pass over the duodenum (Fig. 12-18B). These bands and the volvulus usually cause **duodenal obstruction.** This type of malrotation results from failure of the midgut loop to complete the final 90 degrees of rotation (Fig. 12-11D); consequently, the terminal part of the ileum returns to the abdomen first.

REVERSED ROTATION

In very unusual cases, the midgut loop rotates in a clockwise rather than a counterclockwise direction (Fig. 12-18C). As a result, the duodenum lies anterior to the superior mesenteric artery rather than posterior to it, and the transverse colon lies posterior to the superior mesenteric artery instead of anterior to it. In these infants, the transverse colon may be obstructed by pressure from the superior mesenteric artery.

SUBHEPATIC CECUM AND APPENDIX

If the cecum adheres to the inferior surface of the liver when it returns to the abdomen (Fig. 12-11D), it is drawn superiorly with the liver. As a result, the cecum remains in its fetal position (Fig. 12-18D). Subhepatic cecum and appendix are more common in males than in females. Subhepatic cecum is not common in adults; when it occurs, it may create problems in the diagnosis and surgical removal of the appendix.

INTERNAL HERNIA

In the case of an internal hernia, the small intestine passes into the mesentery of the midgut loop during the return of the intestines to the abdomen (Fig. 12-18E). As a result, a hernia-like sac forms. This very uncommon condition usually does not produce symptoms and is often detected at autopsy or during an anatomical dissection.

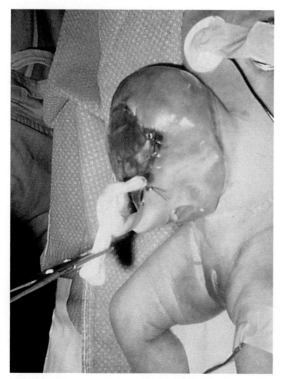

Figure 12–15 An infant with an omphalocele. The defect resulted in herniation of intra-abdominal structures (liver and intestine) into the proximal end of the umbilical cord. The omphalocele is covered by a membrane composed of peritoneum and amnion. *(Courtesy of Dr. N.E. Wiseman, Department of Surgery, Children's Hospital, Winnipeg, Manitoba, Canada.)*

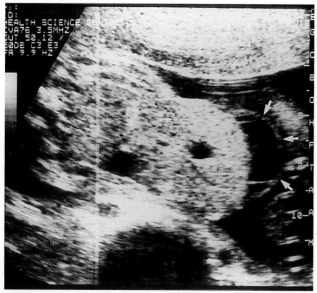

Figure 12–16 Ultrasonogram of the abdomen of a fetus (28 weeks' gestation), showing a large omphalocele, with much of the liver protruding from the abdominal wall. The mass also contains a small, membrane-covered sac *(arrows)*. The umbilical cord was integrally involved in the anomaly. *(Courtesy of Dr. C.R. Harman, Department of Obstetrics, Gynecology and Reproductive Sciences, Women's Hospital and University of Maryland, Baltimore, MD.)*

MIDGUT VOLVULUS

Midgut volvulus is an anomaly in which the small intestine does not enter the abdominal cavity normally and the mesenteries do not undergo normal fixation. As a result, twisting (volvulus) of the intestines occurs (Fig. 12-18F). Only two parts of the intestine—the duodenum and the proximal colon—are attached to the posterior abdominal wall. The small intestine hangs by a narrow stalk that contains the superior mesenteric artery and vein. These vessels are usually twisted in this stalk and become obstructed at or near the duodenojejunal junction. The circulation to the twisted intestine is often restricted; if the vessels are completely obstructed, necrosis develops.

STENOSIS AND ATRESIA OF INTESTINE

Partial occlusion (stenosis) and complete occlusion (atresia) of the intestinal lumen (Fig. 12-5) account for approximately one third of cases of intestinal obstruction. The obstructive lesion occurs most often in the ileum (50%) and duodenum (25%). *These anomalies result from failure of recanalization of the intestine.* Most atresias of the ileum are probably caused by infarction of the fetal bowel as a result of impairment of its blood supply secondary to volvulus. This impairment most likely occurs during the 10th week as the intestines return to the abdomen.

ILEAL DIVERTICULUM AND OTHER OMPHALOENTERIC DUCT REMNANTS

A congenital **ileal diverticulum** (Meckel diverticulum) (Fig. 12-19) occurs in 2% to 4% of infants and is three to five times more prevalent in males than in females. It represents a remnant of the proximal portion of the omphaloenteric duct. It typically appears as a finger-like pouch approximately 3 to 6 cm long that arises from the *antimesenteric border of the ileum*, 40 to 50 cm from the ileocecal junction. *An ileal diverticulum is of clinical significance because it sometimes becomes inflamed and causes symptoms that mimic appendicitis.* The wall of the diverticulum contains all layers of the ileum and may also contain small patches of gastric and pancreatic tissues. The gastric mucosa often secretes acid, producing ulceration and bleeding (Fig. 12-20A to C). An ileal diverticulum may be connected to the umbilicus by a fibrous cord or an **omphaloenteric fistula** (Fig. 12-20B and C); other possible remnants of the omphaloenteric duct are shown in Fig. 12-20D to F.

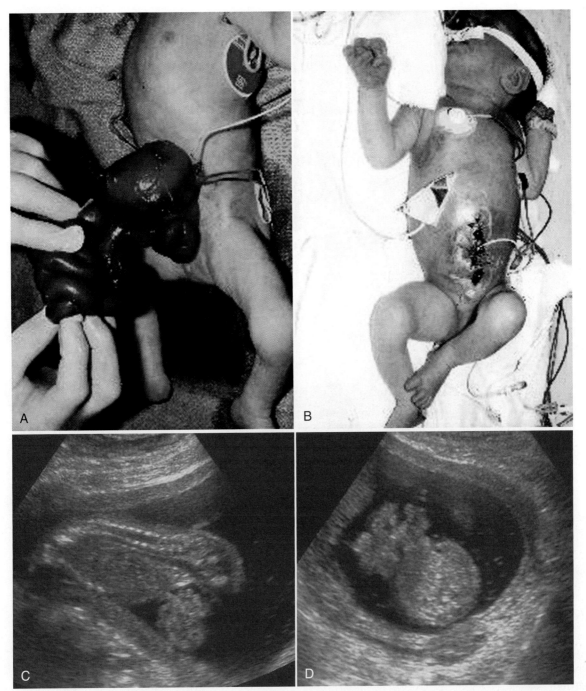

Figure 12–17 **A,** A newborn infant with an anterior abdominal wall defect—gastroschisis. The defect was relatively small (2-4 cm long) and involved all layers of the abdominal wall. It was located to the right of the umbilicus. **B,** The same infant after the viscera were returned to the abdomen and the defect was surgically closed. **C, D,** Sonogram of an 18-week fetus with gastroschisis. Loops of bowel can be seen in the amniotic fluid ventral to the fetus on the sagittal scan **(C)** and the axial scan **(D)** of the fetal abdomen. *(Courtesy of A.E. Chudley, M.D., Section of Genetics and Metabolism, Department of Pediatrics and Child Health, Children's Hospital, Winnipeg, Manitoba, Canada. C and D, Courtesy of Dr. E. A. Lyons, Professor of Radiology, Obstetrics and Gynecology, and Anatomy, Health Sciences Centre, University of Manitoba, Winnipeg, Manitoba, Canada.)*

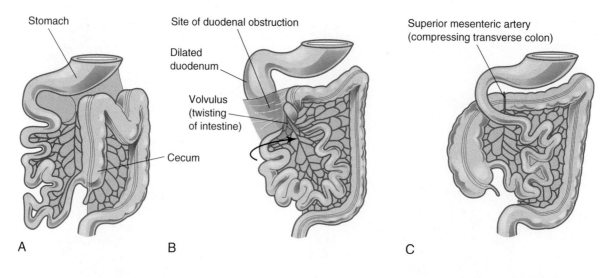

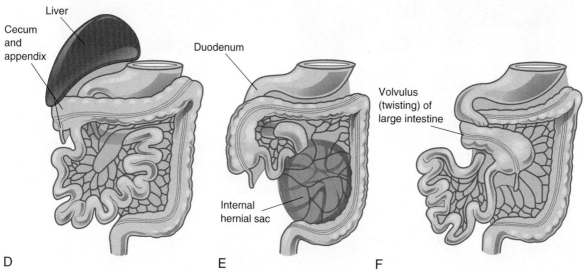

Figure 12–18 Various abnormalities of midgut rotation. **A,** Nonrotation. **B,** Mixed rotation and volvulus. The *arrow* indicates the twisting of the intestine. **C,** Reversed rotation. **D,** Subhepatic cecum and appendix. **E,** Internal hernia. **F,** Midgut volvulus with duodenal obstruction.

Cloaca

The expanded terminal part of the hindgut, the **cloaca**, is an endoderm-lined chamber that is in contact with the surface ectoderm at the cloacal membrane (Fig. 12-21*A* and *B*). This membrane is composed of the endoderm of the cloaca and the ectoderm of the proctodeum (Fig. 12-21*C* and *D*). The cloaca receives the allantois ventrally (Fig. 12-21*A*).

Partitioning of Cloaca

The cloaca is divided into dorsal and ventral parts by mesenchyme—the **urorectal septum**—that develops in the angle between the allantois and the hindgut (Fig. 12-21*C* and *D*). As the septum grows toward the cloacal membrane, it develops forklike extensions that produce infoldings of the lateral walls of the cloaca (Fig. 12-21*B₁*). These folds grow toward each other and fuse, forming a partition that divides the cloaca into two parts (Fig. 12-21*D* to *F₁*)—the rectum and the cranial part of the **anal canal** dorsally, and the **urogenital sinus** ventrally.

By the seventh week, the urorectal septum has fused with the cloacal membrane, dividing it into a smaller, dorsal **anal membrane** and a larger, ventral urogenital membrane (Fig. 12-21*E* and *F*). The area of fusion of the urorectal septum with the cloacal membrane is represented in the adult by the **perineal body**, the tendinous center of the perineum.

Mesenchymal proliferations produce elevations of the surface ectoderm around the **anal membrane**. As a result, this membrane is soon located at the bottom of an ectodermal depression—the *proctodeum* (Fig. 12-21*F*). The

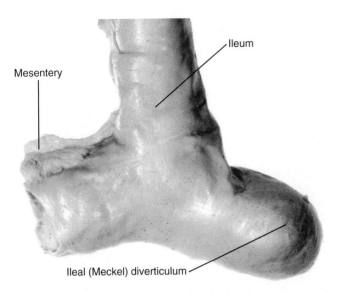

Figure 12–19 A typical ileal diverticulum (cadaveric specimen), commonly referred to clinically as *Meckel diverticulum*. *(From Moore KL, Persaud TVN, Shiota K: Color Atlas of Clinical Embryology, 2nd ed. Philadelphia, WB Saunders, 2000.)*

anal membrane usually ruptures at the end of the eighth week of development.

Anal Canal

The superior two thirds of the adult anal canal are derived from the **hindgut**; the inferior one third develops from the **proctodeum** (Fig. 12-22). The junction of the epithelium derived from the ectoderm of the proctodeum and that derived from the endoderm of the hindgut is roughly indicated by an irregular **pectinate line** located at the inferior limit of the anal valves (Fig. 12-22). This line also indicates the approximate former site of the anal membrane. At the anus, the epithelium is keratinized and continuous with the skin around it. The other layers of the wall of the anal canal are derived from splanchnic mesenchyme.

Because of its hindgut origin, the superior two thirds of the anal canal are supplied mainly by the *superior rectal artery*, the continuation of the *inferior mesenteric artery*. Its nerves are from the autonomic nervous system.

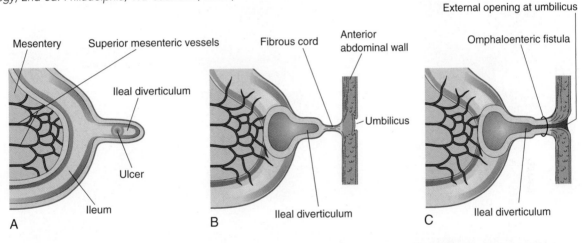

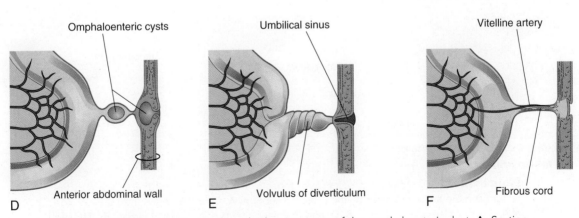

Figure 12–20 Ileal diverticula and other remnants of the omphaloenteric duct. **A,** Section of the ileum and a diverticulum with an ulcer. **B,** A diverticulum connected to the umbilicus by a fibrous cord. **C,** Omphaloenteric fistula resulting from persistence of the entire intra-abdominal portion of the omphaloenteric duct. **D,** Omphaloenteric cysts at the umbilicus and in a fibrous remnant of the omphaloenteric duct. **E,** Umbilical sinus resulting from the persistence of the omphaloenteric duct near the umbilicus. **F,** The omphaloenteric duct has persisted as a fibrous cord connecting the ileum with the umbilicus. A persistent vitelline artery extends along the fibrous cord to the umbilicus.

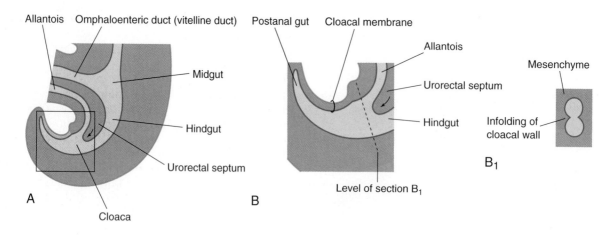

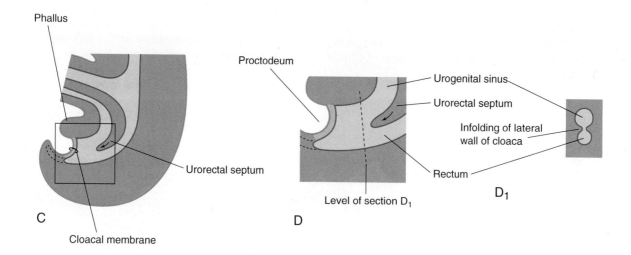

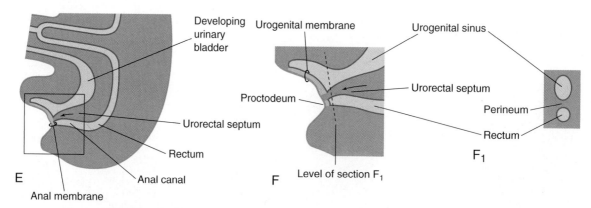

Figure 12–21 Illustrations of successive stages in the partitioning of the cloaca into the rectum and the urogenital sinus by the urorectal septum. **A, C,** and **E,** Views from the left side at 4, 6, and 7 weeks, respectively. **B, D,** and **F,** Enlargements of the cloacal region. **B₁, D₁,** and **F₁,** Transverse sections of the cloaca at the levels shown in **B, D,** and **F,** respectively. Note that the postanal gut, or tailgut (shown in **B**), degenerates and disappears as the rectum forms from the dorsal part of the cloaca (shown in **C**). The *arrows* indicate the growth of the urorectal septum.

The inferior one third of the anal canal, because of its origin from the proctodeum, is supplied mainly by the *inferior rectal arteries*, branches of the internal pudendal artery. The inferior part of the anal canal is supplied by the inferior rectal nerve and is sensitive to pain, temperature, touch, and pressure.

The differences in blood supply, nerve supply, and venous and lymphatic drainage of the two parts of the anal canal are important clinically because the characteristics of carcinomas involving the two parts differ. Tumors in the superior part are painless and arise from the columnar epithelium, whereas those in the inferior part are painful and arise from the squamous epithelium.

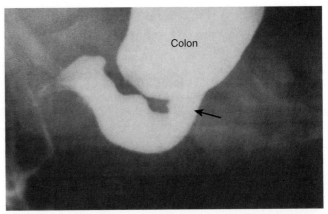

Figure 12–23 Radiograph of the colon, after a barium enema, in a 1-month-old infant with megacolon (Hirschsprung disease). The distal aganglionic segment is narrow, with a dilated proximal colon full of fecal material. Note the transition zone *(arrow)*. *(Courtesy of Dr. Martin H. Reed, Department of Radiology, University of Manitoba and Children's Hospital, Winnipeg, Manitoba, Canada.)*

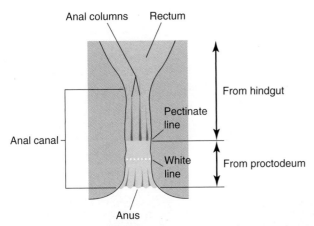

Figure 12–22 The rectum and anal canal, showing their developmental origins. Note that the superior two thirds of the anal canal are derived from the hindgut, whereas the inferior one third of the anal canal is derived from the proctodeum. Because of their different embryologic origins, the superior and inferior parts of the anal canal are supplied by different arteries and nerves and have different venous and lymphatic drainages.

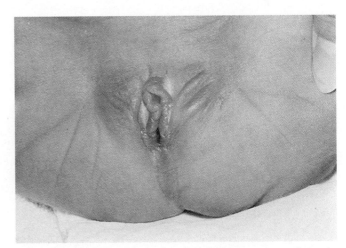

Figure 12–24 Female neonate with membranous anal atresia (imperforate anus). In most cases of anal atresia, a thin layer of tissue separates the anal canal from the exterior. *(Courtesy of A.E. Chudley, M.D., Section of Genetics and Metabolism, Department of Pediatrics and Child Health, Children's Hospital, Winnipeg, Manitoba, Canada.)*

CONGENITAL MEGACOLON

In infants with congenital megacolon, or **Hirschsprung disease** (Fig. 12-23), a part of the colon is dilated because of the *absence of autonomic ganglion cells* in the myenteric plexus distal to the dilated segment of colon. The enlarged colon—**megacolon**—has the normal number of ganglion cells. The dilation results from failure of peristalsis in the aganglionic segment, which prevents movement of the intestinal contents. Males are affected more than females (4 to 1). Congenital megacolon results from failure of neural crest cells to migrate into the wall of the colon during the fifth to seventh weeks of development. Of the genes involved in the pathogenesis of Hirschsprung disease, the *RET proto-oncogene* accounts for most cases.

IMPERFORATE ANUS AND ANORECTAL ANOMALIES

Imperforate anus occurs in approximately 1 in 5000 newborn infants, and it is more common in boys (Figs. 12-24 and 12-25C). *Most anorectal anomalies result from abnormal development of the urorectal septum*, resulting in incomplete separation of the cloaca into urogenital and anorectal parts (Fig. 12-25A). Lesions are classified as low or high, depending on whether the rectum ends superior or inferior to the puborectalis muscle.

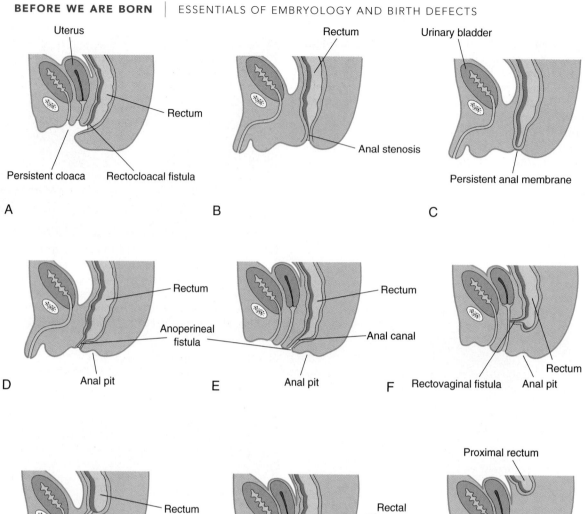

Figure 12–25   Illustrations of various types of anorectal anomalies. **A,** Persistent cloaca. Note the common outlet of the intestinal, urinary, and reproductive tracts. **B,** Anal stenosis. **C,** Membranous anal atresia. **D** and **E,** Anal agenesis with a perineal fistula. **F,** Anorectal agenesis with a rectovaginal fistula. **G,** Anorectal agenesis with a rectourethral fistula. **H** and **I,** Rectal atresia.

LOW RECTAL ANOMALIES

ANAL AGENESIS, WITH OR WITHOUT A FISTULA

The anal canal may end blindly or there may be an **ectopic anus** or an **anoperineal fistula** that opens into the perineum (Fig. 12-25D and E). The abnormal canal may, however, open into the vagina or the urethra in males (Fig. 12-25F and G). Most low anorectal anomalies are associated with an external fistula. **Anal agenesis with a fistula** results from incomplete separation of the cloaca by the urorectal septum.

ANAL STENOSIS

In anal stenosis, the anus is in a normal position but the anus and the anal canal are narrow (Fig. 12-25B). This anomaly is

probably caused by a slight dorsal deviation of the urorectal septum as it grows caudally to fuse with the cloacal membrane.

MEMBRANOUS ATRESIA OF ANUS

In membranous anal atresia, the anus is in the normal position but a thin layer of tissue separates the anal canal from the exterior (Figs. 12-24 and 12-25C). The anal membrane is thin enough to bulge on straining. This anomaly results from failure of the anal membrane to perforate at the end of the eighth week.

HIGH ANORECTAL ANOMALIES

ANORECTAL AGENESIS, WITH OR WITHOUT A FISTULA

In anorectal agenesis, the rectum ends superior to the puborectalis muscle. This is the most common type of anorectal anomaly, and it accounts for approximately two thirds of anorectal defects. Although the rectum ends blindly, there is usually a fistula to the bladder (rectovesical fistula) or the urethra (rectourethral fistula) in males, or to the vagina (rectovaginal fistula) or the vestibule of the vagina (rectovestibular fistula) (Fig. 12-25F and G). Anorectal agenesis with a fistula is the result of incomplete separation of the cloaca by the urorectal septum.

RECTAL ATRESIA

In rectal atresia, the anal canal and the rectum are present but are separated (Fig. 12-25H and I). Sometimes the two segments of bowel are connected by a fibrous cord, the remnant of the atretic portion of the rectum. The cause of rectal atresia may be abnormal recanalization of the colon or, more likely, a defective blood supply.

CLINICALLY ORIENTED QUESTIONS

1. About 2 weeks after birth, an infant began to vomit shortly after feeding. Each time, the vomitus was propelled approximately 2 feet. The physician told the mother that the infant had an obstructing benign growth that causes a narrow outlet from the stomach. Is there an embryologic basis for this anomaly?

2. Do infants with Down syndrome have an increased incidence of duodenal atresia? Can the condition be corrected?

3. A man claimed that his appendix was on his left side. Is this possible and, if so, how could this happen?

4. A patient reported that she had two appendices and separate operations to remove them. Do people ever have two appendices?

5. What is Hirschsprung disease? Some sources state that it is a congenital condition resulting from large bowel obstruction. Is this correct? If so, what is its embryologic basis?

6. A nurse observed what appeared to be feces being expelled from a baby's umbilicus. How could this happen? What conditions would likely be present?

The answers to these questions are at the back of the book.

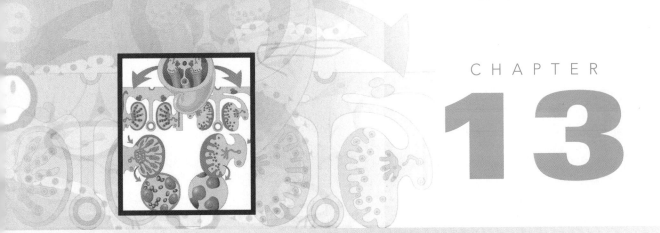

Urogenital System

T he urogenital system is divided functionally into the urinary system and the genital system. Embryologically, these systems are closely associated with one another, especially during their early stages of development.

The urogenital system develops from the intermediate mesenchyme derived from the dorsal wall of the embryo (Fig. 13-1*A* and *B*). During folding of the embryo in the horizontal plane (see Chapter 6), the intermediate mesenchyme (embryonic connective tissue in the mesoderm) is carried ventrally and loses its connection with the somites (Fig. 13-1*C* and *D*). A longitudinal elevation of the mesenchyme—the **urogenital ridge**—forms on each side of the dorsal aorta (Fig. 13-1*F*). The part of the urogenital ridge that gives rise to the urinary system is the **nephrogenic cord** (Fig. 13-1*C* to *F*); the part that gives rise to the genital system is the **gonadal ridge** (see Fig. 13-18*C*).

DEVELOPMENT OF URINARY SYSTEM

The urinary system begins to develop before the genital system; it consists of the kidneys, ureters, urinary bladder, and urethra.

Development of Kidneys and Ureters

Three sets of excretory organs, or kidneys, develop in human embryos. The first set—the *pronephroi*—is rudimentary and never functions. The second set—the *mesonephroi*—is well developed and functions for a brief period. The third set—the *metanephroi*—becomes the permanent kidneys.

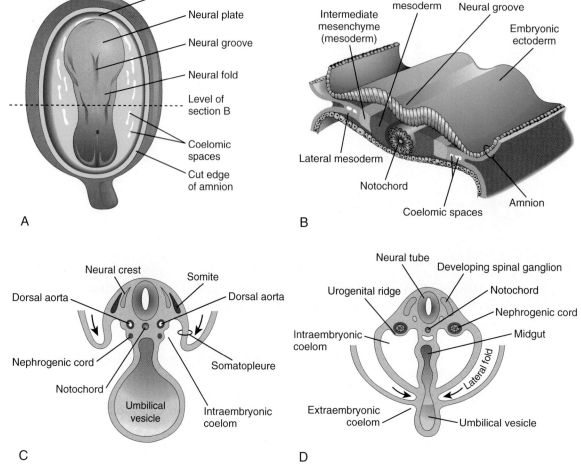

Figure 13–1 A, Dorsal view of an embryo during the third week (approximately 18 days). **B,** Transverse section of the embryo, showing the position of the intermediate mesenchyme before lateral folding occurs. **C,** Transverse section of the embryo after the commencement of folding. **D,** Transverse section of the embryo, showing the lateral folds meeting each other ventrally.

Pronephroi

The transitory pronephroi appear early in the fourth week of development. They are represented by a few cell clusters in the neck region (Fig. 13-2A). The pronephric ducts run caudally and open into the *cloaca* (Fig. 13-2B). The pronephroi degenerate but most of the pronephric ducts persist and are used by the next set of kidneys.

Mesonephroi

The large mesonephroi appear late in the fourth week caudal to the pronephroi (Fig. 13-2) and function as interim kidneys until the permanent kidneys develop (Fig. 13-3). The mesonephroi consist of **glomeruli** and **mesonephric tubules** (Fig. 13-3C to F). The tubules open into the **mesonephric ducts**, originally the pronephric ducts. The mesonephric ducts open into the cloaca. The mesonephroi degenerate toward the end of the first trimester; however, their tubules become the efferent ductules of the testes, and the mesonephric ducts have several adult derivatives in the male (Table 13-1).

Metanephroi

The metanephroi—the **primordia of the permanent kidneys**—begin to develop early in the fifth week and start to function approximately 4 weeks later. Urine formation continues throughout fetal life. The urine is excreted into the amniotic cavity and mixes with the amniotic fluid. The permanent kidneys develop from two sources of mesodermal origin (Fig. 13-4A):

● The ureteric bud
● The metanephric blastema

The **ureteric bud** is an outgrowth from the mesonephric duct, near its entrance into the cloaca, and is the primordium of the ureter, renal pelvis, calices, and collecting tubules (Fig. 13-4B to E). The elongating bud penetrates the **metanephrogenic blastema**—a mass of cells derived from the **nephrogenic cord**—that forms the nephrons (Fig. 13-4B). The stalk of the ureteric bud becomes the **ureter**, and the cranial part of the diverticulum undergoes repetitive branching. The

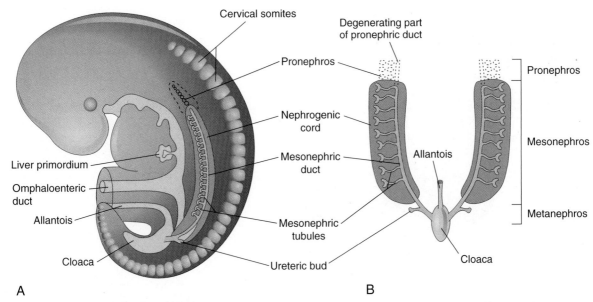

Figure 13–2 The three sets of excretory organs in an embryo during the fifth week. **A,** Lateral view. **B,** Ventral view. In this diagram, the mesonephric tubules have been pulled laterally; their normal position is shown in **A.**

branches form the **collecting tubules** (Figs. 13-4C to E and 13-5).

The **straight collecting tubules** undergo repeated branching, forming successive generations of collecting tubules. The first four generations of tubules enlarge and coalesce to form the **major calices** (Fig. 13-4C to E); the second four generations coalesce to form the **minor calices.** The end of each **arched collecting tubule** induces clusters of mesenchymal cells in the metanephrogenic blastema to form small **metanephric vesicles** (Fig. 13-5A). These vesicles elongate and become the **renal tubules** (Fig. 13-5B and C). The proximal ends of these tubules are invaginated by **glomeruli.** The renal corpuscle (glomerulus and glomerular capsule) and its proximal convoluted tubule, **nephron loop** (of Henle), and distal convoluted tubule constitute a **nephron** (Fig. 13-5D). Each distal convoluted tubule contacts an arched collecting tubule. The tubules become confluent, forming a **uriniferous tubule.**

Branching of the metanephric diverticulum depends on an inductive signal from the metanephric mesoderm—differentiation of the nephrons depends on induction by the collecting tubules. The **molecular aspects** of the reciprocal interactions between the metanephric mesenchyme and the collecting tubules are shown in Figure 13-6.

The **fetal kidneys** are subdivided into lobes. The lobulation usually disappears during infancy as the nephrons increase and grow. At term, nephron formation is complete—each kidney containing approximately 2 million nephrons. Functional maturation of the kidneys occurs after birth.

Positional Changes of Kidneys

The metanephric kidneys lie close to each other in the pelvis (Fig. 13-7A). As the abdomen and pelvis grow, the kidneys gradually come to lie in the abdomen and move

ACCESSORY RENAL ARTERIES

The common variations in the blood supply to the kidneys reflect the manner in which the blood supply continually changes during embryonic and early fetal life (Fig. 13-7). Approximately 25% of adult kidneys have accessory (supernumerary) renal arteries, usually arising from the aorta, superior or inferior to the main renal artery (Fig. 13-8A and B). An accessory artery to the inferior pole (polar renal artery) may cross anterior to the ureter and obstruct it, causing **hydronephrosis,** or distention of the pelvis and calices with urine (Fig. 13-8B). Renal arteries are end arteries; consequently, if an accessory artery is damaged or ligated, the part of the kidney supplied by it will become ischemic. Accessory arteries are approximately twice as common as accessory veins.

farther apart (Fig. 13-7B and C). The caudal part of the embryo grows away from the kidneys so that the kidneys occupy progressively higher cranial levels. As the kidneys change their positions "ascend," they rotate medially almost 90 degrees. By the ninth week, the kidneys come in contact with the suprarenal glands as they attain their adult position (Fig. 13-7C and D).

Changes in Blood Supply of Kidneys

Initially, the renal arteries are branches of the common iliac arteries (Fig. 13-7A and B). Later, the kidneys receive their blood supply from the distal end of the aorta (Fig. 13-7C). The kidneys receive their most cranial arterial branches from the abdominal aorta which become the renal arteries. Normally, the caudal primordial branches undergo involution and disappear.

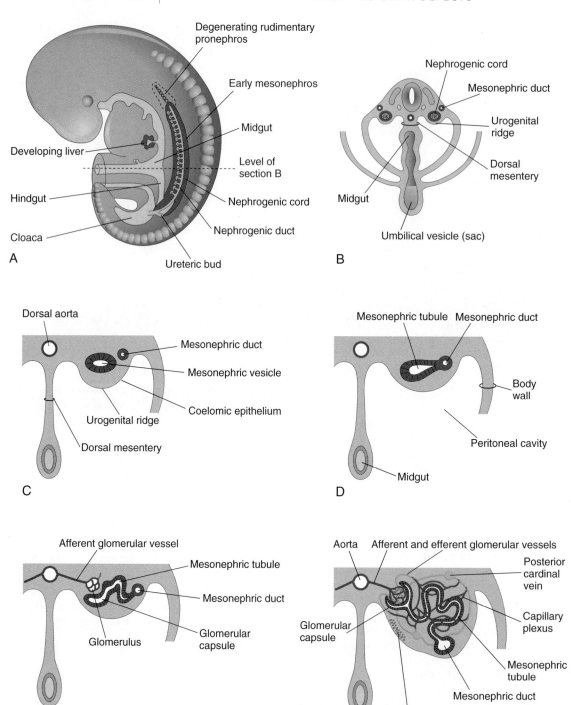

Figure 13–3 **A,** Lateral view of a 5-week embryo showing the extent of the mesonephros and the primordium of the metanephros—permanent kidney. **B,** Transverse section of the embryo showing the nephrogenic cords from which the mesonephric tubules develop. **C** to **F,** Transverse sections showing successive stages in the development of a mesonephric tubule between the 5th and 11th weeks. Note in **C** that the mesenchymal cell cluster in the nephrogenic cord has developed a lumen, thereby forming a mesonephric vesicle. The vesicle soon becomes an S-shaped mesonephric tubule and extends laterally to join the mesonephric duct. The expanded medial end of the mesonephric tubule is invaginated by blood vessels to form a glomerular capsule. The cluster of capillaries projecting into this capsule is the glomerulus.

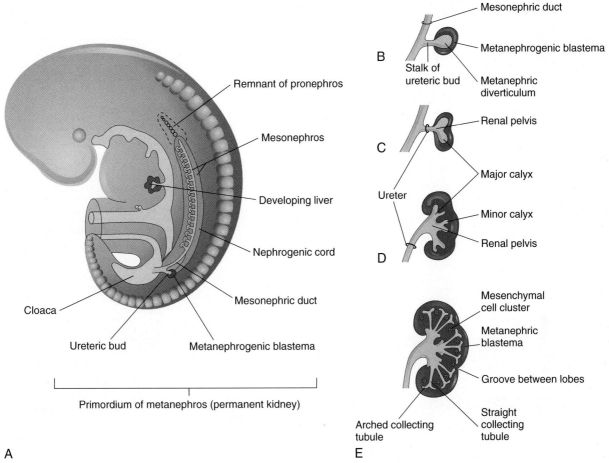

Figure 13–4 Development of the metanephros, the primordium of the permanent kidney. **A,** Lateral view of a 5-week embryo, showing the primordium of the metanephros. **B** to **E,** Successive stages in the development of the ureteric bud (fifth to eighth weeks). Observe the development of the ureter, the renal pelvis, the calices, and the collecting tubules.

CONGENITAL ANOMALIES OF KIDNEYS AND URETERS

Unilateral renal agenesis occurs in approximately 1 in 1000 newborn infants (Fig. 13-9A). Boys are affected more often than girls, and the left kidney is usually the one that is absent. The other kidney usually undergoes compensatory hypertrophy and performs the function of the missing kidney.

Bilateral renal agenesis *is associated with oligohydramnios* (small amount of amniotic fluid) because little or no urine is excreted into the amniotic cavity. This condition occurs in approximately 1 in 3000 births, is three times more common in males, and is incompatible with postnatal life. These infants also have pulmonary hypoplasia. Failure of the metanephric diverticulum to penetrate the metanephric blastema results in absence of renal development because no nephrons are induced by the collecting tubules to develop from the metanephric blastema.

MALROTATION OF KIDNEYS

If the kidney does not rotate, the hilum faces anteriorly (embryonic position) (Figs. 13-7 and 13-9C). If the hilum faces posteriorly, then rotation has progressed too far; if it faces laterally, medial rotation has occurred. Abnormal rotation of the kidneys is often associated with ectopic kidneys.

ECTOPIC KIDNEYS

One or both kidneys may be in an abnormal position (Fig. 13-9B and E). Most ectopic kidneys are located in the pelvis, but some lie in the inferior part of the abdomen. Pelvic kidneys and other forms of ectopia result from failure of the kidneys to "ascend."

Table 13–1 Adult Derivatives and Vestigial Remains of Embryonic Urogenital Structures*

MALE	EMBRYONIC STRUCTURE	FEMALE
Testis	Indifferent gonad	*Ovary*
Seminiferous tubules	Cortex	*Ovarian follicles*
Rete testis	Medulla	Rete ovarii
Gubernaculum	Gubernaculum	*Ovarian ligament*
		Round ligament of the uterus
Efferent ductules of testis	Mesonephric tubules	Epoophoron
Paradidymis		Paroophoron
Appendix of epididymis	Mesonephric duct	Appendix vesiculosa
Duct of epididymis		Duct of epoophoron
Ductus deferens		Longitudinal duct, Gartner duct
Ureter, pelvis, calices, and collecting tubules		*Ureter, pelvis, calices, and collecting tubules*
Ejaculatory duct and seminal gland		
Appendix of testis	Paramesonephric duct	Hydatid (of Morgagni)
		Uterine tube
		Uterus
Urinary bladder	Urogenital sinus	*Urinary bladder*
Urethra (except navicular fossa)		*Urethra*
Prostatic utricle		*Vagina*
Prostate		*Urethral and paraurethral glands*
Bulbourethral glands		*Greater vestibular glands*
Seminal colliculus	Sinus tubercle	Hymen
Penis	Phallus	*Clitoris*
Glans of penis		*Glans of clitoris*
Corpora cavernosa of penis		*Corpora cavernosa of clitoris*
Corpus spongiosum of penis		*Bulb of vestibule*
Ventral aspect of penis	Urogenital folds	*Labia minora*
Scrotum	Labioscrotal swellings	*Labia majora*

*Functional derivatives are shown in italics.

FUSION ANOMALIES

CROSSED FUSED ECTOPIA
Sometimes a kidney crosses to the other side, resulting in crossed renal ectopia, with or without fusion. An unusual kidney abnormality is unilateral fused kidneys (Fig. 13-9D). In such cases, the developing kidneys fuse while they are in the pelvis, and one kidney moves to its normal position, carrying the other one with it.

HORSESHOE KIDNEY
In approximately 1 in 500 persons, the poles of the kidneys are fused (usually the inferior poles) (Fig. 13-10). Normal ascent of the fused kidneys is prevented because they are caught by the root of the inferior mesenteric artery. The function of these kidneys is preserved and each has a normal ureter and blood supply.

DUPLICATIONS OF URINARY TRACT

Duplications of the abdominal part of the ureter and the renal pelvis are common, but a kidney in excess of the normal number (**supernumerary kidney**) is rare (Fig. 13-9C and F). These duplicates result from division of a metanephric diverticulum. Incomplete division of the ureteric primordium results in a divided kidney with a bifid ureter (Fig. 13-9B). Complete division results in a double kidney with a bifid ureter or with separate ureters (Fig. 13-11). A supernumerary kidney with its own ureter probably results from the formation of two metanephric diverticula.

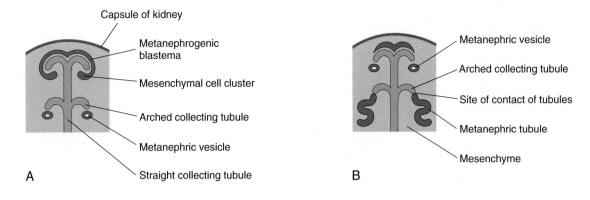

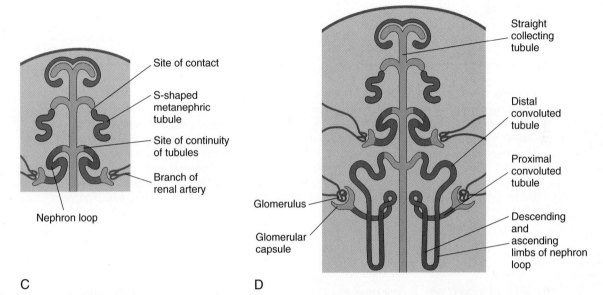

Figure 13–5 Illustrations of stages in nephrogenesis—the development of nephrons. **A,** Nephrogenesis commences approximately at the beginning of the eighth week. **B** and **C,** Note that the metanephric tubules, the primordia of the nephrons, become continuous with the collecting tubules to form uriniferous tubules. **D,** The number of nephrons more than doubles from 20 weeks to 38 weeks. Observe that nephrons are derived from the metanephric mass of the mesoderm and that the collecting tubules are derived from the metanephric diverticulum.

Development of Urinary Bladder

Division of the cloaca by the **urorectal septum** into a dorsal rectum and a ventral **urogenital sinus** is described in Chapter 12. For descriptive purposes, the urogenital sinus is divided into three parts (Fig. 13-11A and C):

- A cranial *vesical part* that forms most of the bladder and is continuous with the allantois
- A middle *pelvic part* that becomes the urethra in the neck of the bladder, the prostatic part of the urethra in males, and the entire urethra in females
- A caudal *phallic part* that grows toward the genital tubercle—the primordium of the penis or the clitoris

Initially, the bladder is continuous with the **allantois** (Fig. 13-11C). The allantois soon constricts and becomes

a thick, fibrous cord, the **urachus** (Fig. 13-11G). In adults, the urachus is represented by the **median umbilical ligament**. As the bladder enlarges, distal parts of the mesonephric ducts are incorporated into its dorsal wall (Fig. 13-11B to H) and contribute to the formation of the connective tissue in the *trigone of the bladder*. The epithelium of the entire bladder is derived from the endoderm of the urogenital sinus. The other layers of the bladder wall develop from the adjacent splanchnic mesenchyme. As the mesonephric ducts are absorbed, the ureters come to open separately into the urinary bladder (Fig. 13-11C to H). In males, the orifices of the mesonephric ducts move close together and enter the prostatic part of the urethra as the caudal ends of these ducts become the *ejaculatory ducts*. In females, the distal ends of the mesonephric ducts degenerate.

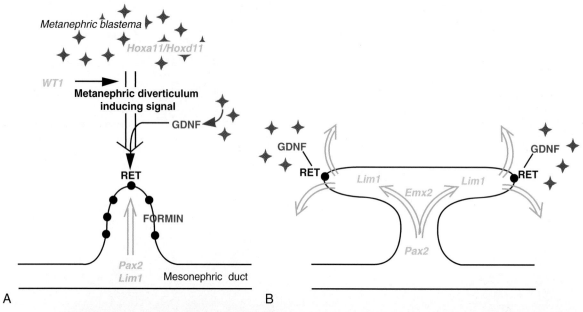

Figure 13–6 Molecular control of kidney development. **A,** Formation of the metanephric diverticulum requires inductive signals derived from the metanephric blastema under the control of transcription factors (*yellow text*), such as WT1, and signaling molecules (*red text*), including GDNF and its epithelial receptor, RET. Normal metanephric diverticulum response to these inductive signals is under the control of transcription factors, such as Pax2, Pax8, Lim1, and the FORMIN gene. **B,** Branching of the metanephric diverticulum is initiated and maintained by interaction with the mesenchyme under the regulation of genes such as Emx2 and specified expression of GDNF and RET at the tips of the invading metanephric diverticulum. *(From Piscione TD, Rosenblum ND: The malformed kidney: disruption of the glomerular and tubular development. Clin Genet 56:342, 1999.)*

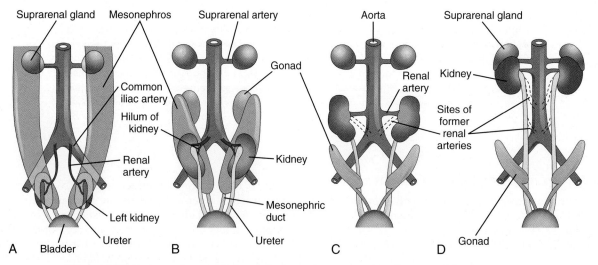

Figure 13–7 Ventral views of the abdominopelvic region of embryos and fetuses (sixth to ninth weeks) showing medial rotation and "ascent" of the kidneys from the pelvis to the abdomen. **A** and **B,** Observe also the decrease in size of the mesonephroi. **C** and **D,** Note that as the kidneys "ascend," they are supplied by arteries at successively higher levels, and that the hilum of the kidney (where the vessels and nerves enter) is eventually directed anteromedially.

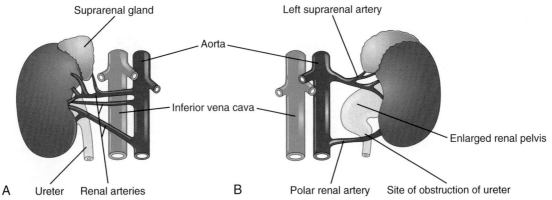

Figure 13–8 Common variations of the renal vessels. **A** and **B,** Multiple renal arteries. The polar renal artery shown in **B** has obstructed the ureter and produced an enlarged renal pelvis.

ECTOPIC URETER

In males, an ectopic ureter may open into the neck of the bladder, the prostatic part of the urethra, the ductus deferens, the prostatic utricle, or the seminal gland. In females, an ectopic ureter may enter the neck of the bladder, the urethra, the vagina, or the vestibule of the vagina. An ectopic ureter results when the ureter is carried caudally with the mesonephric duct and is incorporated into the caudal portion of the vesical part of the urogenital sinus.

URACHAL ANOMALIES

A remnant of the lumen usually persists in the inferior part of the urachus in infants. In approximately 50% of cases, the lumen is continuous with the cavity of the bladder. Remnants of the epithelial lining of the urachus may give rise to **urachal cysts** (Fig. 13-12A). The patent inferior end of the urachus may dilate to form a **urachal sinus** that opens into the bladder. The lumen in the superior part of the urachus may also remain patent and form a urachal sinus that opens at the umbilicus (Fig. 13-12B). Very rarely, the entire urachus remains patent and forms a **urachal fistula** that allows urine to escape from its umbilical orifice (Fig. 13-12C).

EXSTROPHY OF BLADDER

Exstrophy of the bladder is a severe anomaly that occurs in approximately 1 in 10,000 to 1 in 40,000 births, predominantly affecting males (Fig. 13-13). *Exposure and protrusion of the mucosal surface of the posterior wall of the bladder* characterize this congenital anomaly. The trigone of the bladder and the ureteric orifices are exposed, and urine dribbles intermittently from the everted bladder.

Epispadias, in which the urethra opens on the dorsum of the penis, and wide separation of the pubic bones are associated with complete exstrophy of the bladder. In some cases, the penis is divided into two parts, and the scrotum is bifid (split). Exstrophy of the bladder is believed to be caused by failure of the mesenchymal cells to migrate between the ectoderm and the endoderm of the infra-abdominal wall (cloacal membrane) during the fourth week (Fig. 13-14B and C). As a result, no muscle or connective tissue forms in the abdominal wall over the urinary bladder. Rupture of the fragile cloacal membrane results in wide communication between the exterior and the mucous membrane of the bladder. Rupture of the membrane before division of the cloaca by the urorectal septum leads to exstrophy of the cloaca, resulting in exposure of both the bladder and the hindgut.

Development of Urethra

The epithelium of most of the male urethra and the entire female urethra is derived from the endoderm of the urogenital sinus (Figs. 13-11 and 13-15). The distal part of the urethra in the glans of the penis is derived from a solid cord of ectodermal cells that grows from the tip of the glans penis to meet the part of the spongy urethra derived from the phallic part of the urogenital sinus (Fig. 13-15A to C). The ectodermal cord canalizes and joins the rest of the spongy urethra; consequently, the epithelium of the terminal part of the urethra is derived from

the surface ectoderm. The connective tissue and the smooth muscle of the urethra in both sexes are derived from the splanchnic mesenchyme.

DEVELOPMENT OF SUPRARENAL GLANDS

The **cortex** of the suprarenal (adrenal) gland develops from the mesenchyme lining the posterior abdominal wall, whereas the **medulla** differentiates from the

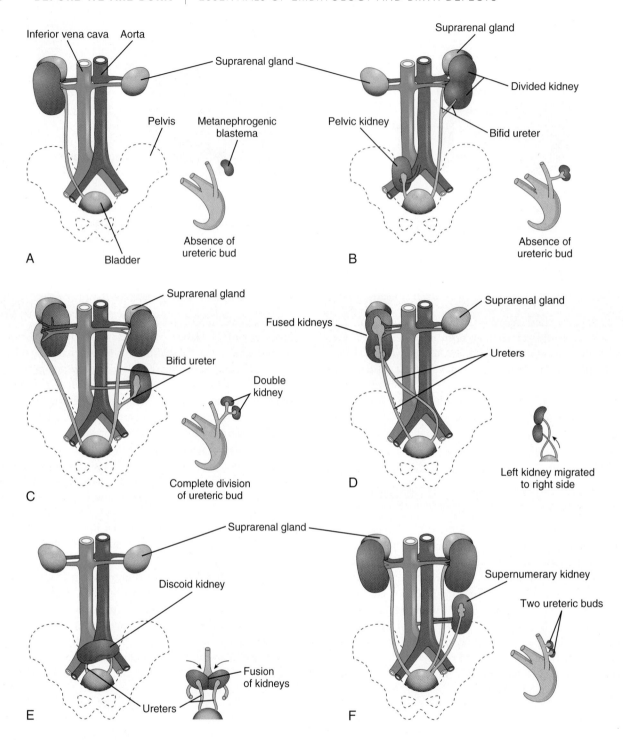

Figure 13–9 Various anomalies of the urinary system. The small sketch at the *lower right* of each illustration shows the probable embryologic basis of the anomaly. **A,** Unilateral renal agenesis. **B,** On the right side of the fetus, a pelvic kidney; on the left side of the fetus, a divided kidney with a bifid ureter. **C,** On the right side of the fetus, malrotation of the kidney; on the left side of fetus, a bifid ureter and a supernumerary kidney. **D,** Crossed fused renal ectopia. The left kidney has crossed over and fused with the right kidney. **E,** Discoid kidney resulting from fusion of the kidneys while they were in the pelvis. **F,** Supernumerary left kidney resulting from the development of two metanephric diverticula.

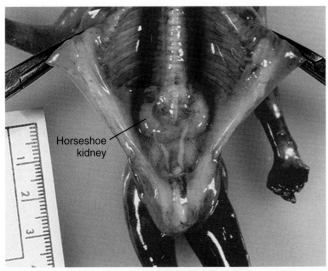

Figure 13–10 Horseshoe kidney in a female fetus (13 weeks). This anomaly resulted from fusion of the inferior poles of the kidneys while they were in the pelvis. *(Courtesy of Dr. D.K. Kalousek, Department of Pathology, University of British Columbia, Children's Hospital, Vancouver, British Columbia, Canada.)*

CONGENITAL ADRENAL HYPERPLASIA: ADRENOGENITAL SYNDROME

Congenital adrenal hyperplasia represents a group of *autosomal recessive disorders* in which an abnormal increase in the cells of the suprarenal cortex results in excessive androgen production during the fetal period. In female infants, this usually causes masculinization of the external genitalia and enlargement of the clitoris (Fig. 13-17). Affected male infants have normal external genitalia and may remain undiagnosed in early infancy. Later in childhood, in both sexes, excess androgen leads to rapid growth and accelerated skeletal maturation. Congenital adrenal hyperplasia (CAH) is usually caused by a genetically determined mutation in the cytochrome-P450c 21-steroid, 21-hydroxylase gene, which results in a deficiency of suprarenal cortical enzymes. These are necessary for the biosynthesis of various steroid hormones. The reduced hormone output results in increased release of adrenocorticotrophic hormone by the anterior pituitary, which causes CAH and overproduction of androgens by the hyperplastic suprarenal glands.

adjacent sympathetic ganglion derived from the **neural crest cells** (Fig. 13-16*A* and *B*). These cells differentiate into the secretory cells of the suprarenal medulla. The cortex is evident during the sixth week as an aggregation of mesenchymal cells seen bilaterally between the root of the dorsal mesentery and the developing gonad (see Fig. 13-18*C*). Differentiation of the characteristic suprarenal cortical zones begins during the late fetal period (Fig. 13-16*C* to *E*). The *zona glomerulosa* and the *zona fasciculata* are present at birth, but the *zona reticularis* is not recognizable until the end of the third year (Fig. 13-16*H*). Relative to body weight, the fetal suprarenal glands are 10 to 20 times larger than the adult glands because of the extensive size of the fetal cortex. The suprarenal medulla remains small until after birth (Fig. 13-16*F*). The suprarenal glands rapidly become smaller as the cortex regresses during the first year of infancy (Fig. 13-16*G*).

DEVELOPMENT OF GENITAL SYSTEM

The early genital systems in the two sexes are similar; therefore, the initial period of genital development is referred to as the *indifferent state of sexual development.*

Development of Gonads

The gonads (testes and ovaries) are derived from three sources (Fig. 13-18):

● Mesothelium (mesodermal epithelium) lining the posterior abdominal wall
● Underlying mesenchyme
● Primordial germ cells

Indifferent Gonads

Gonadal development begins during the fifth week, when a thickened area of mesothelium develops on the medial side of the mesonephros (Fig. 13-18*A* to *C*). Proliferation of this epithelium and the underlying mesenchyme produces a bulge on the medial side of the mesonephros—**gonadal ridge** (Fig. 13-18*A* and *C*). Finger-like epithelial cords—**gonadal cords**—soon grow into the underlying mesenchyme (Fig. 13-18*D*). The **indifferent gonads** now consist of an external cortex and an internal medulla. In embryos with an XX sex chromosome complex, the cortex of the gonad differentiates into an ovary and the medulla regresses. In embryos with an XY sex chromosome complex, the medulla differentiates into a testis and the cortex regresses, except for vestigial remnants (Table 13-1).

Primordial Germ Cells

The **primordial germ cells** originate in the wall of the umbilical vesicle (yolk sac) and migrate along the dorsal mesentery of the gut to the gonadal ridges (Fig. 13-18*A*). During the sixth week, the primordial germ cells enter the underlying mesenchyme and are incorporated into the **gonadal cords** (see Fig. 13-18*D* and *E*). They eventually differentiate into oocytes or sperms.

Sex Determination

Chromosomal and genetic sex, established at fertilization, depends on whether an X-bearing or a Y-bearing sperm fertilizes the X-bearing oocyte. The type of gonads that develop is determined by the sex chromosome complex of the embryo (XX or XY). Before the seventh week, the gonads of the two sexes are identical in appearance and are called **indifferent gonads** (Fig. 13-19).

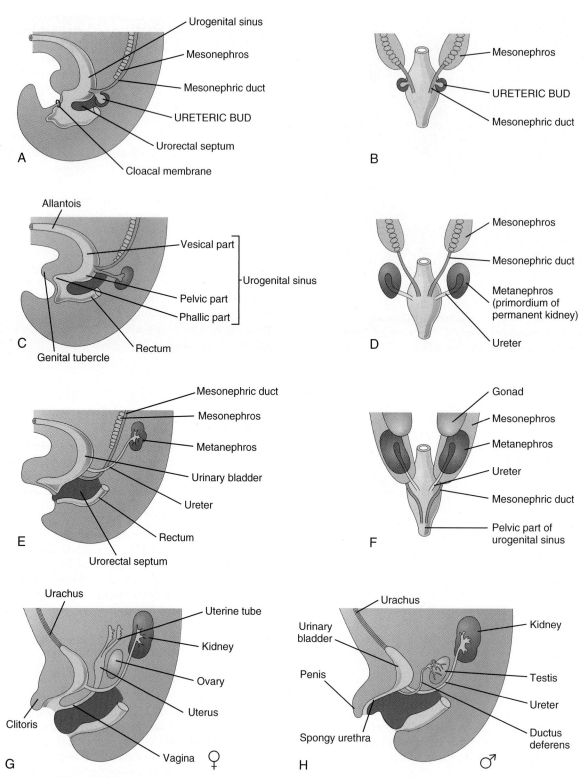

Figure 13–11   Division of the cloaca into the urogenital sinus and rectum; absorption of the mesonephric ducts; development of the urinary bladder, urethra, and urachus; and changes in the location of the ureters. **A,** Lateral view of the caudal half of a 5-week embryo. **B, D,** and **F,** Dorsal views. **C, E, G,** and **H,** Lateral views. The stages shown in **G** and **H** are reached by the 12th week of development.

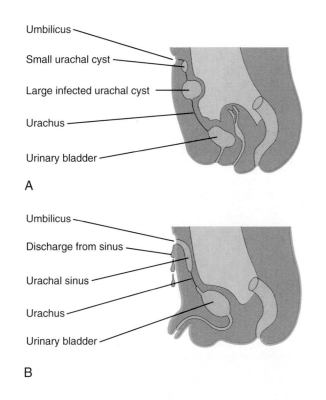

A

B

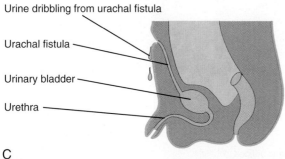

C

Figure 13–12   Urachal anomalies. **A,** Urachal cysts. The most common site for these cysts is in the superior end of the urachus, just inferior to the umbilicus. **B,** Two types of urachal sinuses are shown: one that opens into the bladder and one that opens at the umbilicus. **C,** Patent urachus or urachal fistula connecting the bladder and umbilicus.

Labels in A: Umbilicus, Small urachal cyst, Large infected urachal cyst, Urachus, Urinary bladder

Labels in B: Umbilicus, Discharge from sinus, Urachal sinus, Urachus, Urinary bladder

Labels in C: Urine dribbling from urachal fistula, Urachal fistula, Urinary bladder, Urethra

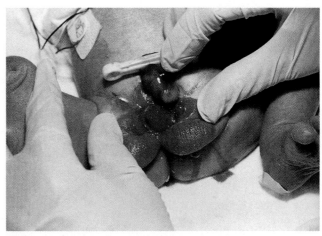

Figure 13–13   A male infant with exstrophy of the bladder. Because of defective closure of the inferior part of the anterior abdominal wall and the anterior wall of the bladder, the urinary bladder appears as an everted, bulging mass inferior to the umbilicus. *(Courtesy of A.E. Chudley, MD, Department of Pediatrics and Child Health, University of Manitoba, Children's Hospital, Winnipeg, Manitoba, Canada.)*

ABNORMAL SEX CHROMOSOME COMPLEXES

In embryos with abnormal sex chromosome complexes, such as XXX or XXY, the number of X chromosomes appears to be unimportant in sex determination. If a normal Y chromosome is present, the embryo develops as a male. If no Y chromosome is present or if the testis-determining region of the Y chromosome has been lost, female development occurs. The loss of an X chromosome does not appear to interfere with the migration of primordial germ cells to the gonadal ridges because some germ cells have been observed in the fetal gonads of 45, XO females with Turner syndrome. Two X chromosomes are needed, however, to bring about complete ovarian development.

Development of a male phenotype requires a Y chromosome. Two X chromosomes are required for the development of the female phenotype.

Development of Testes

A coordinated sequence of genes induces the development of testes. The SRY gene for the testis-determining factor (TDF) on the short arm of the Y chromosome acts as the switch that directs the development of the indifferent gonad into a testis. Expression of the transcription factor SOX9 is also essential for testicular determination. TDF induces the gonadal cords to condense and extend into the medulla of the indifferent gonad, where they branch and anastomose to form the **rete testis** (Fig. 13-19). The connection of the prominent gonadal cords—the **seminiferous cords**—with the surface epithelium is lost when

the **tunica albuginea** develops. This dense tunica, a thick, fibrous capsule, is a characteristic feature of testicular development. Gradually, the testis separates from the degenerating mesonephros and becomes suspended by its own mesentery, the **mesorchium**. The seminiferous cords develop into the seminiferous tubules, the straight tubules (tubuli recti), and the rete testis.

The **seminiferous tubules** are separated by the mesenchyme, giving rise to the **interstitial cells** (of Leydig). By the eighth week, these cells secrete **androgenic hormones**—*testosterone* and *androstenedione*—that induce masculine differentiation of the mesonephric ducts and the external genitalia. Testosterone production is stimulated by **human chorionic gonadotropin**, which reaches peak amounts during the 8- to 12-week period of embryonic and fetal development. The fetal testes also produce a

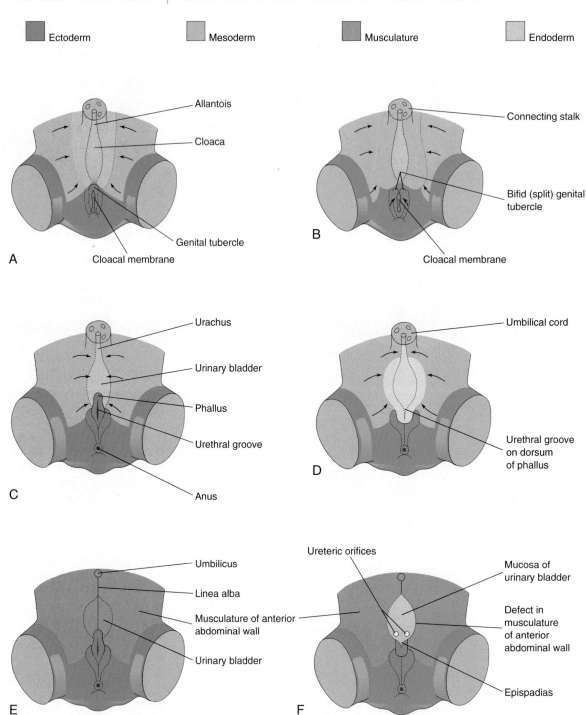

| ■ Ectoderm | ■ Mesoderm | ■ Musculature | ■ Endoderm |

A
- Allantois
- Cloaca
- Genital tubercle
- Cloacal membrane

B
- Connecting stalk
- Bifid (split) genital tubercle
- Cloacal membrane

C
- Urachus
- Urinary bladder
- Phallus
- Urethral groove
- Anus

D
- Umbilical cord
- Urethral groove on dorsum of phallus

E
- Umbilicus
- Linea alba
- Musculature of anterior abdominal wall
- Urinary bladder

F
- Ureteric orifices
- Mucosa of urinary bladder
- Defect in musculature of anterior abdominal wall
- Epispadias

Figure 13–14 **A, C,** and **E,** Normal stages in the development of the infraumbilical abdominal wall and the penis during the fourth to eighth weeks. Note that mesoderm and (later) muscle reinforce the ectoderm of the developing anterior abdominal wall. **B, D,** and **F,** Probable stages in the development of exstrophy of the bladder and epispadias. In **B** and **D,** note that the mesenchyme (embryonic connective tissue) does not extend into the anterior abdominal wall anterior to the urinary bladder. Also note that the genital tubercle is located in a more caudal position than usual, and that the urethral groove has formed on the dorsal surface of the penis. In **F,** the surface ectoderm and the anterior wall of the bladder have ruptured, resulting in exposure of the posterior wall of the bladder. Note that the musculature of the anterior abdominal wall is present on each side of the defect. *(Adapted from Patten BM, Barry A: The genesis of exstrophy of the bladder and epispadias. Am J Anat 90:35, 1952.)*

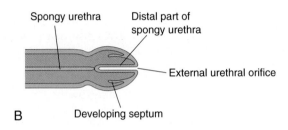

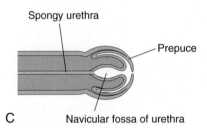

Figure 13–15 Schematic longitudinal sections of the distal part of the developing penis, showing the development of the prepuce and the distal part of the spongy urethra. **A,** At 11 weeks. **B,** At 12 weeks. **C,** At 14 weeks.

glycoprotein known as **müllerian-inhibiting substance** (**MIS**) or antimüllerian hormone. MIS is produced by the sustentacular (Sertoli) cells, which are present until puberty, at which time the levels of MIS decrease. MIS suppresses the development of the paramesonephric ducts, which form the uterus and uterine tubes. The seminiferous tubules remain until puberty (i.e., without lumina), when lumina begin to develop. The walls of the seminiferous tubules are composed of two kinds of cells (Fig. 13-19):

- Sertoli cells, supporting cells derived from the surface epithelium of the testis
- Spermatogonia, primordial sperms derived from the primordial germ cells

Sertoli cells constitute most of the seminiferous epithelium in the fetal testis (Fig. 13-19). The **rete testis** becomes continuous with 15 to 20 mesonephric tubules that become **efferent ductules**. These ductules are connected with the mesonephric duct, which becomes the **ductus epididymis** (Figs. 13-19 and 13-20A).

Development of Ovaries

The X chromosomes have genes for ovarian development; autosomal genes also appear to play a role in ovarian organogenesis. The ovary is not identifiable by histologic examination until approximately the 10th week of development. **Gonadal cords** extend into the medulla of the ovary and form a rudimentary *rete ovarii* (Figs. 13-18D and 13-19). The rete ovarii normally degenerate. **Cortical cords** extend from the surface epithelium of the developing ovary into the underlying mesenchyme during the early fetal period. As the cortical cords increase in size, **primordial germ cells** are incorporated into them. At approximately 16 weeks,

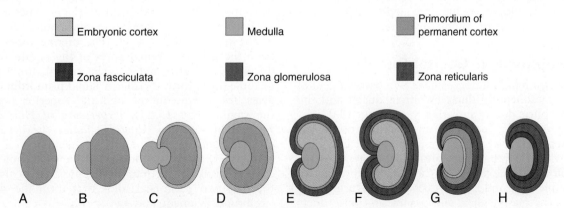

Figure 13–16 Illustrations of the development of the suprarenal glands. **A,** At 6 weeks, showing the mesodermal primordium of the fetal cortex. **B,** At 7 weeks, showing the addition of neural crest cells. **C,** At 8 weeks, showing the fetal cortex and the early permanent cortex beginning to encapsulate the medulla. **D** and **E,** Later stages of encapsulation of the medulla by the cortex. **F,** Neonatal period, showing the fetal cortex and two zones of the permanent cortex. **G,** At 1 year of age. Note that the fetal cortex has almost disappeared. **H,** At 4 years of age. Note the adult pattern of cortical zones. Observe that the fetal cortex has disappeared and that the gland is smaller than it was at birth (**F**).

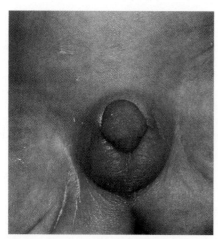

Figure 13–17 External genitalia of a newborn female infant with congenital adrenal hyperplasia (CAH). The virilization was caused by excessive androgens produced by the suprarenal glands during the fetal period. Note the enlarged clitoris and fusion of the labia majora to form a scrotum. (*Courtesy of Dr. Heather Dean, Department of Pediatrics and Child Health, University of Manitoba, Winnipeg, Manitoba, Canada.*)

these cortical cords begin to break up into isolated cell clusters—**primordial follicles**—each of which consists of an **oogonium** (derived from a primordial germ cell), surrounded by a single layer of follicular cells derived from the surface epithelium (see Fig. 13-19). Active mitosis produces many oogonia during fetal life.

No oogonia form postnatally. Although many oogonia degenerate before birth, 2 million or so enlarge to become **primary oocytes** before birth. After birth, the surface epithelium of the ovary flattens to a single layer of cells that is continuous with the mesothelium of the peritoneum at the hilum of the ovary. The surface epithelium becomes separated from the follicles in the cortex by a thin, fibrous capsule, the **tunica albuginea**. As the ovary separates from the regressing mesonephros, it is suspended by its mesentery, the **mesovarium**.

Development of Genital Ducts

Both male and female embryos have two pairs of genital ducts: the **mesonephric ducts** (Wolffian ducts) and the **paramesonephric ducts** (müllerian ducts) (Fig. 13-21A).

The mesonephric ducts play an essential role in the development of the male reproductive system (Fig. 13-20A) while the paramesonephric ducts play an essential role in the development of the female reproductive system (Table 13-1 and Fig. 13-20B and C). During conversion of the mesonephric and paramesonephric ducts into adult structures, some parts of the ducts remain as vestigial structures. These vestiges are rarely seen unless pathologic changes develop in them.

Development of Male Genital Ducts

The fetal testes produce testosterone and müllerian-inhibiting substance (MIS). **Testosterone** stimulates the mesonephric ducts to form male genital ducts; **MIS**

causes the paramesonephric ducts to disappear by epithelial-mesenchymal transformation. As the mesonephros degenerates, some mesonephric tubules persist and are transformed into **efferent ductules** (Fig. 13-20A). These ductules open into the mesonephric duct, which has been transformed into the **duct of the epididymis** in this region. Distal to the epididymis, the mesonephric duct acquires a thick investment of smooth muscle and becomes the **ductus deferens**. The part of the mesonephric duct between the duct of this gland and the urethra becomes the **ejaculatory duct**.

Seminal Gland A lateral outgrowth from the caudal end of each mesonephric duct gives rise to the **seminal gland** (vesicle). The secretions of this pair of glands nourish the sperms.

Prostate Multiple endodermal outgrowths arise from the prostatic part of the urethra and grow into the surrounding mesenchyme (Fig. 13-22). The glandular epithelium of the prostate differentiates from these endodermal cells and the associated mesenchyme differentiates into the dense stroma and the smooth muscle of the prostate. Secretions from the prostate make up a portion of the fluid in the ejaculate.

Bulbourethral Glands The bulbourethral glands are pea-sized structures that develop from paired outgrowths from the spongy part of the urethra (Fig. 13-20A). The smooth muscle fibers and the stroma differentiate from the adjacent mesenchyme. The secretions of these glands and the previous ones, mix with the sperms to form the semen (ejaculate).

Development of Female Genital Ducts and Glands

In female embryos, the mesonephric ducts regress because of lack of testosterone, and the paramesonephric ducts develop because of the absence of MIS. Female sexual development does not depend on the presence of ovaries or hormones. The **paramesonephric ducts** form most of the female genital tract. The **uterine tubes** develop from the unfused cranial parts of the paramesonephric ducts (Fig. 13-20B and C). The caudal, fused portions of these ducts form the **uterovaginal primordium**, which gives rise to the uterus and the superior portion of the vagina (Fig. 13-21). *Expression of Hox genes in the paramesonephric ducts regulates the development of the female genital ducts.* The endometrial stroma and myometrium are derived from splanchnic mesenchyme. Fusion of the paramesonephric ducts also brings together two peritoneal folds that form the right and left **broad ligament** and two peritoneal compartments, the **rectouterine pouch** and the **vesicouterine pouch** (Fig. 13-23B to D).

Development of Vagina The vaginal epithelium is derived from the endoderm of the urogenital sinus. The fibromuscular wall of the vagina develops from the surrounding mesenchyme. Contact of the *uterovaginal primordium* with the urogenital sinus, forming the

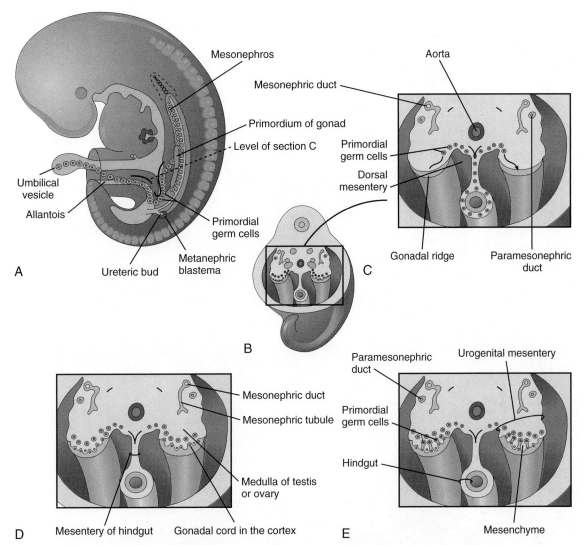

Mesonephros

Mesonephric duct

Primordium of gonad

Level of section C

Umbilical
vesicle

Allantois

Primordial
germ cells

Ureteric bud

Metanephric
blastema

A

B

Aorta

Mesonephric duct

Primordial
germ cells

Dorsal
mesentery

Gonadal ridge

Paramesonephric
duct

C

Mesonephric duct

Mesonephric tubule

Medulla of testis
or ovary

Mesentery of hindgut   Gonadal cord in the cortex

D

Paramesonephric
duct

Urogenital mesentery

Primordial
germ cells

Hindgut

Mesenchyme

E

Figure 13–18 **A,** A 5-week embryo, showing migration of primordial germ cells from the umbilical vesicle into the embryo. **B,** Three-dimensional sketch of the caudal region of the 5-week embryo, showing the location and extent of the gonadal ridges. **C,** Transverse section, showing the gonadal ridges and the migration of primordial germ cells into the developing gonads. **D,** Transverse section of a 6-week embryo, showing the gonadal cords. **E,** Similar section at a later stage, showing the indifferent gonads and the paramesonephric ducts.

sinus tubercle (Fig. 13-21B), induces the formation of paired endodermal outgrowths—**sinovaginal bulbs** (Fig. 13-23A). They extend from the urogenital sinus to the caudal end of the uterovaginal primordium. The sinovaginal bulbs fuse to form a **vaginal plate** (Fig. 13-20B). The central cells of this plate break down, forming the lumen of the vagina. The peripheral cells of the plate form the vaginal epithelium or lining (see Fig. 13-20C). Until late in fetal life, the lumen of the vagina is separated from the cavity of the urogenital sinus by a membrane—the **hymen** (Fig. 13-24H; see also Fig. 13-20C). The hymen is formed by invagination of the posterior wall of the urogenital sinus.

Female Auxiliary Genital Glands Buds grow from the urethra into the surrounding mesenchyme, forming the mucus-secreting **urethral and paraurethral glands**

(Fig. 13-20B). Outgrowths from the urogenital sinus form bilateral **greater vestibular glands** (of Bartholin) in the lower one third of the labia majora. These tubuloalveolar glands also secrete mucus (see Table 13-1).

Development of External Genitalia

From the fourth week to the early part of the seventh week, the external genitalia are sexually undifferentiated (Fig. 13-24A and B). Distinguishing sexual characteristics begin to appear during the 9th week, but the external genitalia are not fully differentiated until the 12th week. Early in the fourth week, the proliferating mesenchyme produces a **genital tubercle** in both sexes at the cranial end of the cloacal membrane. *Fgf8 is involved in the signaling pathways in the early development of the*

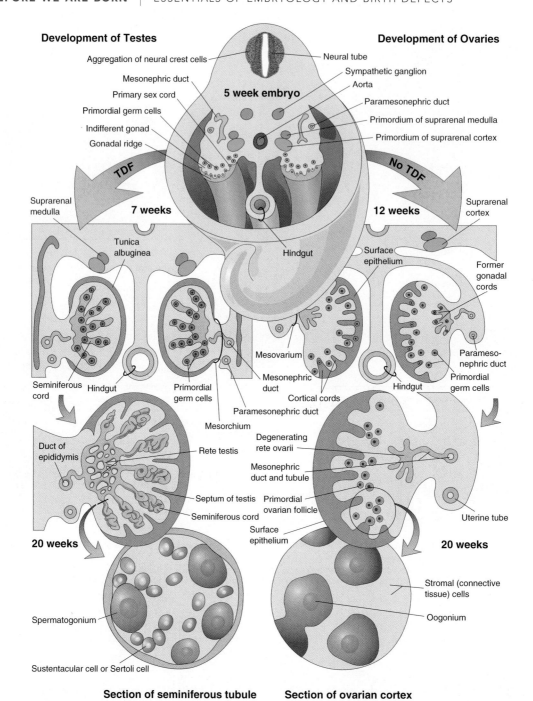

Figure 13–19   Differentiation of the indifferent gonads of a 5-week embryo (*top*) into ovaries or testes. The *left side* of the drawing shows the development of testes resulting from the effects of the testis-determining factor (TDF) located on the Y chromosome. Note that the gonadal cords become seminiferous cords, the primordia of the seminiferous tubules. The parts of the gonadal cords that enter the medulla of the testis form the rete testis. In the section of the testis at the *bottom left,* observe that there are two kinds of cells: spermatogonia, derived from the primordial germ cells and Sertoli cells, derived from the mesenchyme. The *right side* shows the development of ovaries in the absence of TDF. Cortical cords have extended from the surface epithelium of the gonad, and primordial germ cells have entered them. They are the primordia of the oogonia. Follicular cells are derived from the surface epithelium of the ovary. The *arrows* indicate the changes that occur as the gonads (testes and ovaries) develop.

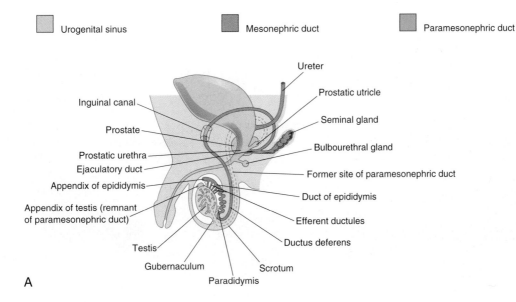

Urogenital sinus   Mesonephric duct   Paramesonephric duct

A

Ureter
Prostatic utricle
Inguinal canal
Seminal gland
Prostate
Bulbourethral gland
Prostatic urethra
Ejaculatory duct
Former site of paramesonephric duct
Appendix of epididymis
Duct of epididymis
Appendix of testis (remnant of paramesonephric duct)
Efferent ductules
Testis
Ductus deferens
Gubernaculum
Scrotum
Paradidymis

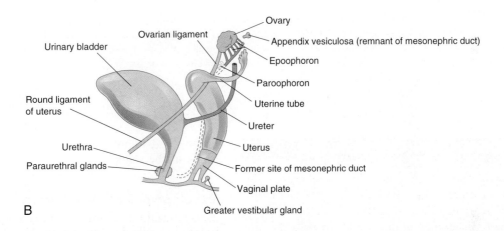

B

Ovary
Ovarian ligament
Appendix vesiculosa (remnant of mesonephric duct)
Urinary bladder
Epoophoron
Paroophoron
Round ligament of uterus
Uterine tube
Ureter
Urethra
Uterus
Paraurethral glands
Former site of mesonephric duct
Vaginal plate
Greater vestibular gland

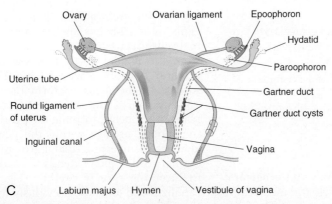

C

Ovary   Ovarian ligament   Epoophoron
Hydatid
Uterine tube
Paroophoron
Round ligament of uterus
Gartner duct
Gartner duct cysts
Inguinal canal
Vagina
Labium majus   Hymen   Vestibule of vagina

Figure 13–20 Development of male and female reproductive systems from the genital ducts and the urogenital sinus. Vestigial structures are also shown. **A,** Reproductive system in a newborn male infant. **B,** Female reproductive system in a 12-week fetus. **C,** Reproductive system in a newborn female infant.

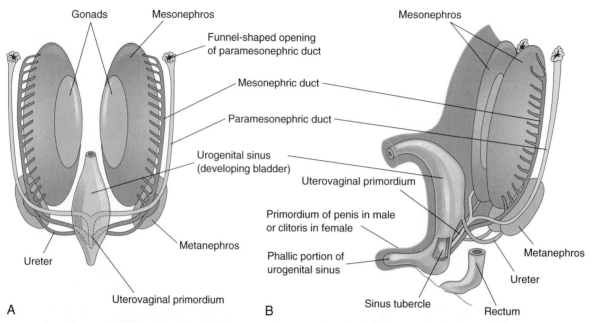

Figure 13–21 **A,** Ventral view of a 7-week embryo, showing the two pairs of genital ducts that are present during the indifferent state of sexual development. **B,** Lateral view of a 9-week fetus, showing the sinus tubercle on the posterior wall of the urogenital sinus. It becomes the hymen in females (Fig. 13-20C) and the seminal colliculus in males.

DETERMINATION OF FETAL SEX

Assessment of fetal sex by transabdominal ultrasound is important for decision making especially in pregnancies at risk of serious X-linked abnormalities. Assessment is based on the direct visualization of the external genitalia. By the 12th week of gestation the genital tubercle has differentiated to form the penis. Several studies indicate that sex assignment is highly accurate in most cases (99%–100%) after 13 weeks of gestation providing the external genitalia are not malformed. The accuracy of diagnosis increases with gestational age and depends on the experience of the sonographer, the equipment, the position of the fetus, and the amount of amniotic fluid.

external genitalia. **Labioscrotal swellings** and **urogenital folds** soon develop on each side of the cloacal membrane. The genital tubercle soon elongates to form a **primordial phallus** (Fig. 13-24B). When the urorectal septum fuses with the cloacal membrane at the end of the sixth week, it divides the cloacal membrane into a dorsal anal membrane and a ventral urogenital membrane The **urethral membrane** lies in the floor of a median cleft, the **urethral groove**, which is bound by the urogenital folds (Fig. 13-24C and D). The anal and urogenital membranes rupture approximately 1 week later, forming the anus and the **urogenital orifice**, respectively. In the female fetus, the urethra and vagina open into a common cavity, the **vestibule of the vagina**.

Development of Male External Genitalia

Masculinization of the indifferent external genitalia is induced by **dihydrotestosterone** (Fig. 13-24C, E, and G). As the primordial phallus enlarges and elongates to become the penis, the urogenital folds form the lateral walls of the **urethral groove** on the ventral surface of the penis. This groove is lined by a proliferation of endodermal cells, the **urethral plate** (Fig. 13-24C), which extends from the phallic portion of the urogenital sinus. The **urethral folds** fuse with each other along the ventral surface of the penis to form the **spongy urethra** (Fig. 13-24E_1 to E_3). The surface ectoderm fuses in the median plane of the penis, forming the **penile raphe** and enclosing the spongy urethra within the penis. At the tip of the **glans penis**, an ectodermal ingrowth forms a cellular ectodermal cord, which extends toward the root of the penis to meet the spongy urethra (Fig. 13-15A). This cord canalizes and joins the previously formed spongy urethra (Fig. 13-15B). This juncture completes the terminal part of the urethra and moves the external urethral orifice to the tip of the glans penis (see Fig. 13-15C). During the 12th week, a circular ingrowth of ectoderm occurs at the periphery of the glans penis (Fig. 13-15B). When this ingrowth breaks down, it forms the **prepuce** (foreskin) (Fig. 13-15C). The **corpora cavernosa** penis and the **corpus spongiosum** penis develop from mesenchyme in the phallus. The **labioscrotal swellings** grow toward each other and fuse to form the **scrotum** (Fig. 13-24E). The

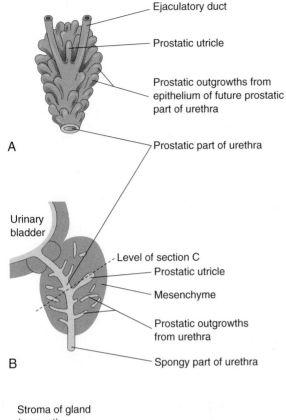

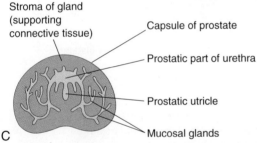

Figure 13–22 **A,** Dorsal view of the developing prostate in an 11-week fetus. **B,** Median section of the developing urethra and prostate. **C,** Section of the prostate (at 16 weeks) at the level shown in *B.*

line of fusion of these folds is clearly visible as the **scrotal raphe** (Fig. 13-24G).

Development of Female External Genitalia

Growth of the primordial phallus in the female fetus gradually decreases as it becomes the **clitoris** (Fig. 13-24D, F, and H). The clitoris develops in the same way as the penis, except that the urogenital folds do not fuse, but for posteriorly, where they join to form the **frenulum of the labia minora**. The unfused parts of the urogenital folds form the **labia minora**. The labioscrotal folds fuse posteriorly to form the **posterior labial commissure** and anteriorly to form the **anterior labial commissure** and the **mons pubis**. Most parts of the **labioscrotal folds** remain unfused and form two large folds of skin, the **labia majora**.

INTERSEX DISORDERS

Advances in molecular genetics have led to a better understanding of abnormal sexual development and ambiguous genitalia. Because of psychosocial stigma and in order to provide better clinical management for infants born with atypical chromosomal constitution or gonads, a new nomenclature has been introduced to describe these conditions, which are now called **disorders of sex development (DSD)**. The new classification avoids using the term "hermaphrodite." (See Lee PA, Houk CP, Ahmed SF, Hughes IA: Consensus statement on management of intersex disorders. *Pediatrics* 118:e488, 2006.)

OVOTESTICULAR DSD (TRUE HERMAPHRODITISM)

Persons with the extremely rare intersexual condition of ovotesticular DSD (true hermaphroditism) usually have a 46, XX sex chromosome constitution. Ovotesticular DSD results from an error in sex determination, and these individuals have both testicular and ovarian tissue. The phenotype may be male or female, but the external genitalia are always ambiguous.

46, XX DSD (FEMALE PSEUDOHERMAPHRODITISM)

Females with 46, XX DSD (female pseudohermaphroditism) result from exposure of a female fetus to excessive androgens, the principal effect of which is virilization of the external genitalia (Fig. 13-25). Persons with this intersexual condition have *chromatin-positive nuclei* and a 46, XX chromosome constitution. The common cause of 46, XX DSD is **congenital adrenal hyperplasia**. There is no ovarian abnormality, but the excessive production of androgens by the fetal suprarenal glands causes masculinization of the external genitalia, varying from enlargement of the clitoris to almost masculine genitalia. Commonly, **clitoral hypertrophy**, partial fusion of the labia majora, and a persistent urogenital sinus are noted.

46, XY DSD (MALE PSEUDOHERMAPHRODITISM)

Males with 46, XY DSD (male pseudohermaphroditism) have sex *chromatin-negative nuclei* and a 46, XY chromosome constitution. The external and internal genitalia are variable, owing to varying degrees of development. These anomalies are caused by inadequate production of testosterone and MIS by the fetal testes. Testicular development ranges from rudimentary to normal.

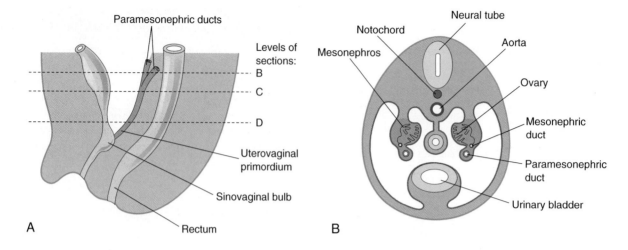

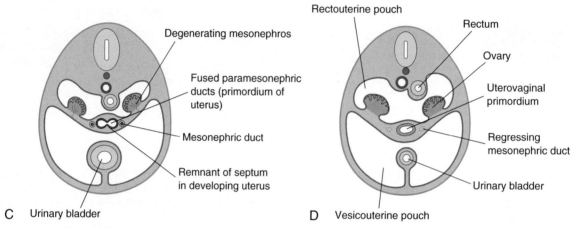

Figure 13–23 Early development of the ovaries and uterus. **A,** Sagittal section of the caudal region of an 8-week female embryo. **B,** Transverse section, showing the paramesonephric ducts approaching each other. **C,** Similar section at a more caudal level, showing fusion of the paramesonephric ducts. **D,** Similar section, showing the uterovaginal primordium, broad ligament, and pouches in the pelvic cavity.

ANDROGEN INSENSITIVITY SYNDROME

Androgen insensitivity syndrome (AIS)—also called **testicular feminization syndrome**—occurs in 1 in 20,000 live births. Individuals with this unusual condition are usually normal-appearing females, despite the presence of testes and a 46, XY chromosome constitution. The external genitalia are female but the vagina usually ends in a blind pouch and the uterus and the uterine tubes are absent or rudimentary. At puberty, there is normal development of breasts and female characteristics, but menstruation does not occur and pubic hair is scanty or absent. In some cases, the external genitalia are abnormal (e.g., enlarged clitoris and a scrotum-like structure; see Fig. 13-25). The failure of masculinization to occur in these individuals results from a resistance to the action of testosterone at the cellular level in the genital tubercle and the labioscrotal and urogenital folds.

HYPOSPADIAS

There are four types of hypospadias: glanular, penile, penoscrotal, and perineal hypospadias. Hypospadias is the most frequent anomaly involving the penis and is found in 1 in 125 male infants. In **glanular hypospadias,** the external urethral orifice is on the ventral surface of the glans penis. In **penile hypospadias** the external urethral orifice is on the ventral surface of the body of the penis. The glanular and penile types of hypospadias are the most common types (Fig. 13-26). In **penoscrotal hypospadias,** the urethral orifice is at the junction of the penis and the scrotum. In **perineal hypospadias,** the external urethral orifice is located between the unfused halves of the scrotum. Hypospadias results from inadequate production of androgens by the fetal testes. It is believed that environmental factors may disrupt testosterone-related gene expression.

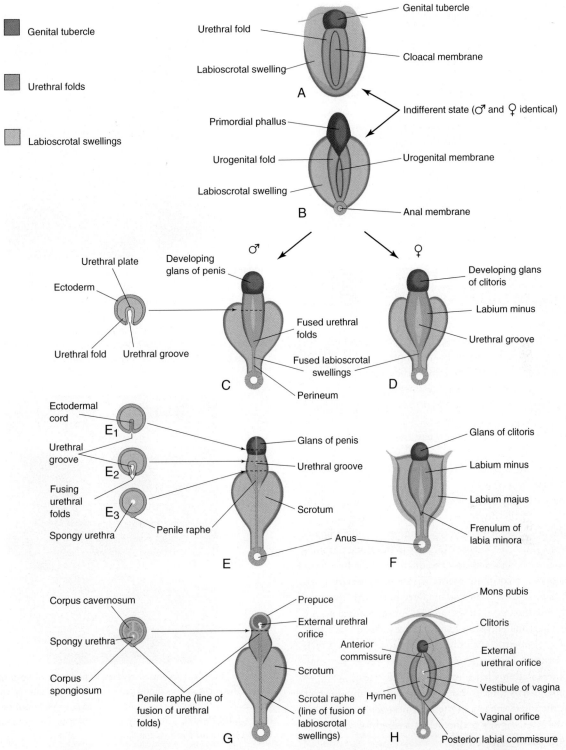

Genital tubercle

Urethral folds

Labioscrotal swellings

Figure 13–24 Development of the external genitalia. **A** and **B,** Appearance of the genitalia during the indifferent state (fourth to seventh weeks). **C, E,** and **G,** Stages in the development of the male external genitalia at 9, 11, and 12 weeks, respectively. On the *left* are schematic transverse sections of the developing penis, showing the formation of the spongy urethra and scrotum. **D, F,** and **H,** Stages in the development of the female external genitalia at 9, 11, and 12 weeks, respectively.

EPISPADIAS

In a rare condition known as **epispadias**, the urethra opens on the dorsal surface of the penis. It is *often associated with exstrophy of the bladder* (see Fig. 13-13). Epispadias may result from inadequate ectodermal-mesenchymal interactions during development of the genital tubercle. As a consequence, the genital tubercle develops more dorsally than in normal embryos. Consequently, when the urogenital membrane ruptures, the urogenital sinus opens on the dorsal surface of the penis. Urine is expelled at the root of the malformed penis.

ANOMALIES OF FEMALE GENITAL TRACT

Various types of uterine duplication and vaginal anomalies result from developmental arrest of the uterovaginal primordium during the eighth week of development (Fig. 13-27B to G). The main developmental anomalies are:

* Incomplete fusion of the paramesonephric ducts
* Incomplete development of one or both paramesonephric ducts
* Failure of parts of one or both paramesonephric ducts to develop
* Incomplete canalization of the vaginal plate that forms the vagina

In some cases, the uterus is divided internally by a septum (Fig. 13-27F). If the duplication involves only the superior part of the body of the uterus, the condition is called **bicornuate uterus** (Fig. 13-27D and E). If growth of one paramesonephric duct is retarded and the duct does not fuse with the other one, a **bicornuate uterus with a rudimentary horn** develops (Fig. 13-27E). The rudimentary horn may not communicate with the cavity of the uterus. A **unicornuate uterus** develops when one paramesonephric duct does not develop; this results in a uterus with one uterine tube (Fig. 13-27G). In many of these cases, the individuals are fertile, but may have an increased incidence of premature delivery.

A **double uterus** (uterus didelphys) results from failure of fusion of the inferior parts of the paramesonephric ducts. It may be associated with a double or a single vagina (Fig. 13-27B and C).

Agenesis of the vagina results from failure of the sinovaginal bulbs to develop and form the vaginal plate (Fig. 13-20B). When the vagina is absent, the uterus is usually absent also, because the developing uterus (uterovaginal primordium) induces the formation of sinovaginal bulbs, which fuse to form the vaginal plate. Failure of canalization of the vaginal plate results in blockage of the vagina. Failure of the inferior end of the vaginal plate to perforate results in an **imperforate hymen** (Fig. 13-20C).

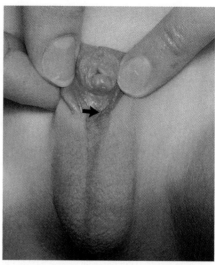

Figure 13–25   External genitalia of a 6-year-old girl, showing an enlarged clitoris and a scrotum-like structure formed by fusion of the labia majora. The *arrow* indicates the opening into the urogenital sinus (see Fig. 13-11C). This extreme masculinization is the result of congenital adrenal hyperplasia. (*Courtesy of Dr. Heather Dean, Department of Pediatrics and Child Health, University of Manitoba, Winnipeg, Manitoba, Canada.*)

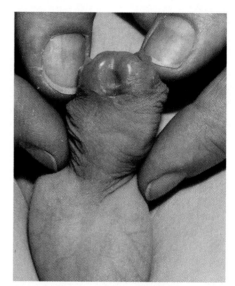

Figure 13–26   Glanular hypospadias in a male infant. There is a shallow pit in the glans penis at the usual site of the urethral orifice. (*Courtesy of A.E. Chudley, M.D., Department of Pediatrics and Child Health, University of Manitoba, Children's Hospital, Winnipeg, Manitoba, Canada.*)

DEVELOPMENT OF INGUINAL CANALS

The inguinal canals form pathways for the testes to descend from their intra-abdominal position through the anterior abdominal wall and into the scrotum. *Inguinal canals develop in both sexes* because of the morphologically indifferent state of sexual development. As the mesonephros degenerates, a ligament called the **gubernaculum** develops on each side of the abdomen from the inferior pole of the gonad (Fig. 13-28A). The

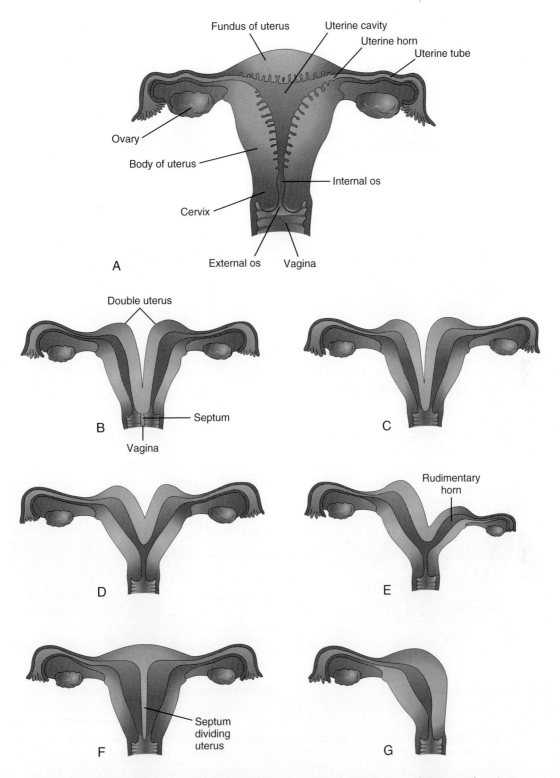

Figure 13–27 Various types of congenital uterine anomalies. **A,** Normal uterus and vagina. **B,** Double uterus (uterus didelphys) and double vagina. Note the septum dividing the vagina. **C,** Double uterus with a single vagina. **D,** Bicornuate uterus (two uterine horns). **E,** Bicornuate uterus with a rudimentary left horn. **F,** Septate uterus. Note the septum dividing the uterus. **G,** Unicornuate uterus. Note that only half of the uterus exists.

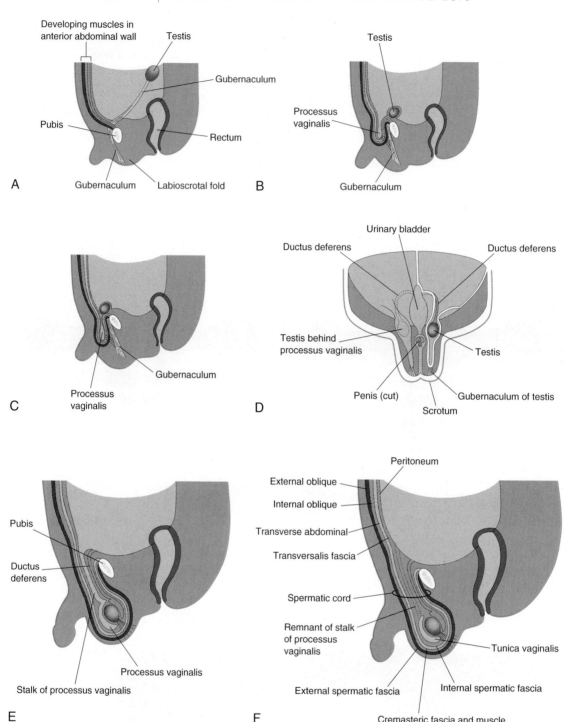

Figure 13–28   Formation of the inguinal canals and descent of the testes. **A,** Sagittal section of a 7-week embryo, showing the testis adjacent to the dorsal abdominal wall. **B** and **C,** Similar sections at approximately 28 weeks, showing the processus vaginalis and the testis beginning to pass through the inguinal canal. Note that the processus vaginalis carries fascial layers of the abdominal wall before it. **D,** Frontal section of a fetus approximately 3 days later, showing descent of the testis posterior to the processus vaginalis. The processus vaginalis has been cut away on the *left side* to show the testis and ductus deferens. **E,** Sagittal section of a newborn male infant, showing the processus vaginalis communicating with the peritoneal cavity by a narrow stalk. **F,** Similar section of a 1-month-old male infant after obliteration of the stalk of the processus vaginalis. Note that the extended fascial layers of the abdominal wall now form the coverings of the spermatic cord.

gubernaculum passes obliquely through the developing anterior abdominal wall at the site of the future inguinal anal. The gubernaculum attaches caudally to the internal surface of the **labioscrotal swellings**.

The **processus vaginalis**, an evagination of peritoneum, develops ventral to the gubernaculum and herniates through the abdominal wall along the path formed by the gubernaculum (Fig. 13-28B to E). The processus vaginalis carries extensions of the layers of the abdominal wall, which form the walls of the inguinal canal. In males, these layers also form the coverings of the spermatic cord and the testis (Fig. 13-28E and F). The opening in the transversalis fascia produced by the vaginal process becomes the **deep inguinal ring**, and the opening created in the external oblique aponeurosis forms the **superficial inguinal ring**.

Descent of Testes

By 26 weeks, the testes have descended retroperitoneally from the posterior abdominal wall to the deep inguinal rings (see Fig. 13-28B and C). This change in position occurs as the fetal pelvis enlarges and the trunk of the embryo elongates. Transabdominal movement of the testes is largely a relative movement that results from growth of the cranial part of the abdomen away from the future pelvic region.

Testicular descent through the inguinal canals and into the scrotum is controlled by androgens (e.g., testosterone) produced by the fetal testes. The gubernaculum appears to guide the testes during their descent. Descent of the testes through the inguinal canals and into the scrotum usually begins during the 26th week and takes 2 to 3 days. When the testis descends, it carries its ductus deferens and vessels with it. As the testis and the ductus deferens descend, they are ensheathed by the fascial extensions of the abdominal wall (Fig. 13-28F):

● The extension of the transversalis fascia becomes the internal spermatic fascia.

● The extensions of the internal oblique muscle and the fascia become the cremasteric muscle and fascia.
● The extension of the external oblique aponeurosis becomes the external spermatic fascia.

Within the scrotum, the testis projects into the distal end of the processus vaginalis. During the perinatal period, the connecting stalk of the process is usually obliterated, isolating the **tunica vaginalis** as a peritoneal sac related to the testis (Fig. 13-28F).

Descent of Ovaries

The ovaries also descend from the posterior abdominal wall to the pelvis, just inferior to the pelvic brim. The gubernaculum is attached to the uterus near the attachment of the uterine tube. The cranial part of the gubernaculum becomes the **ovarian ligament** and the caudal part forms the **round ligament** of the uterus (Fig. 13-20C). The round ligaments pass through the inguinal canals and terminate in the labia majora. The relatively small processus vaginalis in the female is usually obliterated and it disappears long before birth.

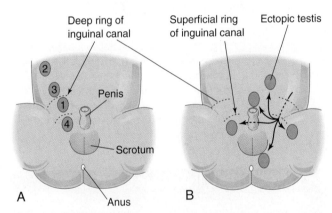

Figure 13–29 Possible sites of cryptorchid and ectopic testes. **A,** Positions of cryptorchid testes, numbered 1 to 4 in order of increasing frequency. **B,** Usual locations of ectopic testes.

CRYPTORCHIDISM

Cryptorchidism (undescended testes) occurs in up to 30% of premature male infants and in approximately 3% to 4% of full-term male infants. Cryptorchidism may be unilateral or bilateral. In most cases, the testes descend into the scrotum by the end of the first year. If both testes remain within or just outside the abdominal cavity, they do not mature and sterility is common. If uncorrected, there is a significantly higher risk for the development of germ cell tumors, especially in cases of abdominal cryptorchidism. **Cryptorchid testes** may be in the abdominal cavity or anywhere along the usual path of descent of the testis, but they are usually in the inguinal canal (Fig. 13-29A). The cause of most cases of cryptorchidism is unknown, but a deficiency of androgen production by the fetal testes is an important factor.

ECTOPIC TESTES

After traversing the inguinal canal, the testis may deviate from its usual path of descent and lodge in various abnormal locations (Fig. 13-29B):
* Interstitial (external to the aponeurosis of the external oblique muscle)
* In the proximal part of the medial thigh
* Dorsal to the penis
* On the opposite side (crossed ectopia)

All types of ectopic testis are rare, but **interstitial ectopia** occurs most frequently. Ectopic testis occurs when a part of the gubernaculum passes to an abnormal location and the testis follows it.

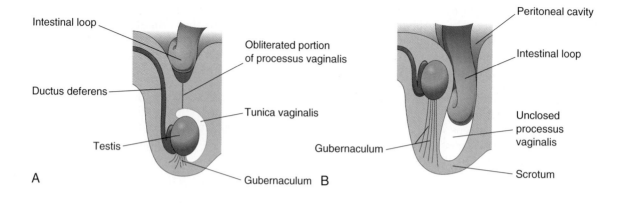

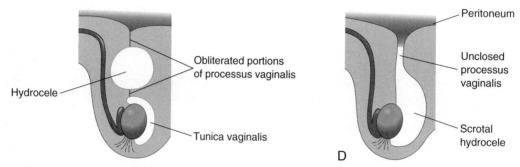

Figure 13–30 Sagittal sections showing conditions resulting from failure of closure of the processus vaginalis. **A,** Incomplete congenital inguinal hernia resulting from persistence of the proximal part of the processus vaginalis. **B,** Complete congenital inguinal hernia entering the unclosed processus in the scrotum. Cryptorchidism, a commonly associated condition is also shown. **C,** Large hydrocele that arose from an unobliterated portion of the processus vaginalis. **D,** Hydrocele of the testis and the spermatic cord resulting from peritoneal fluid passing into a patent processus vaginalis.

CONGENITAL INGUINAL HERNIA

If the communication between the tunica vaginalis and the peritoneal cavity does not close, a **persistent processus vaginalis** occurs. A loop of intestine may herniate through it into the scrotum or labia majora (Fig. 13-30A and B). Embryonic remnants resembling the ductus deferens or the epididymis are often found in inguinal hernial sacs. Congenital inguinal hernia is much more common in males than in females and it is often associated with cryptorchidism and, in females, with androgen insensitivity syndrome.

HYDROCELE

Occasionally, the abdominal end of the processus vaginalis remains open, but is too small to permit herniation of the intestine (Fig. 13-30D). In such cases, peritoneal fluid passes into the patent processus vaginalis and forms a **hydrocele of the testis.** If the middle part of the processus vaginalis remains open, fluid may accumulate and give rise to a **hydrocele of the spermatic cord** (Fig. 13-30C).

CLINICALLY ORIENTED QUESTIONS

1. Does a horseshoe kidney usually function normally? What problems may occur with this anomaly and how can they be corrected?

2. A patient was told that he has two kidneys on one side and none on the other. How did this abnormality probably happen? Are there likely to be any problems associated with this condition?

3. Are individuals with ovotesticular DSD (true hermaphrodites) ever fertile?

4. When a baby is born with ambiguous external genitalia, how long does it take to assign the appropriate sex? What does the physician tell the parents? How is the appropriate sex determined?

5. What is the most common type of disorder that produces ambiguous external genitalia? Will masculinizing, or androgenic, hormones given during the fetal period of development cause ambiguity of the external genitalia in female fetuses?

The answers to these questions are at the back of the book.

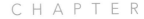
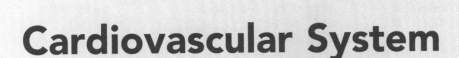

Cardiovascular System

*T*he cardiovascular system is the first major system to function in the embryo. The primordial heart and vascular system appear in the middle of the third week of development (Fig. 14-1). The heart begins to beat at 22 to 23 days (Fig. 14-2). This precocious development is necessary because the rapidly growing embryo can no longer satisfy its nutritional and oxygen requirements by diffusion alone.

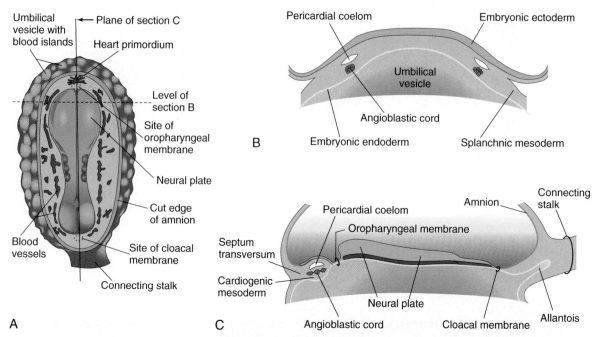

Figure 14–1   Early development of the heart. **A,** Dorsal view of an embryo (approximately 18 days). **B,** Transverse section of the embryo, showing angioblastic cords and their relationship to the pericardial coelom. **C,** Longitudinal section through the embryo, showing the relationship of the angioblastic cords to the oropharyngeal membrane, pericardial coelom, and septum transversum.

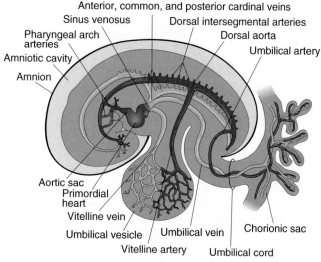

Figure 14–2   The embryonic cardiovascular system (at approximately 26 days), showing vessels on the left side only. The umbilical vein carries well-oxygenated blood and nutrients from the chorion (the embryonic part of the placenta) to the embryo. The umbilical arteries carry poorly oxygenated blood and waste products from the embryo to the chorionic sac.

EARLY DEVELOPMENT OF THE HEART AND BLOOD VESSELS

Paired endothelial strands—**angioblastic cords**—appear in the cardiogenic mesoderm during the third week of development (Fig. 14-1*B* and *C*). These cords canalize to form two **heart tubes** that soon fuse to form a single **heart**

tube late in the third week (see Fig. 14-5). An inductive influence from the anterior endoderm stimulates early formation of the heart. Cardiac morphogenesis is controlled by a cascade of *regulatory genes and transcription factors.*

Development of Embryonic Veins Associated with the Heart

Three paired veins drain into the tubular heart of a 4-week embryo (Fig. 14-2):

- *Vitelline veins* return poorly oxygenated blood from the umbilical vesicle (yolk sac).
- *Umbilical veins* carry well-oxygenated blood from the chorionic sac (primordial placenta); only the left umbilical vein persists.
- *Common cardinal veins* return poorly oxygenated blood from the body of the embryo to the heart.

The **vitelline veins** enter the **sinus venosus** of the primordial heart (Figs. 14-2 to 14-4*A* and *B*). As the liver primordium grows into the septum transversum, the hepatic cords anastomose around preexisting endothelium-lined spaces. These spaces, the primordia of the hepatic sinusoids, later become linked to the vitelline veins. The **hepatic veins** form from the remains of the right vitelline vein in the region of the developing liver. The **portal vein** develops from an anastomotic network of vitelline veins around the duodenum (Fig. 14-4*B*). The fate of the umbilical veins may be summarized as follows (see Fig. 14-4*B*):

- The right umbilical vein and the cranial part of the left umbilical vein between the liver and the sinus venosus degenerate.
- The persistent caudal part of the left umbilical vein becomes the umbilical vein, which carries well-oxygenated blood from the placenta to the embryo.
- A large venous shunt—the ductus venosus—develops within the liver and connects the umbilical vein with the inferior vena cava (IVC).

The **cardinal veins** (Figs. 14-2 and 14-3A) constitute the main venous drainage system of the embryo. The anterior and posterior cardinal veins drain the cranial and caudal parts of the embryo, respectively (Fig. 14-3A). These join the **common cardinal veins**, which enter the **sinus venosus** (Fig. 14-4A). During the eighth week, the **anterior cardinal veins** are connected by an oblique anastomosis (Fig. 14-4B) that shunts blood from the left to the right anterior cardinal vein. This shunt becomes the **left brachiocephalic vein** when the caudal part of the left anterior cardinal vein degenerates (Figs. 14-3D and 14-4C). The **superior vena cava** (SVC) forms from the right anterior cardinal vein and the right common cardinal vein. The only adult derivatives of the posterior cardinal veins are the root of the azygos vein and the common iliac veins.

The subcardinal and supracardinal veins gradually replace and supplement the posterior cardinal veins. The **subcardinal veins** appear first (Fig. 14-3A) and form the stem of the left renal vein, the suprarenal veins, the gonadal veins (testicular and ovarian), and a segment of the inferior vena cava (Fig. 14-3D). The **supracardinal veins** become disrupted in the region of the kidneys (Fig. 14-3C). Cranial to this, they become united by an anastomosis that forms the **azygos** and the **hemiazygos veins** (Figs. 14-3D and 14-4C). Caudal to the kidneys, the left supracardinal vein degenerates but the right supracardinal vein becomes the inferior part of the IVC (Fig. 14-3D). The **IVC** forms as blood returning from the caudal part of the embryo is shifted from the left to the right side of the body.

Pharyngeal Arch Arteries and Other Branches of the Dorsal Aorta

As the *pharyngeal arches* form during the fourth and fifth weeks of development, they are supplied by **pharyngeal arch arteries** that arise from the **aortic sac** and terminate in the **dorsal aortae** (Fig. 14-2). Initially, the paired dorsal aortae run through the entire length of the embryo. Later, the caudal portions of the paired dorsal aortae fuse to form a single lower thoracic/abdominal aorta. Of the remaining paired dorsal aortae, the right regresses and the left becomes the primordial aorta.

Intersegmental Arteries

Thirty or so branches of the dorsal aorta, collectively known as the **intersegmental arteries**, pass between and carry blood to the somites and their derivatives (Fig. 14-2). The intersegmental arteries in the neck join to form the **vertebral arteries**. Most of the original connections of the intersegmental arteries to the dorsal aorta eventually

disappear. In the thorax, the intersegmental arteries persist as **intercostal arteries**. Most of the intersegmental arteries in the abdomen become **lumbar arteries**; however, the fifth pair of lumbar intersegmental arteries remains as the **common iliac arteries**. In the sacral region, the intersegmental arteries form the lateral sacral arteries. The caudal end of the dorsal aorta becomes the median sacral artery.

Fate of Vitelline and Umbilical Arteries

The unpaired ventral branches of the dorsal aorta supply the umbilical vesicle, allantois, and chorion (Fig. 14-2). The **vitelline arteries** supply the umbilical vesicle (yolk sac) and later, the primordial gut, which forms from the incorporated part of the umbilical vesicle. Only three vitelline arteries remain: the *celiac arterial trunk* to the foregut; the *superior mesenteric artery* to the midgut, and the *inferior mesenteric artery* to the hindgut.

The paired **umbilical arteries** pass through the connecting stalk (primordial umbilical cord) and join the vessels in the chorion. The umbilical arteries carry poorly oxygenated fetal blood to the placenta (Fig. 14-2). The proximal parts of these arteries become the internal iliac arteries and the superior vesical arteries, whereas the distal parts are obliterated after birth and become the medial umbilical ligaments.

LATER DEVELOPMENT OF THE HEART

As the heart tubes fuse, the external layer of the embryonic heart, the **primordial myocardium** is formed from the splanchnic mesoderm surrounding the **pericardial coelom** (Figs. 14-5 and 14-6B and C). At this stage, the developing heart is composed of a thin tube, separated from a thick primordial myocardium by gelatinous connective tissue called **cardiac jelly** (Fig. 14-6C and D). The endothelial tube becomes the internal endothelial lining of the heart, the **endocardium**, and the primordial myocardium becomes the muscular wall of the heart, the **myocardium**. The epicardium is derived from the mesothelial cells that arise from the external surface of the sinus venosus (Fig. 14-6F).

As folding of the head region occurs, the heart and the pericardial cavity appear ventral to the foregut and caudal to the oropharyngeal membrane (Fig. 14-7A to C). Concurrently, the tubular heart elongates and develops alternate dilations and constrictions (Fig. 14-5C to E): the **bulbus cordis** (composed of the **truncus arteriosus**, conus arteriosus, and conus cordis), ventricle, the atrium, and the sinus venosus.

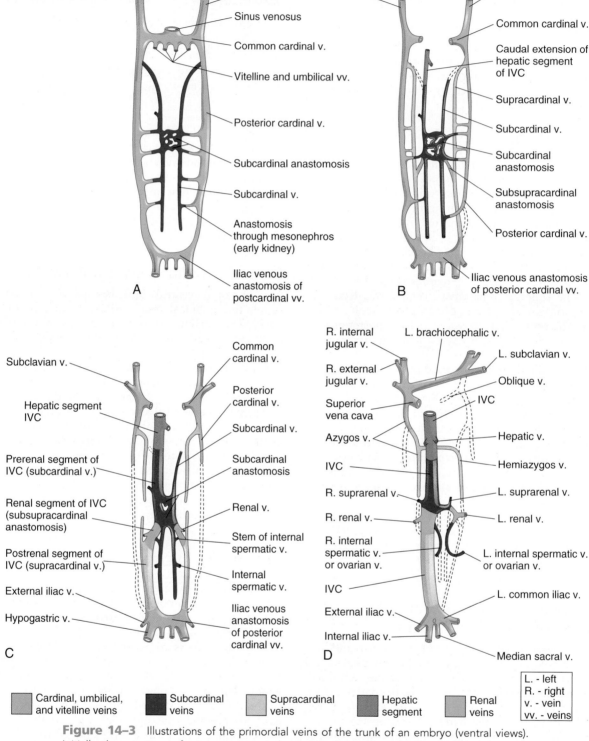

Figure 14–3 legend:
- Cardinal, umbilical, and vitelline veins
- Subcardinal veins
- Supracardinal veins
- Hepatic segment
- Renal veins

L. - left
R. - right
v. - vein
vv. - veins

Figure 14–3 Illustrations of the primordial veins of the trunk of an embryo (ventral views). Initially, three systems of veins are present: the umbilical veins from the chorionic sac, the vitelline veins from the umbilical vesicle, and the cardinal veins from the body of the embryo. Next, the subcardinal veins appear, and finally the supracardinal veins develop. **A,** At 6 weeks. **B,** At 7 weeks. **C,** At 8 weeks. **D,** Adult, showing the transformations that produce the adult venous pattern. *(Modified from Arey LB: Developmental Anatomy, rev. 7th ed. Philadelphia, WB Saunders, 1974).*

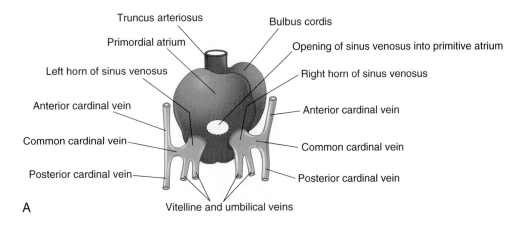

Truncus arteriosus

Primordial atrium

Left horn of sinus venosus

Anterior cardinal vein

Common cardinal vein

Posterior cardinal vein

Bulbus cordis

Opening of sinus venosus into primitive atrium

Right horn of sinus venosus

Anterior cardinal vein

Common cardinal vein

Posterior cardinal vein

A

Vitelline and umbilical veins

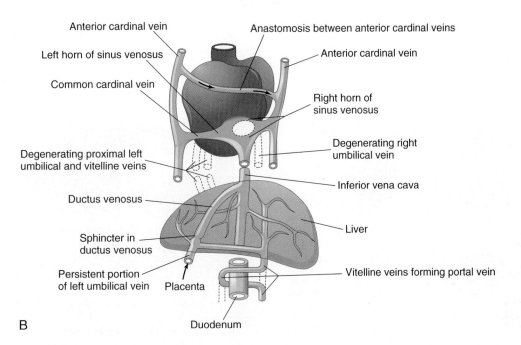

Anterior cardinal vein

Left horn of sinus venosus

Common cardinal vein

Degenerating proximal left umbilical and vitelline veins

Ductus venosus

Sphincter in ductus venosus

Persistent portion of left umbilical vein

Placenta

B

Duodenum

Anastomosis between anterior cardinal veins

Anterior cardinal vein

Right horn of sinus venosus

Degenerating right umbilical vein

Inferior vena cava

Liver

Vitelline veins forming portal vein

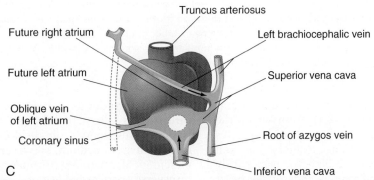

Future right atrium

Future left atrium

Oblique vein of left atrium

Coronary sinus

C

Truncus arteriosus

Left brachiocephalic vein

Superior vena cava

Root of azygos vein

Inferior vena cava

Figure 14–4   Dorsal views of the developing heart. **A,** During the fourth week (approximately 24 days); the primordial atrium and the sinus venosus, as well as the veins draining into them, are evident. **B,** At 7 weeks, the right sinual horn is enlarged and the venous circulation through the liver is established. (The organs are not drawn to scale.) **C,** At 8 weeks, showing the adult derivatives of the cardinal veins. *Arrows* indicate the flow of blood.

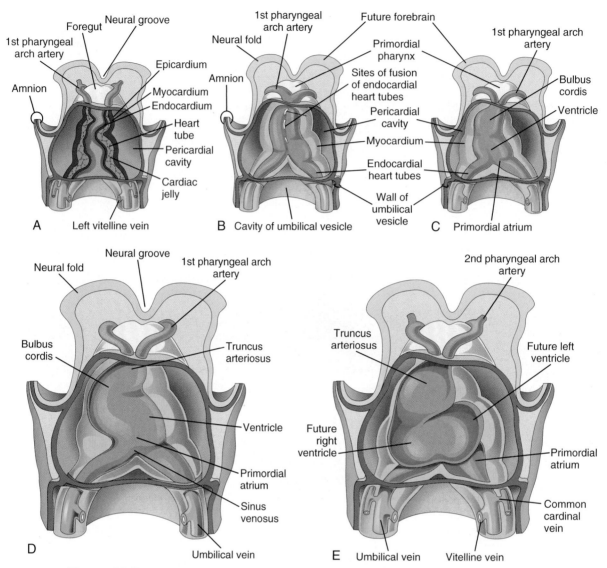

Figure 14–5 **A** to **C,** Ventral views of the developing heart and the pericardial region (22–35 days). The ventral pericardial wall has been removed to show the developing myocardium and fusion of the two heart tubes to form a single heart tube. Fusion begins at the cranial ends of the tubes and extends caudally until a single tubular heart is formed. **D** and **E,** As the tubular heart elongates, it bends on itself, forming an S-shaped heart.

The tubular **truncus arteriosus** (TA) is continuous cranially with the aortic sac (Fig. 14-8*A*), from which the pharyngeal arch arteries arise. The **sinus venosus** receives the umbilical, vitelline, and common cardinal veins from the chorion, umbilical vesicle, and embryo, respectively (Fig. 14-4*A*). The arterial and venous ends of the heart are fixed by the pharyngeal arches and the septum transversum, respectively. Because the **bulbus cordis** and ventricle grow faster than the other regions, the heart bends on itself, forming a U-shaped **bulboventricular loop** (Fig. 14-6*E*). *Transforming growth factor β nodal is involved in looping of the heart tube.* As the primordial heart bends, the atrium and sinus venosus appear dorsal to the truncus arteriosus, bulbus cordis, and ventricle (Fig. 14-8*A* and *B*). By this stage, the sinus venosus has developed lateral expansions, the right and left **horns of the sinus venosus.**

As the heart develops, it gradually invaginates the **pericardial cavity** (Figs. 14-6*C* and *D* and 14-7*C*). The heart is initially suspended from the dorsal wall by a mesentery, the **dorsal mesocardium.** However, the central part of this mesentery degenerates, forming a communication—the **transverse pericardial sinus**—between the right and left sides of the pericardial cavity (Fig. 14-6*E* and *F*). At this stage, the heart is attached only at its cranial and caudal ends.

Circulation through Primordial Heart

Blood enters the sinus venosus (Fig. 14-8*A* and 14-4*A*) from the:

● Embryo through the common cardinal veins
● Developing placenta through the umbilical veins
● Umbilical vesicle through the vitelline veins

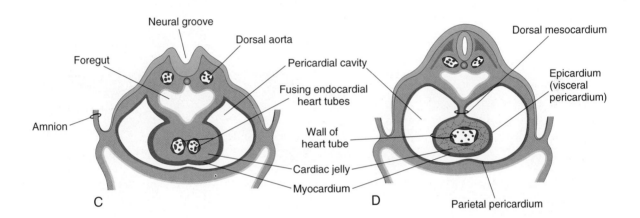

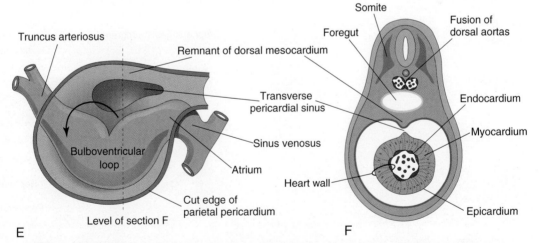

Figure 14–6 **A,** Dorsal view of an embryo (approximately 20 days). **B,** Schematic transverse section of the heart region of the embryo illustrated in **A,** showing the two endocardial heart tubes and the lateral folds of the body. **C,** Transverse section of a slightly older embryo, showing the formation of the pericardial cavity and the fusing heart tubes. **D,** Similar section (approximately 22 days), showing the single heart tube suspended by the dorsal mesocardium. **E,** Schematic drawing of the heart (approximately 28 days), showing degeneration of the central part of the dorsal mesocardium and formation of the transverse sinus of the pericardium. The *arrow* shows bending of the primordial heart. **F,** Transverse section of the embryo at the level seen in **E,** showing the layers of the heart wall.

Figure 14–7 Longitudinal sections through the cranial half of human embryos during the fourth week of development. The effect of the head fold (*arrows*) on the position of the heart and other structures is shown. **A** and **B,** As the head fold develops, the heart tube and the pericardial cavity come to lie ventral to the foregut and caudal to the oropharyngeal membrane. **C,** Note that the positions of the pericardial cavity and the septum transversum have reversed with respect to each other. The septum transversum now lies posterior to the pericardial cavity, where it will form the central tendon of the diaphragm.

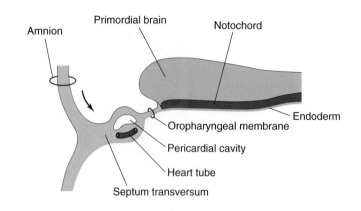

A

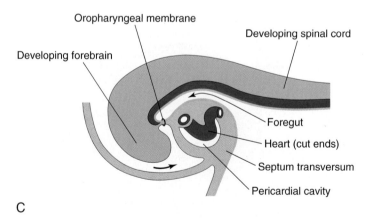

B

C

Blood from the sinus venosus enters the **primordial atrium;** flow from it is controlled by **sinuatrial valves** (Fig. 14-8*A*). The blood then passes through the **atrioventricular canal** into the **primordial ventricle.** When the ventricle contracts, blood is pumped through the **bulbus cordis** and **truncus arteriosus** into the **aortic sac,** from which it is distributed to the pharyngeal arch arteries (Fig. 14-8*B*). The blood then passes into the dorsal aortae for distribution to the embryo, umbilical vesicle, and placenta.

Partitioning of Primordial Heart

Partitioning of the atrioventricular (AV) canal, primordial atrium, and ventricle begins at approximately the middle of the fourth week and is essentially completed by the end of the eighth week.

Toward the end of the fourth week, **endocardial cushions** form on the dorsal and ventral walls of the AV canal (Fig. 14-8*A*). These cushions approach each other and fuse, dividing the AV canal into right and left AV canals

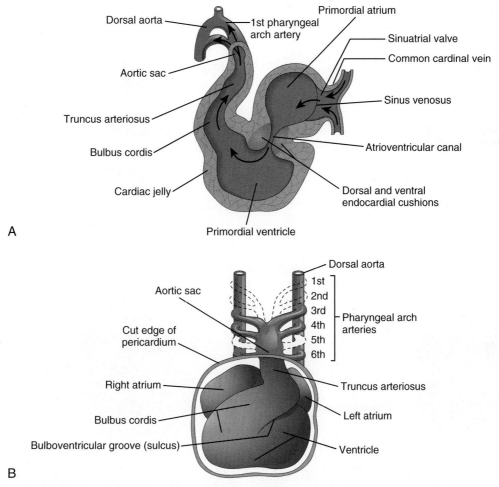

Figure 14–8 **A,** Sagittal section of the primordial heart (approximately 24 days), showing blood flowing through it (*arrows*). **B,** Ventral view of the heart and the pharyngeal arch arteries (approximately 35 days). The ventral wall of the pericardial sac has been removed to show the heart in the pericardial cavity.

(Fig. 14-9*B*). These canals partially separate the primordial atrium from the ventricle, and the cushions function as AV valves. The endocardial cushions develop from a specialized extracellular matrix related to the myocardium. *Its formation is associated with the expression of transforming growth factor b2 and bone morphogenetic factors 2A and 4.*

Partitioning of Primordial Atrium

The primordial atrium is divided into right and left atria by the formation and subsequent modification and fusion of two septa, the septum primum and the septum secundum (Figs. 14-9*A* to *E* and 14-10).

The **septum primum** grows toward the fusing endocardial cushions from the roof of the primordial atrium, partially dividing the atrium into right and left halves. As this curtain-like septum develops, a large opening—the **foramen primum**—forms between its free edge and the endocardial cushions (Figs. 14-9*C* and 14-10*A* to *C*). The foramen allows shunting of oxygenated blood from the right to the left atrium. The foramen becomes progressively smaller and disappears as the septum primum

fuses with the fused endocardial cushions to form the **primordial AV septum** (see Fig. 14-10*D* and *D₁*).

Before the foramen primum disappears, perforations, produced by **apoptosis** (**programmed cell death**), appear in the central part of the septum primum. As the free edge of the septum primum fuses with the left side of the fused endocardial cushions, obliterating the foramen primum (Figs. 14-9*D* and 14-10*D*), the perforations coalesce to form another opening—the **foramen secundum** (Fig. 14-10*C*). The foramen secundum ensures continued shunting of oxygenated blood from the right to the left atrium.

The **septum secundum** grows from the ventrocranial wall of the atrium, immediately to the right of the septum primum (Fig. 14-10*D₁*). As this crescentic, muscular septum grows during the fifth and sixth weeks, it gradually overlaps the foramen secundum in the septum primum (Fig. 14-10*E* and *F*). The septum secundum forms an incomplete partition between the atria; the opening in the foramen secundum is called the **oval foramen** (*foramen ovale*). The cranial part of the septum primum gradually disappears (Fig. 14-10*G₁*).

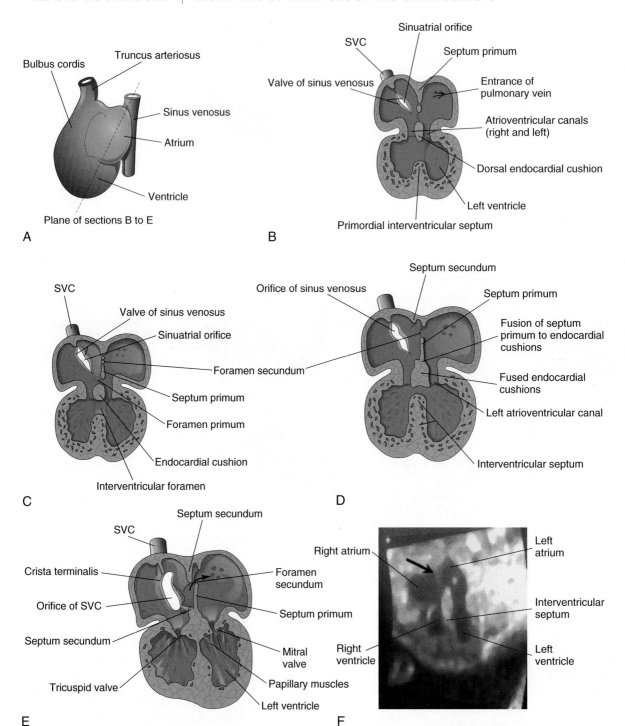

Figure 14–9   The developing heart, showing partitioning of the atrioventricular canal, the primordial atrium, and the ventricle. **A,** The plane of sections **B** to **E. B,** At the fourth week (approximately 28 days), showing the early appearance of the septum primum, the interventricular septum, and the dorsal endocardial cushion. **C,** Frontal section of the heart (approximately 32 days), showing perforations in the dorsal part of the septum primum. **D,** Frontal section of the heart (approximately 35 days), showing the foramen secundum. **E,** At approximately 8 weeks, the heart is partitioned into four chambers. The *arrow* indicates the flow of well-oxygenated blood from the right to the left atrium. **F,** Sonogram of a second-trimester fetus, showing the four chambers of the heart. Note the septum secundum (*arrow*) and the descending aorta. *(F, Courtesy of Dr. G.J. Reid, Department of Obstetrics, Gynecology and Reproductive Sciences, University of Manitoba, Women's Hospital, Winnipeg, Manitoba, Canada.)*

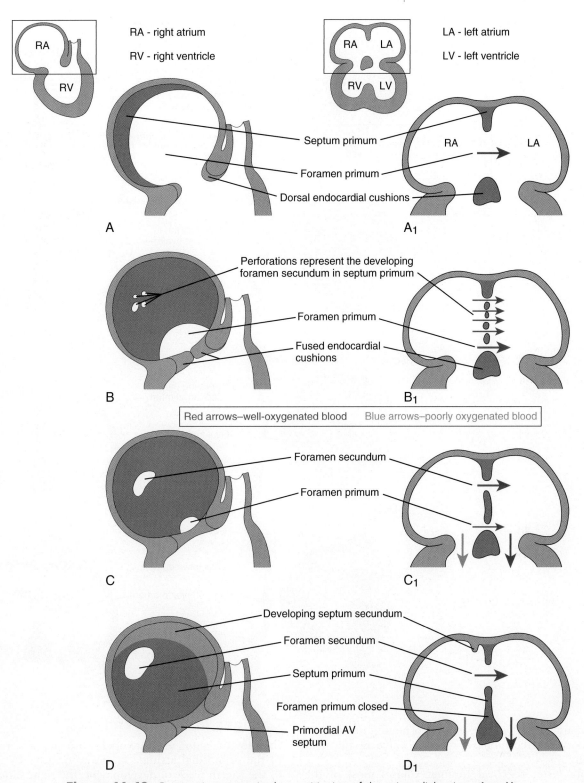

RA - right atrium

RV - right ventricle

LA - left atrium

LV - left ventricle

RA — LA

RV — LV

Septum primum

Foramen primum

Dorsal endocardial cushions

RA → LA

A

A₁

Perforations represent the developing
foramen secundum in septum primum

Foramen primum

Fused endocardial
cushions

B

B₁

Red arrows—well-oxygenated blood   Blue arrows—poorly oxygenated blood

Foramen secundum

Foramen primum

C

C₁

Developing septum secundum

Foramen secundum

Septum primum

Foramen primum closed

Primordial AV
septum

D

D₁

Figure 14–10 Progressive stages in the partitioning of the primordial atrium. **A** to **H,**
Views of the developing interatrial septum, as viewed from the right side. **A₁** to **H₁,** Frontal
sections of the developing interatrial septum. As the septum secundum grows, note that it
overlaps the opening (foramen secundum) in the septum primum Observe the valve of the
oval foramen in **G₁** and **H₁**.   *Continued*

Figure 14–10, cont'd

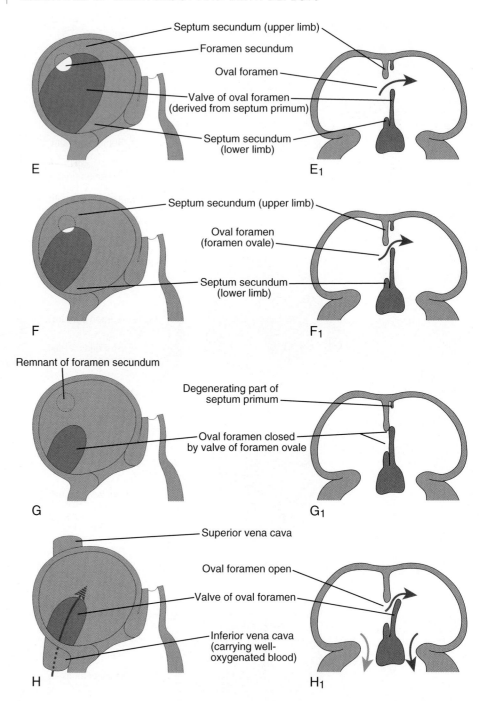

The remaining part of the septum primum, attached to the endocardial cushions, forms the **valve of the oval foramen.**

Before birth, the oval foramen allows most of the oxygenated blood entering the right atrium from the IVC to pass into the left atrium (Fig. 14-10H_1). It also prevents the passage of blood in the opposite direction—the septum primum would close against the relatively rigid septum secundum (Fig. 14-10G_1). *After birth*, the oval foramen functionally closes due to higher pressure in the left atrium, and the valve of the oval foramen fuses with the septum secundum, forming the oval fossa (fossa ovalis). As a result, the interatrial septum becomes a complete partition between the atria.

Changes in Sinus Venosus

Initially, the sinus venosus opens into the posterior wall of the primordial atrium (sinuatrial orifice). By the end of the fourth week of development, the right sinual horn becomes larger than the left sinual horn (Fig. 14-11*A* and *B*). As this occurs, the sinuatrial orifice moves to the right and opens in the part of the primordial atrium that will become the adult right atrium (Fig. 14-12*C*). As the right sinual horn enlarges, it receives all of the blood from the head and neck through the SVC, and from the placenta and the caudal regions of the body through the IVC.

The left sinual horn becomes the **coronary sinus,** and the right sinual horn is incorporated into the wall of the

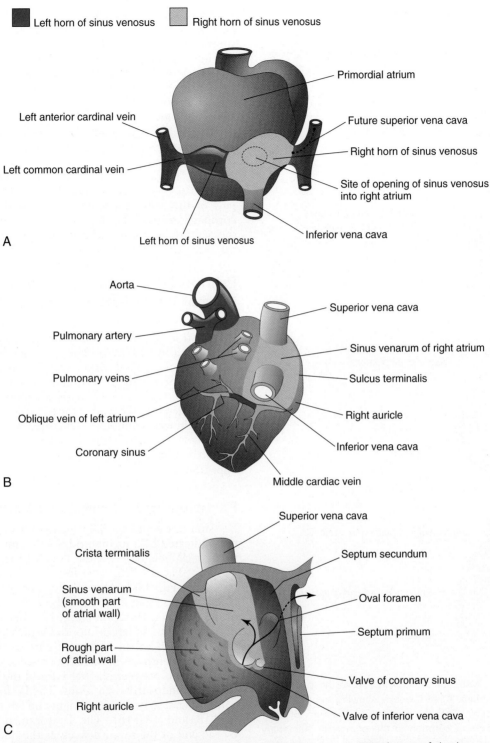

■ Left horn of sinus venosus   ■ Right horn of sinus venosus

A

Primordial atrium

Left anterior cardinal vein

Future superior vena cava

Right horn of sinus venosus

Left common cardinal vein

Site of opening of sinus venosus into right atrium

Inferior vena cava

Left horn of sinus venosus

B

Aorta

Superior vena cava

Pulmonary artery

Sinus venarum of right atrium

Pulmonary veins

Sulcus terminalis

Oblique vein of left atrium

Right auricle

Coronary sinus

Inferior vena cava

Middle cardiac vein

C

Superior vena cava

Crista terminalis

Septum secundum

Sinus venarum (smooth part of atrial wall)

Oval foramen

Septum primum

Rough part of atrial wall

Valve of coronary sinus

Right auricle

Valve of inferior vena cava

Figure 14–11 Illustrations of the fate of the sinus venosus. **A,** Dorsal view of the heart (approximately 26 days), showing the primordial atrium and sinus venosus. **B,** Dorsal view at 8 weeks, after incorporation of the right sinual horn into the right atrium. The left sinual horn has become the coronary sinus. **C,** Internal view of the fetal right atrium, showing the smooth part of the wall of the right atrium (sinus venarum), derived from the right sinual horn. The crista terminalis and the valves of the inferior vena cava and the coronary sinus, derived from the right sinuatrial valve are also shown. The primordial right atrium becomes the right auricle, a conical muscular pouch. *Arrows* indicate the flow of blood.

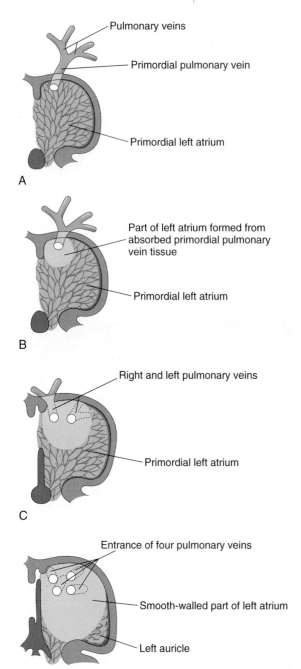

Figure 14–12 Illustrations of absorption of the pulmonary vein into the left atrium. **A,** At 5 weeks, showing the primordial pulmonary vein opening into the primordial left atrium. **B,** Later stage, showing partial absorption of the primordial pulmonary vein. **C,** At 6 weeks, showing the openings of two pulmonary veins into the left atrium as a result of absorption of the primordial pulmonary vein. **D,** At 8 weeks, showing four pulmonary veins with separate atrial orifices. The primordial left atrium becomes the left auricle, a tubular pouch of the atrium. Most of the left atrium is formed by absorption of the primordial pulmonary vein and its branches.

right atrium (Fig. 14-11*B* and *C*) and becomes the smooth part of the internal wall of the right atrium is called the **sinus venarum** (Fig. 14-11*B* and *C*). The remainder of the anterior internal surface of the wall of the right atrium, as well as that of the **auricle**, has a rough, trabeculated appearance. These latter two parts are derived from the primordial atrium. The smooth part and the rough part are demarcated internally in the right atrium by a vertical ridge, termed the **crista terminalis**, or terminal crest (Fig. 14-11*C*), and externally by a shallow groove, the **sulcus terminalis**, or terminal groove (Fig. 14-11*B*). The crista terminalis represents the cranial part of the right **sinuatrial valve** (Fig. 14-11*C*); the caudal part of this valve forms the valves of the IVC and the coronary sinus. The left sinuatrial valve fuses with the septum secundum and is incorporated with it into the interatrial septum.

Primordial Pulmonary Vein and Formation of Left Atrium

Most of the wall of the left atrium is smooth because it is formed by the incorporation of the primordial pulmonary vein (Fig. 14-12*A*). This vein develops as an outgrowth of the dorsal atrial wall, just to the left of the septum primum. As the atrium expands, the primordial pulmonary vein and its main branches are gradually incorporated into the wall of the left atrium (Fig. 14-12*B*). As a result, four pulmonary veins are formed (Fig. 14-12*C* and *D*). The small left auricle is derived from the primordial atrium; its internal surface has a rough, trabeculated appearance.

Partitioning of Primordial Ventricle

Division of the primordial ventricle into two ventricles is first indicated by a median ridge—the **muscular interventricular (IV) septum**—in the floor of the ventricle, near its apex (Fig. 14-9*B*). This fold has a concave superior free edge (Fig. 14-13*A*). Initially, most of its increase in height results from dilation of the ventricles on each side of the muscular IV septum (Fig. 14-13*B*). Myocytes from both the right and left primordial ventricles contribute to the formation of the *muscular part of the IV septum*. Until the seventh week, there is a crescent-shaped opening (**IV foramen**) between the free edge of the IV septum and the fused endocardial cushions. The IV foramen permits communication between the right and left ventricles (Figs. 14-13*B* and 14-14*B*). The IV foramen usually closes by the end of the seventh week as the bulbar ridges fuse with the endocardial cushion (Fig. 14-14*C* to *E*). **Closure of the IV foramen** and formation of the membranous part of the IV septum result from the fusion of tissues from three sources: the right bulbar ridge, the left bulbar ridge, and the endocardial cushion.

The **membranous part of the IV septum** is derived from an extension of tissue from the right side of the endocardial cushion to the muscular part of the IV septum. This tissue merges with the **aorticopulmonary septum** and the thick, muscular part of the IV septum (Fig. 14-15*B*). Closure of the IV foramen and formation of the membranous part of the IV septum results in communication of

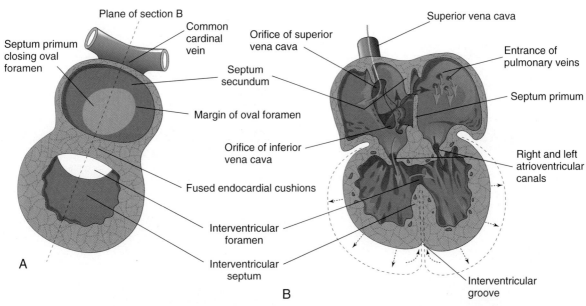

Figure 14–13   Illustrations of partitioning of the primordial heart. **A,** Sagittal section late in the fifth week, showing the cardiac septa and foramina. **B,** Frontal section at a slightly later stage, showing the directions of blood flow through the heart (*blue arrows*) and the expansion of the ventricles (*dotted arrows*).

the pulmonary trunk with the right ventricle and the aorta communicates with the left ventricle (Fig. 14-14*E*). A process of cavitation in the ventricular walls forms a sponge-like mass of muscular bundles. Some bundles remain as the **trabeculae carneae**. Other bundles become the **papillary muscles** and **tendinous cords** (Latin *chordae tendineae*). The tendinous cords run from the papillary muscles to the AV valves (Fig. 14-15*B*).

Partitioning of Bulbus Cordis and Truncus Arteriosus

During the fifth week, active proliferation of the mesenchymal cells in the walls of the bulbus cordis results in the formation of **bulbar ridges** (Figs. 14-14*C* and *D* and 14-16*B* and *C*). Similar ridges form in the truncus arteriosus; these are continuous with the bulbar ridges. The bulbar and **truncal ridges** are derived mainly from the neural crest mesenchyme. *Bone morphogenetic protein and other signaling systems, such as Wnt and fibroblast growth factor, have been implicated in the induction and migration of neural crest cells through the primordial pharynx and the pharyngeal arches.* Concurrently, the bulbar and truncal ridges undergo 180-degree spiraling. The spiral orientation of the bulbar and truncal ridges, possibly caused in part by the streaming of blood from the ventricles, results in the formation of a spiral **aorticopulmonary septum** when the ridges fuse (Fig. 14-16*D* to *G*). This septum divides the bulbus cordis and the truncus arteriosus into two arterial channels, the **aorta**, and the **pulmonary trunk**. Because of the spiraling of the aorticopulmonary septum, the pulmonary trunk twists around the ascending aorta (see Fig. 14-16*H*).

FETAL CARDIAC ULTRASONOGRAPHY

Echocardiography and Doppler ultrasonography have made it possible for sonographers to recognize normal and abnormal fetal cardiac anatomy. Most studies are performed at 18 to 22 weeks gestation, when the heart is large enough to be examined easily; however, real-time ultrasound images of the fetal heart can be obtained at 16 weeks.

The **bulbus cordis** is incorporated into the walls of the definitive ventricles in several ways (see Fig. 14-14*A* and *B*):

● In the right ventricle, the bulbus cordis is represented by the conus arteriosus (infundibulum), which gives origin to the pulmonary trunk.
● In the left ventricle, the bulbus cordis forms the walls of the aortic vestibule, the part of the ventricular cavity just inferior to the aortic valve.

Development of Cardiac Valves

The semilunar valves develop from three swellings of subendocardial tissue around the orifices of the aorta and pulmonary trunk (Fig. 14-17*B* to *F*). These swellings are hollowed out and reshaped to form three thin-walled cusps. The **AV valves** (tricuspid and mitral valves) develop similarly from localized proliferations of tissue around the AV canals.

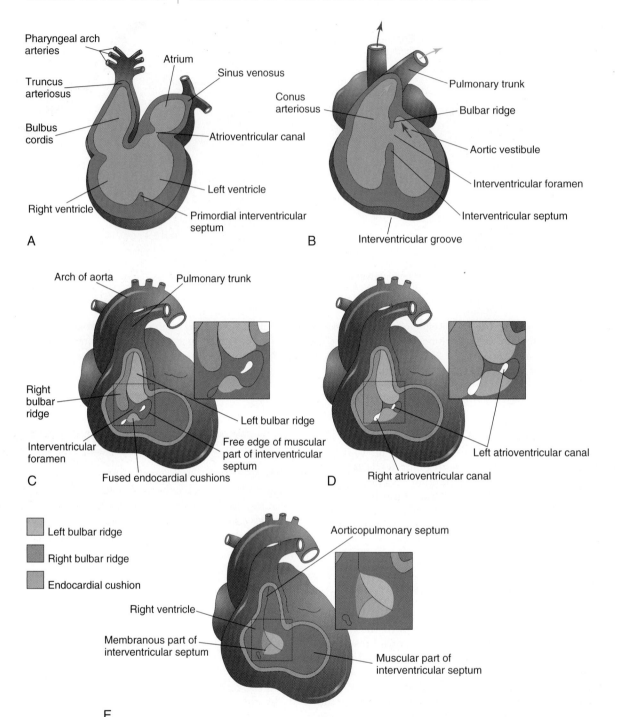

Figure 14–14 Illustrations of the incorporation of the bulbus cordis into the ventricles and partitioning of the bulbus cordis and truncus arteriosus into the aorta and the pulmonary trunk. **A,** Sagittal section at 5 weeks, showing the bulbus cordis as one of the chambers of the primordial heart. **B,** Schematic coronal section at 6 weeks, after the bulbus cordis has been incorporated into the ventricles to become the conus arteriosus (infundibulum) of the right ventricle and the aortic vestibule of the left ventricle. The *arrows* indicate blood flow. **C to E,** Closure of the interventricular (IV) foramen and formation of the membranous part of the IV septum. The walls of the truncus arteriosus, the bulbus cordis, and the right ventricle have been removed. **C,** At 5 weeks, showing the bulbar ridges and fused endocardial cushions. **D,** At 6 weeks, showing how the proliferation of subendocardial tissue diminishes the IV foramen. **E,** At 7 weeks, showing the fused bulbar ridges, the membranous part of the IV septum formed by extensions of tissue from the right side of the endocardial cushions, and closure of the IV foramen.

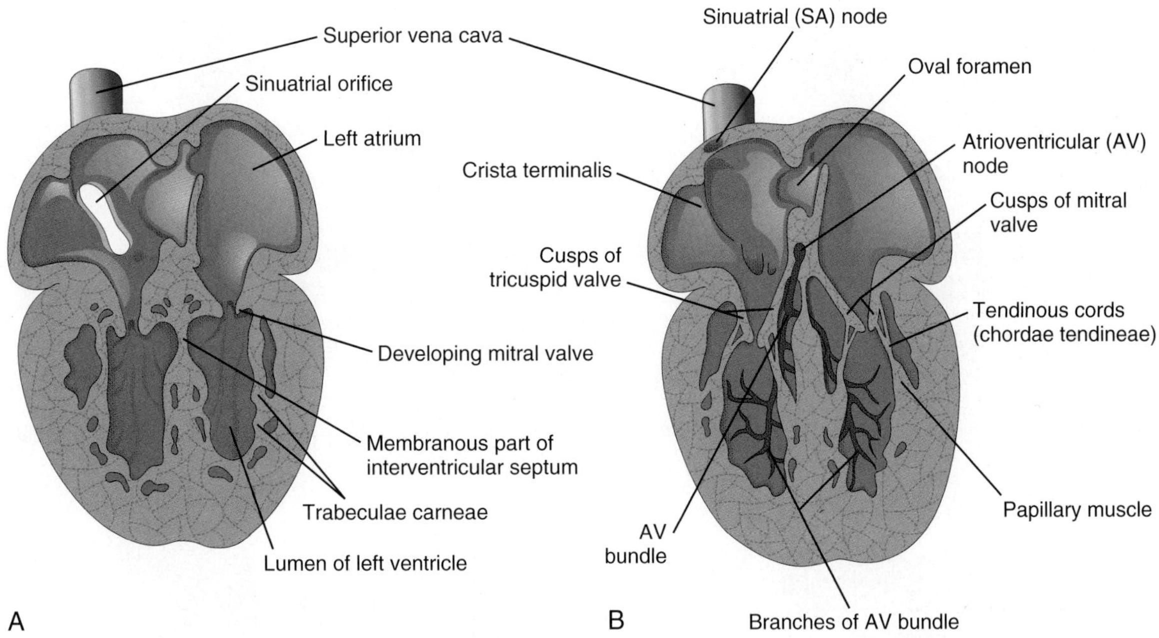

Figure 14–15 Schematic sections of the heart, showing successive stages in the development of the atrioventricular valves, tendinous cords (Latin *chordae tendineae*), and papillary muscles. **A,** At 7 weeks. **B,** At 20 weeks, showing the conducting system of the heart.

ABNORMALITIES OF CONDUCTING SYSTEM

Abnormalities of the conducting tissue may cause unexpected death during infancy, as in "crib death," or **sudden infant death syndrome**. Most likely, no single mechanism is responsible for the sudden, unexpected deaths of apparently healthy infants. A *brainstem developmental abnormality* or maturational delay related to neuroregulation of cardiorespiratory control has been suggested.

DEXTROCARDIA

If the heart tube bends to the left instead of to the right, the heart is displaced to the right (Fig. 14-18), and there is transposition whereby the heart and its vessels are reversed, left to right, as in a mirror image. **Dextrocardia** is the most frequent positional abnormality of the heart. In **dextrocardia with situs inversus** (transposition of abdominal viscera), the incidence of accompanying cardiac defects is low. In isolated dextrocardia, the abnormal position of the heart is not accompanied by displacement of other viscera.

Conducting System of Heart

Initially, the muscle layers of the atrium and the ventricle are continuous. The primordial atrium acts as the interim pacemaker of the heart, but the sinus venosus soon takes over this function. The **sinuatrial node** develops during the fifth week. This node is located in the right atrium, near the entrance of the superior vena cava (SVC) (Fig. 14-15*B*). After incorporation of the sinus venosus into the heart, cells from its left wall are found in the base of the interatrial septum, near the opening of the coronary sinus. Together with cells from the AV region, they form the **AV node and the AV bundle**, located just superior to the endocardial cushions. The fibers arising from the AV bundle pass from the atrium into the ventricle and split into right and left **bundle branches**, which are distributed throughout the ventricular myocardium (Fig. 14-15*B*). The sinuatrial node, AV node,

and AV bundle are richly supplied by nerves; however, the primordial conducting system is developed before these nerves enter the heart.

BIRTH DEFECTS OF THE HEART AND GREAT VESSELS

Congenital heart defects (CHDs) occur with a frequency of 6 to 8 in 1000 births. Some cases of CHD are caused by single-gene or chromosomal mechanisms; others result from exposure to teratogens such as the *rubella virus*. Most CHDs are believed to be caused by multiple factors, both genetic and environmental (i.e., multifactorial inheritance). Recent technology, such as real-time, 3D *echocardiography*, has permitted the detection of fetal CHDs as early as the 17th or 18th week of gestation.

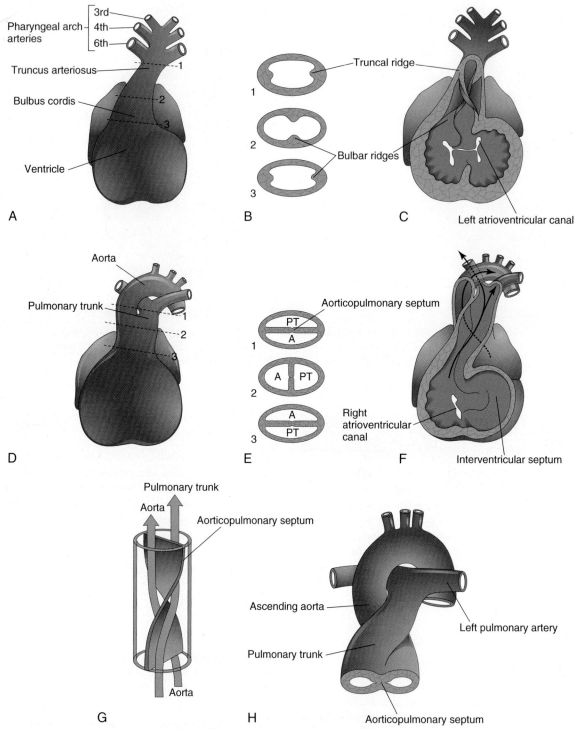

Figure 14–16   Partitioning of the bulbus cordis and truncus arteriosus. **A,** Ventral aspect of the heart at 5 weeks. The *broken lines* and *arrows* indicate the levels of the sections shown in **B. B,** Transverse sections of the truncus arteriosus and bulbus cordis, showing the truncal and bulbar ridges. **C,** The ventral wall of the heart and the truncus arteriosus has been removed to show these ridges. **D,** Ventral aspect of the heart after partitioning of the truncus arteriosus. The *broken lines* and *arrows* indicate the levels of the sections shown in **E. E,** Sections through the newly formed aorta *(A)* and the pulmonary trunk *(PT)* show the aorticopulmonary septum. **F,** At 6 weeks. The ventral wall of the heart and the pulmonary trunk has been removed to show the aorticopulmonary septum. **G,** The spiral form of the aorticopulmonary septum is shown. **H,** The ascending aorta and pulmonary trunk are shown as they twist around each other and they leave the heart.

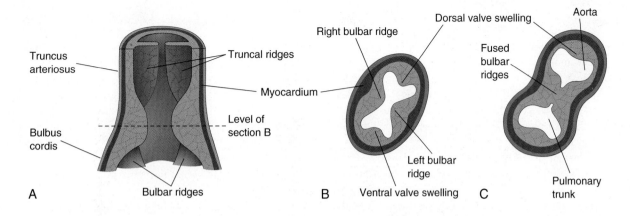

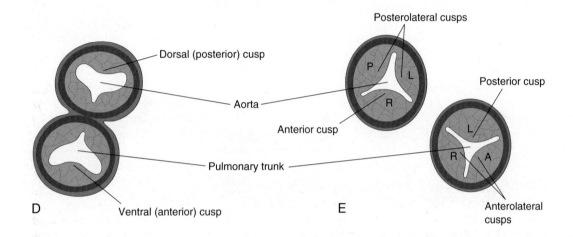

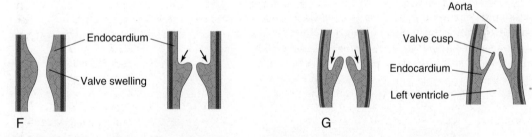

Figure 14–17 Development of the semilunar valves of the aorta and pulmonary trunk. **A,** Section of the truncus arteriosus and the bulbus cordis, showing the valve swellings. **B,** Transverse section of the bulbus cordis. **C,** Similar section after fusion of the bulbar ridges. **D,** Formation of the walls and valves of the aorta and the pulmonary trunk. **E,** Rotation of the vessels has established the adult positions of the valves in relation to each other. **F** and **G,** Longitudinal sections of the aorticoventricular junction, showing successive stages in the hollowing (*arrows*) and thinning of the valve swellings to form the valve cusps. *L,* left; *P,* posterior; *R,* right.

ECTOPIA CORDIS

In ectopia cordis, an extremely rare condition, the heart is located outside the thoracic cavity. The most common thoracic form of ectopia cordis results from faulty development of the sternum and pericardium secondary to incomplete fusion of the lateral folds in the formation of the thoracic wall during the fourth week. Death occurs in most cases during the first few days after birth, usually as a result of infection, cardiac failure, or hypoxemia. If no severe cardiac defects are present, surgical therapy usually consists of covering the heart with skin.

ATRIAL SEPTAL DEFECTS

Atrial septal defects (ASDs) occur more frequently in girls than in boys. The most common form of ASD is a **patent oval foramen** (Figs. 14-19A and 14-20A to D). A small, isolated patent oval foramen is of no hemodynamic significance. However, if other defects are present (e.g., pulmonary atresia), blood is shunted through the oval foramen into the left atrium, producing **cyanosis.**

A **probe patent oval foramen** is present in up to 25% of people. In this abnormality, a probe can be passed from one atrium to the other through the superior part of the floor of the oval fossa; the defect is not clinically significant. A probe patent oval foramen results from incomplete adhesion between the flap of the valve of the oval foramen and the septum secundum after birth.

There are four clinically significant types of ASD (Fig. 14-20), of which the first two are relatively common:

* Ostium secundum defect
* Endocardial cushion defect with a foramen primum defect
* Sinus venosus defect
* Common atrium

Ostium secundum ASDs (Fig. 14-20A to D) occur in the area of the oval fossa and include defects of both the septum primum and the septum secundum. Females with ASDs outnumber males 3 to 1. Ostium secundum ASDs are one of the most common, yet least severe types of congenital heart disease (CHD). The patent oval foramen usually results from abnormal resorption of the septum primum during the formation of the foramen secundum. If resorption occurs in abnormal locations, the septum primum is fenestrated, or net-like (Fig. 14-20A). If excessive resorption of the septum primum occurs, the resulting short septum primum does not close the oval foramen (Fig. 14-20B). If an abnormally large oval foramen develops as a result of defective development of the septum secundum, a normal septum primum does not close the abnormal oval foramen at birth. Large ostium secundum ASDs may also occur because of a combination of excessive resorption of the septum primum and a large oval foramen.

Endocardial cushion defects with a patent foramen primum (Fig. 14-20E) are less common forms of ASD. The septum primum does not fuse with the endocardial cushions, resulting in a patent foramen primum. Usually, there is also a cleft in the anterior cusp of the mitral valve.

Sinus venosus ASDs are located in the superior part of the interatrial septum, close to the entry of the SVC (Fig. 14-20F). These defects result from incomplete absorption of the sinus venosus into the right atrium, abnormal development of the septum secundum, or both. **Common atrium** occurs in patients with all three types of defects: ostium secundum, ostium primum, and sinus venosus.

VENTRICULAR SEPTAL DEFECTS

Ventricular septal defects (VSDs) are the most common type of CHD, accounting for approximately 25% of cases. VSDs occur more frequently in males than in females. *Most VSDs involve the membranous part of the IV septum* (Fig. 14-21B). Many small VSDs close spontaneously, usually during the first year of life. Most people with a large VSD have massive left to right shunting of blood. *Muscular VSD* is a less common type of defect that may appear anywhere in the muscular part of the IV septum. **Transposition of the great arteries** (Fig. 14-22) and a rudimentary outlet chamber are present in most infants with this severe type of CHD.

PERSISTENT TRUNCUS ARTERIOSUS

Persistent truncus arteriosus results from failure of the truncal ridges and the aorticopulmonary septum to develop normally and to divide the truncus arteriosus into the aorta and the pulmonary trunk (Fig. 14-21). The most common type of persistent truncus arteriosus is a **single arterial** trunk (truncus arteriosus) that branches to form the pulmonary trunk and the ascending aorta (Fig. 14-21A and B) supplying the systemic, pulmonary, and coronary circulations. A VSD is always present with truncus arteriosus, and the truncus arteriosus straddles the VSD (Fig. 14-21B).

NORMAL

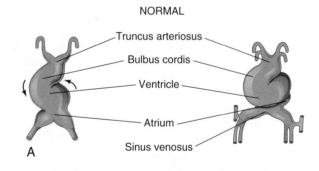

DEXTROCARDIA

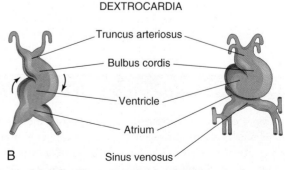

Figure 14–18   The primordial heart during the fourth week. **A,** Normal bending to the right (*arrows*). **B,** Abnormal bending to the left (*arrows*).

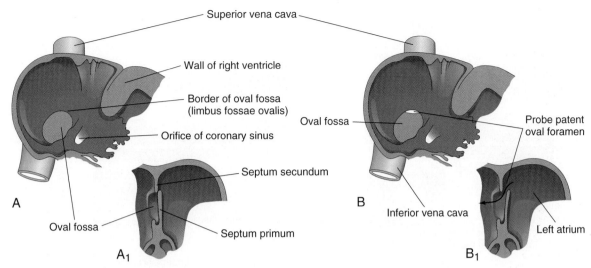

Figure 14–19 **A,** Normal postnatal appearance of the right side of the interatrial septum after adhesion of the septum primum to the septum secundum. **A₁,** Section of the interatrial septum, showing the formation of the oval fossa in the interatrial septum. Note that the floor of this fossa is formed by the septum primum. **B** and **B₁,** Similar views of a probe patent oval foramen resulting from incomplete adhesion of the septum primum to the septum secundum.

TRANSPOSITION OF GREAT ARTERIES

Transposition of the great arteries is the most common cause of cyanotic heart disease in newborn infants (Fig. 14-22). In typical cases, the aorta lies anterior and to the right of the pulmonary trunk and arises anteriorly from the morphologic right ventricle, whereas the pulmonary trunk arises from the morphologic left ventricle. There is also an ASD, with or without an associated patent ductus arteriosus (PDA) and VSD. This defect is believed to result from failure of the conus arteriosus to develop normally during incorporation of the bulbus cordis into the ventricles. Defective neural crest cell migration may also be involved.

TETRALOGY OF FALLOT

The classic group of four cardiac defects known as *tetralogy of Fallot* (see Fig. 14-23*A* and *B*) consists of the following:
* Pulmonary stenosis (obstructed right ventricular outflow)
* Ventricular septal defect
* Dextroposition of the aorta (straddling or overriding both ventricles)
* Right ventricular hypertrophy

The pulmonary trunk is usually small, and there may be varying degrees of pulmonary artery stenosis as well.

UNEQUAL DIVISION OF TRUNCUS ARTERIOSUS

Unequal division of the truncus arteriosus (Figs. 14-21 and 14-23*A* and *B*) results when partitioning of the truncus arteriosus superior to the valves is disparate, producing one large great artery and one small one. As a result, the aorticopulmonary septum is not aligned with the IV septum, and a VSD results. The larger vessel (aorta or pulmonary trunk) usually straddles the VSD (Fig. 14-23*A* and *B*). In **pulmonary valve stenosis**, the cusps of the pulmonary valve are fused together to form a dome with a narrow central opening. In **infundibular stenosis**, the conus arteriosus of the right ventricle is underdeveloped. The two types of pulmonary stenosis may be concurrent. Depending on the degree of obstruction to blood flow, there is a variable degree of hypertrophy of the right ventricle (see Fig. 14-23*B*).

AORTIC STENOSIS AND AORTIC ATRESIA

In **aortic valve stenosis**, the edges of the valve are usually fused to form a dome with a narrow opening. This anomaly may be present at birth (congenital), or it may develop after birth (acquired). The valvular stenosis causes extra work for the heart and results in hypertrophy of the left ventricle and abnormal heart sounds (**heart murmurs**). In *subaortic stenosis*, there is often a band of fibrous tissue just inferior to the aortic valve. The narrowing of the aorta results from persistence of tissue that normally degenerates as the valve forms. **Aortic atresia** is present when obstruction of the aorta or its valve is complete.

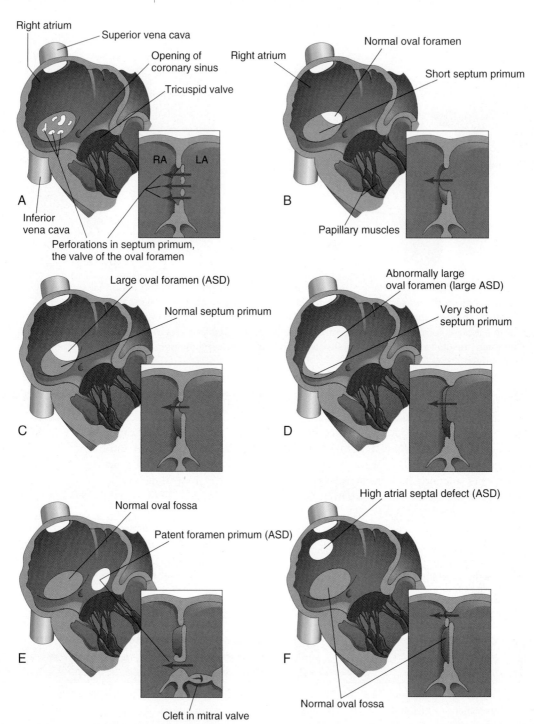

Figure 14–20   Illustrations of the right aspect of the interatrial septum. The adjacent sketches of sections of the septa show various types of atrial septal defects (ASD). **A,** Patent oval foramen resulting from resorption of the septum primum in abnormal locations. **B,** Patent oval foramen caused by excessive resorption of the septum primum ("short flap defect"). **C,** Patent oval foramen resulting from an abnormally large oval foramen. **D,** Patent oval foramen resulting from an abnormally large oval foramen and excessive resorption of the septum primum. **E,** Endocardial cushion defect with a primum-type ASD. The adjacent section shows the cleft in the anterior cusp of the mitral valve. **F,** Sinus venosus ASD. The high septal defect resulted from abnormal absorption of the sinus venosus into the right atrium. In **E** and **F,** note that the oval fossa has formed normally. *Arrows* indicate the direction of flow of blood.

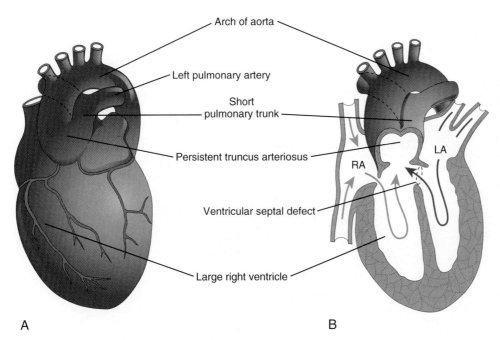

Figure 14–21 The main types of persistent truncus arteriosus (PTA). **A,** The common trunk divides into the aorta and a short pulmonary trunk. **B,** Frontal section of the heart shown in **A.** Observe the circulation in this heart (*arrows*) and the ventricular septal defect (VSD). *LA,* left atrium; *RA,* right atrium.

Labels in Figure 14–21: Arch of aorta; Left pulmonary artery; Short pulmonary trunk; Persistent truncus arteriosus; Ventricular septal defect; Large right ventricle; RA; LA; A; B

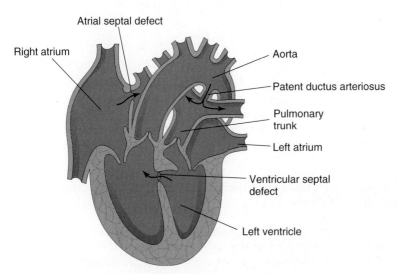

Labels in Figure 14–22: Atrial septal defect; Right atrium; Aorta; Patent ductus arteriosus; Pulmonary trunk; Left atrium; Ventricular septal defect; Left ventricle

Figure 14–22 Frontal section of a malformed heart, showing transposition of the great arteries. The ventricular septal defect (VSD) and the atrial septal defect (ASD) allow mixing of the arterial and venous blood. Transposition of the great arteries is the most common single cause of cyanotic heart disease in newborn infants. As is shown here, it is often associated with other cardiac anomalies (VSD and ASD). The *arrows* indicate the flow of blood. In TGA, when there is an ASD, blood flows from the right atrium to the left atrium.

DERIVATIVES OF PHARYNGEAL ARCH ARTERIES

As the pharyngeal arches develop during the fourth week, they are supplied by **pharyngeal arch arteries** that arise from the *aortic sac* (Fig. 14-24B). The pharyngeal arch arteries terminate in the dorsal aorta on the ipsilateral side. Although six pairs of pharyngeal arch arteries usually develop, they are not all present at the same time (Fig. 14-6).

Derivatives of First Pair of Pharyngeal Arch Arteries

The first pair of arteries largely disappears but remnants of them form parts of the **maxillary arteries**, which supply the ears, teeth, muscles of the eyes and face.

Derivatives of Second Pair of Pharyngeal Arch Arteries

Dorsal parts of the second pair of pharyngeal arch arteries persist and form the stems of the small **stapedial arteries**, which run through the ring of the stapes (but undergo atrophy before birth).

Derivatives of Third Pair of Pharyngeal Arch Arteries

Proximal parts of the third pair of pharyngeal arch arteries form the **common carotid arteries**, which supply structures in the head (Fig. 14-25D). Distal parts of the third pair of pharyngeal arch arteries join with the dorsal aortas to form the **internal carotid arteries**, and they supply the ears, the orbits, and the brain and its meninges.

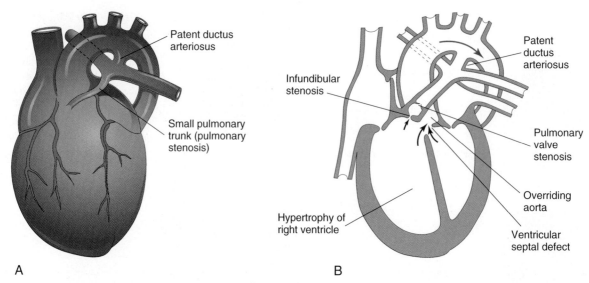

Figure 14–23 **A,** An infant's heart showing a small pulmonary trunk (pulmonary stenosis) and a large aorta resulting from unequal partitioning of the truncus arteriosus. There is also hypertrophy of the right ventricle and a patent ductus arteriosus. **B,** Frontal section of a heart, showing a tetralogy of Fallot. Observe the four cardiac defects of this tetralogy: pulmonary valve stenosis, ventricular septal defect, overriding aorta, and hypertrophy of the right ventricle. In this case, infundibular stenosis is also shown. The *arrows* indicate the flow of blood into the great vessels (aorta and pulmonary trunk).

Derivatives of Fourth Pair of Pharyngeal Arch Arteries

The left fourth pharyngeal arch artery forms part of the arch of the aorta (Fig. 14-25C and D). The proximal part of the arch artery develops from the aortic sac, whereas the distal part is derived from the left dorsal aorta. The right fourth pharyngeal arch artery becomes the proximal part of the **right subclavian artery**. The distal part of the subclavian artery forms from the right dorsal aorta and the right seventh intersegmental artery. The left subclavian artery is not derived from a pharyngeal arch artery; it forms from the left seventh intersegmental artery (Fig. 14-25A). As development proceeds, differential growth shifts the origin of the left subclavian artery cranially. Consequently, it comes to lie close to the origin of the left common carotid artery (Fig. 14-25D).

Fate of Fifth Pair of Pharyngeal Arch Arteries

In approximately 50% of embryos, the fifth pair of pharyngeal arch arteries comprises rudimentary vessels that soon degenerate, leaving no vascular derivatives. In other embryos, these arches do not develop.

Derivatives of Sixth Pair of Pharyngeal Arch Arteries

The **left sixth pharyngeal arch artery** develops as follows (Fig. 14-25B and C):

- The proximal part of the artery persists as the proximal part of the left pulmonary artery.
- The distal part of the artery passes from the left pulmonary artery to the dorsal aorta and forms a prenatal shunt, the ductus arteriosus.

The right sixth pharyngeal arch artery develops as follows:

- The proximal part of the artery persists as the proximal part of the right pulmonary artery.
- The distal part of the artery degenerates.

The transformation of the sixth pair of pharyngeal arch arteries explains why the course of the **recurrent laryngeal nerves** differs on the two sides. These nerves supply the sixth pair of pharyngeal arches and hook around the sixth pair of pharyngeal arch arteries on their way to the developing larynx (Fig. 14-26A). **On the right,** because the distal part of the right sixth pharyngeal arch artery degenerates, the right recurrent laryngeal nerve moves superiorly and hooks around the proximal part of the right subclavian artery, the derivative of the fourth pharyngeal arch artery (Fig. 14-26B). **On the left,** the left recurrent laryngeal nerve hooks around the ductus arteriosus formed by the distal part of the sixth pharyngeal arch artery. When this arterial shunt involutes after birth, the nerve remains around the **ligamentum arteriosum** (remnant of the ductus arteriosus) and the arch of the aorta (Fig. 14-26C).

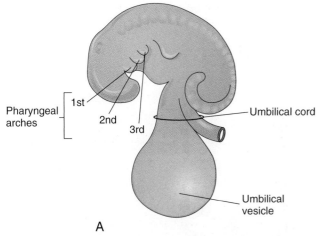

Pharyngeal arches
- 1st
- 2nd
- 3rd

Umbilical cord

Umbilical vesicle

A

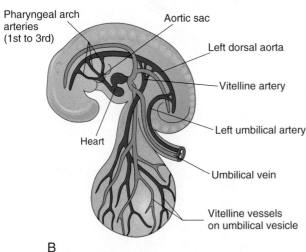

Pharyngeal arch arteries (1st to 3rd)

Aortic sac

Left dorsal aorta

Vitelline artery

Left umbilical artery

Heart

Umbilical vein

Vitelline vessels on umbilical vesicle

B

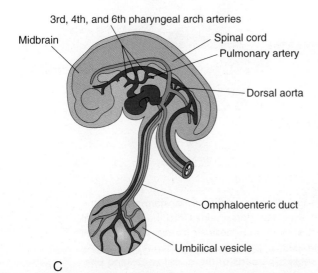

3rd, 4th, and 6th pharyngeal arch arteries

Midbrain

Spinal cord

Pulmonary artery

Dorsal aorta

Omphaloenteric duct

Umbilical vesicle

C

Figure 14–24 The pharyngeal arches and pharyngeal arch arteries. **A,** Left side of an embryo (approximately 26 days). **B,** Illustration of this embryo, showing the left pharyngeal arch arteries arising from the aortic sac, running through the pharyngeal arches, and terminating in the left dorsal aorta. **C,** An embryo (approximately 37 days). Note the single dorsal aorta and the mostly degenerated first two pairs of pharyngeal arch arteries.

COARCTATION OF AORTA

Aortic coarctation (constriction) occurs in approximately 10% of children and adults with CHDs. Coarctation is characterized by a constriction of the aorta of varying length (Fig. 14-27). Most constrictions occur distal to the origin of the left subclavian artery, at the entrance of the ductus arteriosus (**juxtaductal coarctation**). A classification system of preductal and postductal coarctations is commonly used; however, in most cases, the coarctation is directly opposite the ductus arteriosus. Coarctation of the aorta occurs twice as often in males as in females. Coarctation of the aorta is caused by genetic factors, environmental factors, or both.

DOUBLE PHARYNGEAL ARCH ARTERY

Double pharyngeal arch artery is a rare anomaly that is characterized by a *vascular ring around the trachea and the esophagus* (Fig. 14-28). The vascular ring results from failure of the distal part of the right dorsal aorta to disappear (see Fig. 14-28A); as a result, right and left arches form. Usually, the right arch of the aorta is the larger one and it passes posterior to the trachea and the esophagus (see Fig. 14-28B).

RIGHT ARCH OF AORTA

When the entire right dorsal aorta persists (Fig. 14-29A) and the distal part of the left dorsal aorta involutes, a right pharyngeal arch artery results. There are two main types:

* *Right arch of the aorta without a retroesophageal component* (see Fig. 14-29B). The ductus arteriosus (or ligamentum arteriosum) passes from the right pulmonary artery to the right arch of the aorta.
* *Right arch of the aorta with a retroesophageal component* (see Fig. 14-29C). Originally, a small left arch of the aorta probably involuted, leaving the right arch of the aorta posterior to the esophagus. The ductus arteriosus (or ligamentum arteriosum) attaches to the distal part of the arch of the aorta and forms a ring that may constrict the esophagus and the trachea.

PHARYNGEAL ARCH ARTERY ANOMALIES

Because of the many changes involved in the transformation of the embryonic pharyngeal arch system of arteries into the adult arterial pattern, it is understandable why anomalies may occur. Most irregularities result from the persistence of parts of the pharyngeal arch arteries that usually disappear or from the disappearance of parts that normally persist.

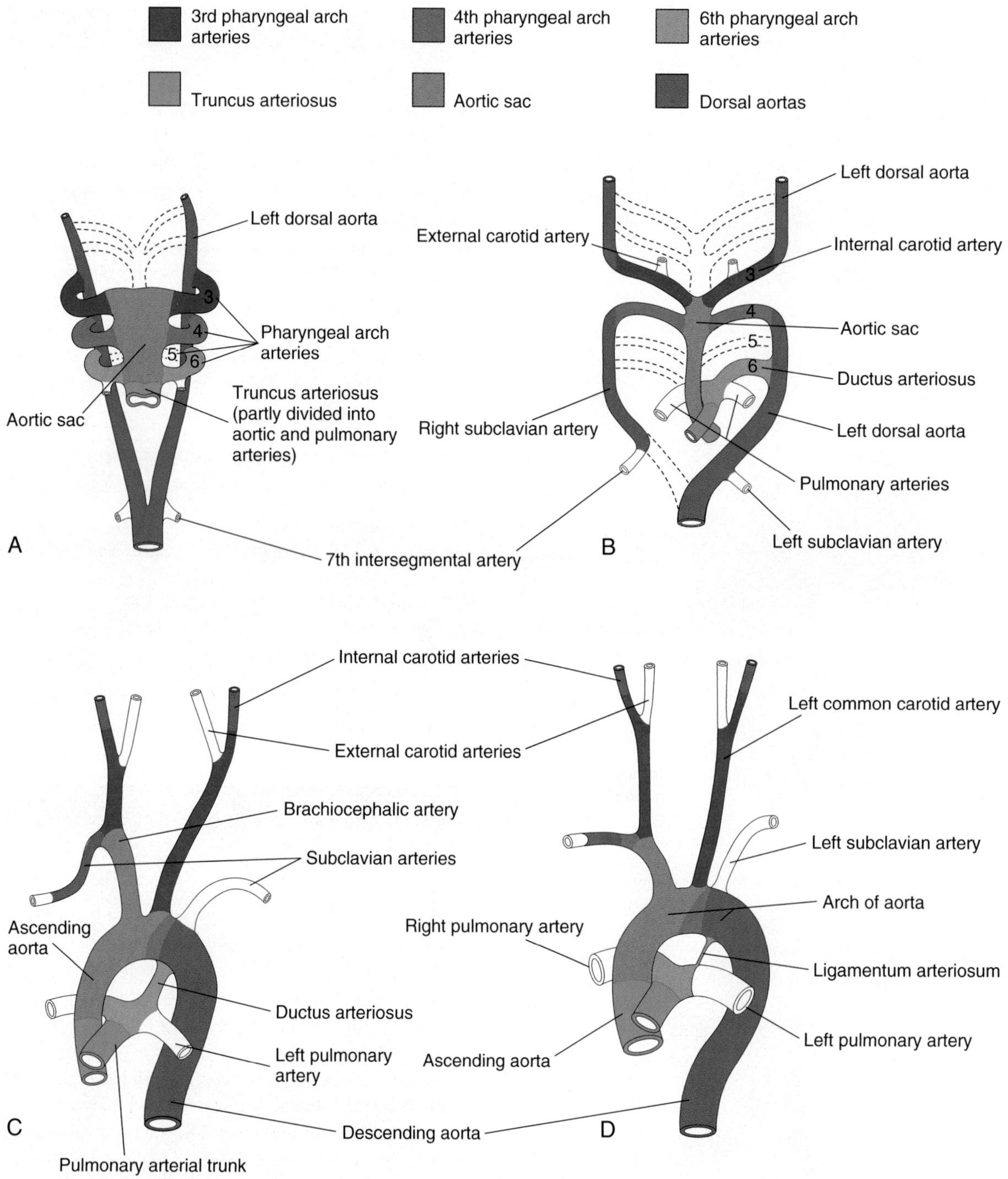

Figure 14–25 Illustration of the arterial changes that occur during transformation of the truncus arteriosus, aortic sac, pharyngeal arch arteries, and dorsal aortas into the adult arterial pattern. The vessels that are not colored are not derived from these structures. **A,** Pharyngeal arch arteries at 6 weeks. By this stage, the first two pairs of pharyngeal arch arteries have largely disappeared. **B,** Pharyngeal arch arteries at 7 weeks. The parts of the dorsal aortas and pharyngeal arch arteries that normally disappear are indicated with *broken lines.* **C,** Arterial arrangement at 8 weeks. **D,** Arterial vessels of a 6-month-old infant. Note that the ascending aorta and the pulmonary arteries are considerably smaller in **C** than in **D.** This represents the relative flow through these vessels at the different stages of development. Observe the large size of the ductus arteriosus in **C;** it is essentially a direct continuation of the pulmonary trunk. Eventually, the ductus arteriosus becomes the ligamentum arteriosum, as shown in **D.**

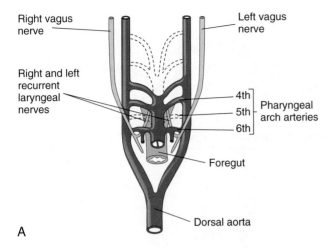

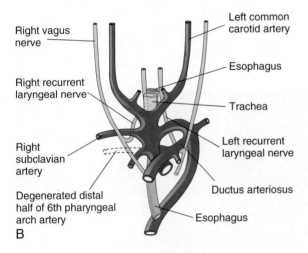

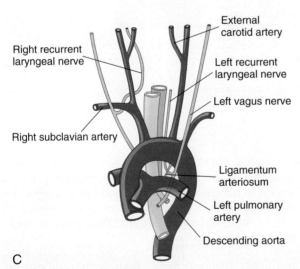

Figure 14–26 The relation of the recurrent laryngeal nerves to the pharyngeal arch arteries. **A,** At 6 weeks, showing that the recurrent laryngeal nerves are hooked around the sixth pair of pharyngeal arch arteries. **B,** At 8 weeks, showing that the right recurrent laryngeal nerve is hooked around the right subclavian artery and the left recurrent laryngeal nerve is hooked around the ductus arteriosus and the arch of the aorta. **C,** In a child, the left recurrent laryngeal nerve is hooked around the ligamentum arteriosum and the arch of the aorta.

ANOMALOUS RIGHT SUBCLAVIAN ARTERY

The right subclavian artery normally arises from the distal part of the arch of the aorta and passes posterior to the trachea and the esophagus to supply the right upper limb (Fig. 14-30). A **retroesophageal right subclavian artery** occurs when the right fourth pharyngeal arch artery and the right dorsal aorta disappear cranial to the seventh intersegmental artery. As a result, the right subclavian artery forms from the right seventh intersegmental artery and the distal part of the right dorsal aorta. As development proceeds, differential growth shifts the origin of the right subclavian artery cranially, until it comes to lie close to the origin of the left subclavian artery.

FETAL AND NEONATAL CIRCULATION

The fetal circulation (Fig. 14-31) is designed to serve prenatal needs. Modifications at birth establish the neonatal pattern (Fig. 14-32). Before birth, the lungs do not provide gas exchange and the pulmonary vessels are vasoconstricted. Three shunts are essential in the transitional circulation: the ductus venosus, oval foramen, and ductus arteriosus.

Fetal Circulation

Highly oxygenated, nutrient-rich blood returns under high pressure from the placenta in the **umbilical vein** (see Fig. 14-31). On approaching the liver, approximately one half of the blood passes directly into the **ductus venosus,** a fetal vessel connecting the umbilical vein to the IVC; consequently this blood bypasses the liver. The other half of the blood in the umbilical vein flows into the sinusoids of the liver and enters the IVC through the **hepatic veins.** Blood flow through the ductus venosus is regulated by a sphincter mechanism close to the umbilical vein. After a short course in the IVC, all of the blood enters the right atrium of the heart. Most blood from the IVC is directed by the inferior border of the septum secundum (**crista dividens**), through the **oval foramen,** and into the left atrium. There, it mixes with the relatively small amount of poorly oxygenated blood returning from the lungs through the pulmonary veins. Fetal lungs use the oxygen from the blood instead of replenishing it. From the left atrium, the blood then passes to the left ventricle and leaves through the ascending aorta. The arteries to the heart, head, neck, and upper limbs receive well-oxygenated blood. The liver also receives well-oxygenated blood from the umbilical vein.

The small amount of well-oxygenated blood from the IVC that remains in the right atrium mixes with poorly oxygenated blood from the SVC and the coronary sinus and passes into the right ventricle. This blood, with medium oxygen content, leaves the heart through the pulmonary trunk. Because of the high pulmonary

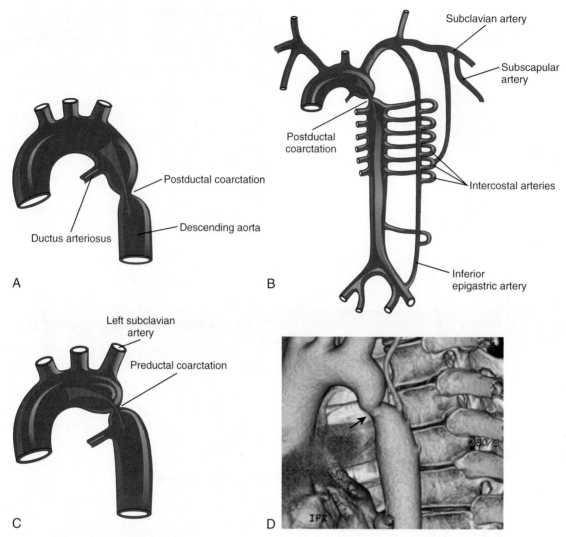

Figure 14–27 **A,** Postductal coarctation of the aorta. **B,** Common routes of the collateral circulation that develop in association with postductal coarctation of the aorta. **C,** Preductal coarctation. *Arrows* indicate flow of blood. **D,** Preductal coarctation (*arrow*) in aorta in an adult. (**D,** *Courtesy of Dr. James Koenig, Department of Radiology, Health Sciences Centre, Winnipeg, Manitoba, Canada.*)

vascular resistance in fetal life, pulmonary blood flow is low. Approximately 10% of the blood goes to the lungs, but most of it passes through the ductus arteriosus into the aorta to the fetal body. It then returns to the placenta through the umbilical arteries (Fig. 14-31). Approximately 10% of blood from the ascending aorta enters the descending aorta to supply the viscera and the inferior part of the body. Most of the blood in the descending aorta passes into the umbilical arteries and is returned to the placenta for reoxygenation.

Transitional Neonatal Circulation

Important circulatory adjustments occur at birth, when the circulation of fetal blood through the placenta ceases and the infant's lungs expand and begin to function (Fig. 14-32). *As soon as the infant is born, the oval foramen, ductus arteriosus, ductus venosus, and umbilical vessels*

are no longer needed. The sphincter in the ductus arteriosus constricts and all blood entering the liver passes through the hepatic sinusoids. This, combined with occlusion of the placental circulation, causes an immediate decrease in blood pressure in the IVC and the right atrium.

Because of increased pulmonary blood flow, the pressure in the left atrium is higher than in the right atrium. **The increased left atrial pressure closes the oval foramen** by pressing the valve of the foramen against the septum secundum (Fig. 14-32). The output from the right ventricle then flows entirely into the pulmonary circulation. Because pulmonary vascular resistance is lower than systemic vascular resistance, blood flow in the ductus arteriosus reverses, passing from the aorta to the pulmonary trunk.

The **ductus arteriosus begins to constrict at birth,** but for a few days there is often a small shunt of blood from

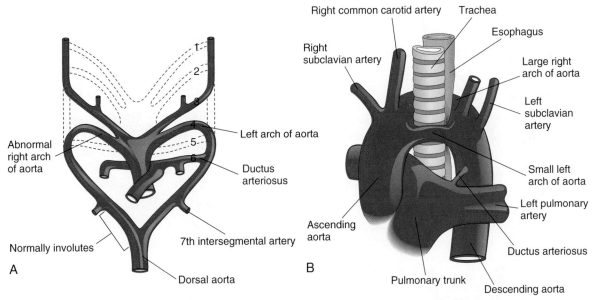

Figure 14–28 **A,** Embryonic pharyngeal arch arteries, showing the embryologic basis of a double arch of the aorta. The distal portion of the right dorsal aorta persists and forms a right pharyngeal arch artery. **B,** A large right arch of the aorta and a small left arch of the aorta arise from the ascending aorta and form a vascular ring around the trachea and the esophagus. Note the compression of the esophagus and the trachea. The right common carotid and subclavian arteries arise separately from the large right arch of the aorta.

the aorta to the pulmonary trunk in healthy, full-term infants. In premature infants and those with persistent hypoxia, the ductus arteriosus may remain open much longer. In full-term infants, oxygen is the most important factor in controlling closure of the ductus arteriosus, and it appears to be mediated by bradykinin and *prostaglandins.*

The **umbilical arteries constrict at birth,** preventing loss of the infant's blood. The umbilical cord is not tied for a minute or so; consequently, blood flow through the umbilical vein continues, transferring fetal blood from the placenta to the infant.

The change from the fetal to the adult pattern of blood circulation is not a sudden occurrence. Some changes occur with the first breath; others take place over hours and days. The closure of fetal shunts and the oval foramen is initially a functional change. Later, anatomical closure results from the proliferation of endothelial and fibrous tissues.

Derivatives of Fetal Vascular Structures

Because of the changes in the cardiovascular system at birth, certain vessels and structures are no longer required after birth.

Umbilical Vein and Round Ligament of the Liver

The intra-abdominal part of the *umbilical vein* eventually becomes the *round ligament of the liver* (Latin *ligamentum teres*) (Fig. 14-32). The umbilical vein remains

PATENT DUCTUS ARTERIOSUS

A common anomaly, PDA occurs two to three times more frequently in females than in males (see Fig. 14-33B). Functional closure of the ductus arteriosus usually occurs soon after birth; however, if it remains patent, aortic blood is shunted into the pulmonary artery. PDA is the most common congenital anomaly associated with maternal rubella infection during early pregnancy. *Premature infants, infants born at high altitude, and those with certain chromosomal anomalies may also have a PDA.* The embryologic basis of PDA is failure of the ductus arteriosus to involute after birth and form the ligamentum arteriosum.

patent for a considerable period and may be used for blood transfusions during early infancy. These transfusions are often performed to prevent brain damage and death in infants with anemia as a result of erythroblastosis fetalis.

Ductus Venosus and Ligamentum Venosum

The ductus venosus becomes the *ligamentum venosum*; however, its closure is more prolonged than that of the ductus arteriosus. The ligamentum venosum passes through the liver from the left branch of the portal vein to the IVC, to which it is attached (Fig. 14-33).

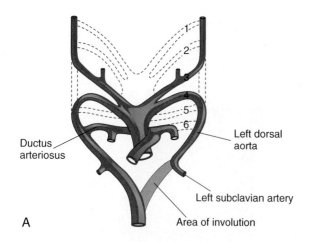

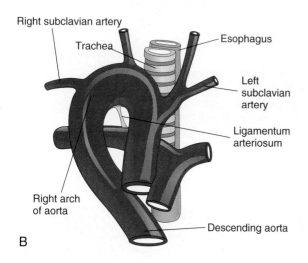

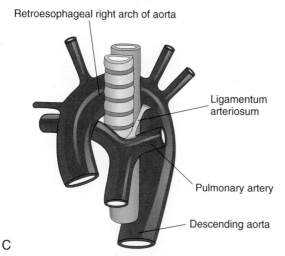

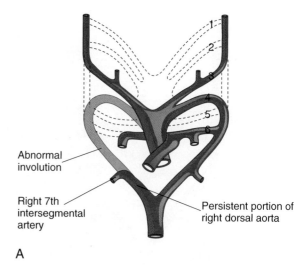

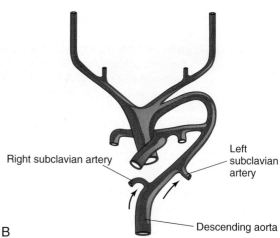

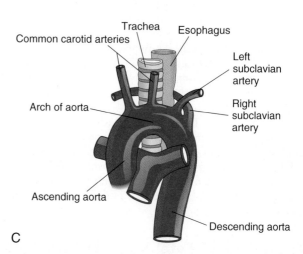

Figure 14–29 **A,** Pharyngeal arch arteries showing abnormal involution of the distal portion of the left dorsal aorta. There is also persistence of the entire right dorsal aorta and the distal part of the right sixth pharyngeal arch artery. **B,** Right pharyngeal arch artery without a retroesophageal component. **C,** Right arch of the aorta with a retroesophageal component. The abnormal right arch of the aorta and the ligamentum arteriosum (postnatal remnant of the ductus arteriosus) form a vascular ring that compresses the esophagus and the trachea.

Figure 14–30 The possible embryologic basis for an abnormal origin of the right subclavian artery. **A,** The right fourth pharyngeal arch artery and the cranial part of the right dorsal aorta have involuted. As a result, the right subclavian artery forms from the right seventh intersegmental artery and the distal segment of the right dorsal aorta. **B,** As the arch of the aorta forms, the right subclavian artery is carried cranially (*arrows*) with the left subclavian artery. **C,** The abnormal right subclavian artery arises from the aorta and passes posterior to the trachea and the esophagus.

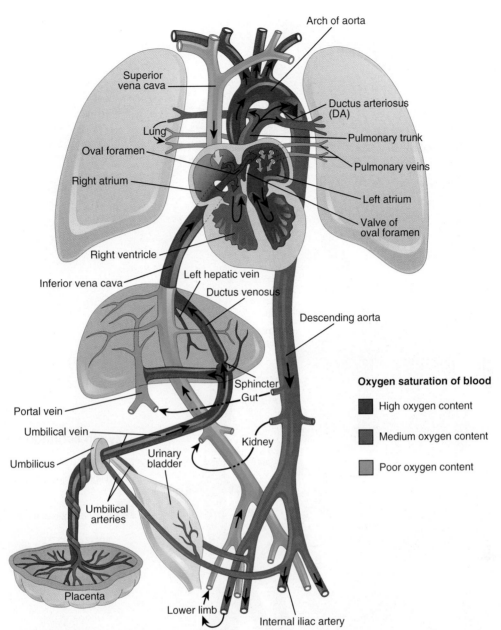

Figure 14–31 Fetal circulation. The colors indicate the oxygen saturation of the blood, and the *arrows* show the course of the blood from the placenta to the heart. The organs are not drawn to scale. A small amount of highly oxygenated blood from the inferior vena cava remains in the right atrium and mixes with poorly oxygenated blood from the superior vena cava. Observe that three shunts permit most of the blood to bypass the liver and lungs: (1) the ductus venosus, (2) the oval foramen, and (3) the ductus arteriosus. The poorly oxygenated blood returns to the placenta for oxygen and nutrients through the umbilical arteries.

Umbilical Arteries and Abdominal Ligaments

Most of the intra-abdominal parts of the umbilical arteries become the **medial umbilical ligaments** (see Fig. 14-32); the proximal parts of these vessels persist as the **superior vesical arteries,** which supply the urinary bladder.

Oval Foramen and Oval Fossa

The oval foramen normally closes functionally at birth. Anatomical closure occurs by the third month and results from tissue proliferation and adhesion of the septum primum to the left margin of the septum secundum. The septum primum forms the floor of the oval fossa. The inferior edge of the septum secundum forms a rounded fold, the border of the oval fossa (Latin *limbus fossae ovalis*), which marks the former boundary of the oval foramen (Fig. 14-19).

Ductus Arteriosus and Ligamentum Arteriosum

Functional closure of the ductus arteriosus is usually completed 10 to 15 hours after birth. Anatomical closure of the ductus arteriosus and formation of the ligamentum arteriosum usually occurs by the 12th postnatal week.

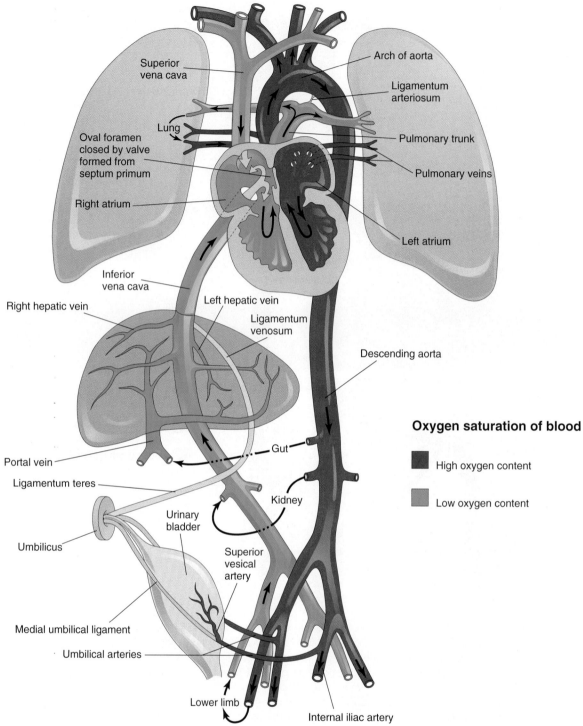

Figure 14–32 Neonatal circulation. The adult derivatives of the fetal vessels and structures that become nonfunctional at birth are shown. The *arrows* indicate the course of the blood in the infant. The organs are not drawn to scale. After birth, the three fetal shunts cease to function, and the pulmonary and systemic circulations become separated.

DEVELOPMENT OF THE LYMPHATIC SYSTEM

The lymphatic system begins to develop at the end of the sixth week. Lymphatic vessels develop in a manner similar to that described for blood vessels, and they make connections with the venous system. The early lymphatic capillaries join each other to form a network of lymphatics. **Six primary lymph sacs** exist at the end of the embryonic period (Fig. 14-34A):

- Two *jugular lymph sacs* near the junction of the subclavian veins with the anterior cardinal veins (future internal jugular veins)

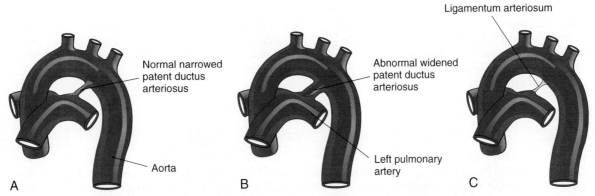

Normal narrowed patent ductus arteriosus

Aorta

Abnormal widened patent ductus arteriosus

Left pulmonary artery

Ligamentum arteriosum

Figure 14–33 Closure of the ductus arteriosus. **A,** The ductus arteriosus of a newborn infant. **B,** Abnormal patent ductus arteriosus in a 6-month-old infant. **C,** The ligamentum arteriosum in a 6-month-old infant.

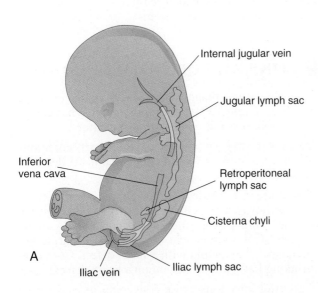

Internal jugular vein

Jugular lymph sac

Inferior vena cava

Retroperitoneal lymph sac

Cisterna chyli

Iliac vein

Iliac lymph sac

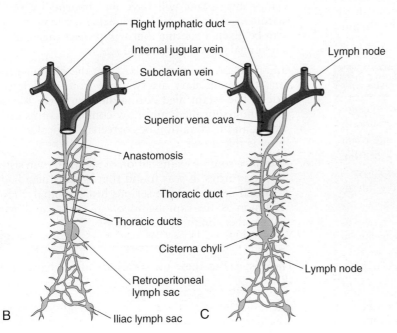

Right lymphatic duct

Internal jugular vein

Subclavian vein

Lymph node

Superior vena cava

Anastomosis

Thoracic duct

Thoracic ducts

Cisterna chyli

Lymph node

Retroperitoneal lymph sac

Iliac lymph sac

Figure 14–34 Development of the lymphatic system. **A,** Left side of a 7-½ week embryo, showing the primary lymph sacs. **B,** Ventral view of the lymphatic system at 9 weeks, showing the paired thoracic ducts. **C,** Later in the fetal period, showing formation of the thoracic duct and the right lymphatic duct.

- Two *iliac lymph sacs* near the junction of the iliac veins with the posterior cardinal veins
- One *retroperitoneal lymph sac* in the root of the mesentery on the posterior abdominal wall
- One *cisterna chyli (chyle cistern)* located dorsal to the retroperitoneal lymph sac

Lymphatic vessels soon join the lymph sacs and accompany main veins; to the head, neck, and upper limbs from the jugular lymph sacs; to the lower trunk and lower limbs from the iliac lymph sacs; and to the primordial gut from the retroperitoneal lymph sac and the **cisterna chyli**. Two large channels (right and left thoracic ducts) connect the jugular lymph sacs with this cistern. Soon, a large anastomosis forms between these channels (Fig. 14-34*B*).

The **thoracic duct** develops from:

- The caudal part of the right thoracic duct
- The anastomosis between the thoracic ducts and the cranial part of the left thoracic duct

The **right lymphatic duct** is derived from the cranial part of the right thoracic duct (Fig. 14-34*C*). The thoracic duct and the right lymphatic duct connect with the venous system at the venous angle between the internal jugular vein and the subclavian vein.

Development of Lymph Nodes

Except for the superior part of the cisterna chyli, the lymph sacs are transformed into groups of lymph nodes during the early fetal period. Mesenchymal cells invade each lymph sac and form a network of lymphatic channels, the primordia of the *lymph sinuses*. Other mesenchymal cells give rise to the capsules and connective tissue framework of the lymph nodes.

The **lymphocytes** are derived originally from primordial stem cells in the umbilical vesicle mesenchyme and later from the liver and spleen. The lymphocytes eventually enter the bone marrow, where they divide to form *lymphoblasts*. The lymphocytes that appear in the lymph nodes before birth are derived from the thymus,

ANOMALIES OF LYMPHATIC SYSTEM

Congenital anomalies of the lymphatic system are uncommon. There may be diffuse swelling of a part of the body, termed **congenital lymphedema**. This condition may result from dilation of the primordial lymphatic channels or from congenital hypoplasia of the lymphatic vessels. **Cystic hygromas** are large swellings that usually appear in the inferolateral part of the neck and consist of large, single or multilocular, fluid-filled cavities. Hygromas may be present at birth, but they often enlarge and become evident during later infancy. Hygromas are believed to arise from parts of a jugular lymph sac that are pinched off, or from lymphatic spaces that do not establish connections with the main lymphatic channels.

a derivative of the third pair of pharyngeal pouches (Chapter 10). Small lymphocytes leave the *thymus* and circulate to other lymphoid organs. Later, some mesenchymal cells in the lymph nodes also differentiate into lymphocytes.

Development of Spleen and Tonsils

The spleen develops from an aggregation of mesenchymal cells in the dorsal mesentery of the stomach (see Chapter 12). The **palatine tonsils** develop primarily from the second pair of pharyngeal pouches and the nearby mesenchyme. The **tubal tonsils** develop from aggregations of lymph nodules around the pharyngeal openings of the pharyngotympanic tubes. The **pharyngeal tonsils** (adenoids) develop from an aggregation of lymph nodules in the wall of the nasopharynx. The **lingual tonsil** develops from an aggregation of lymph nodules in the root of the tongue. Lymph nodules also develop in the mucosa of the respiratory and alimentary systems.

CLINICALLY ORIENTED QUESTIONS

1. A pediatrician diagnosed a heart murmur in a newborn infant. What does this mean? What causes this condition, and what does it indicate?

2. Are congenital anomalies of the heart common? What is the most common congenital heart defect in neonates?

3. What are the causes of congenital anomalies of the cardiovascular system? Can drugs taken by the mother during pregnancy cause congenital cardiac defects? One mother who drank heavily during her pregnancy had a child with a heart defect. Could her drinking have caused her infant's heart defect?

4. Can viral infections cause congenital heart disease? Is it true that if a mother has measles during pregnancy, her infant will have an abnormality of the cardiovascular system? Is it true that pregnant women can be given a vaccine that will protect their unborn child against certain viruses?

5. In an infant, the aorta arose from the right ventricle and the pulmonary artery arose from the left ventricle. The infant died during the first week. What is this anomaly called, and how common is this disorder? Can the condition be corrected surgically? If so, how is this done?

6. During a routine examination of identical twin sisters in their forties, it was found that one of them had a reversed heart. Is this a serious heart anomaly? How common is this among identical twins, and what causes this condition to develop?

The answers to these questions are at the back of the book.

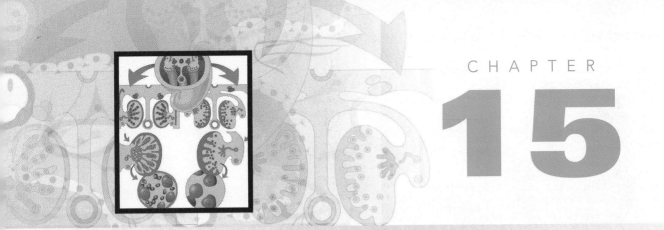

Musculoskeletal System

SKELETAL SYSTEM

As the notochord and neural tube form, the *intraembryonic mesoderm* lateral to these structures thickens to form two longitudinal columns of **paraxial mesoderm** (Fig. 15-1*A* and *B*). Toward the end of the third week, these columns become segmented into blocks, that is, **somites** (Fig. 15-1*C*). Each somite differentiates into two parts (Fig. 15-1*D* and *E*):

- The ventromedial part is the sclerotome; its cells form the vertebrae and ribs.
- The dorsolateral part is the dermomyotome; cells from its *myotome region* form myoblasts (primordial muscle cells), whereas those from its *dermatome* region form the dermis (fibroblasts).

The bones and connective tissue of the craniofacial structures are formed from mesenchyme in the head region that is derived from the neural crests.

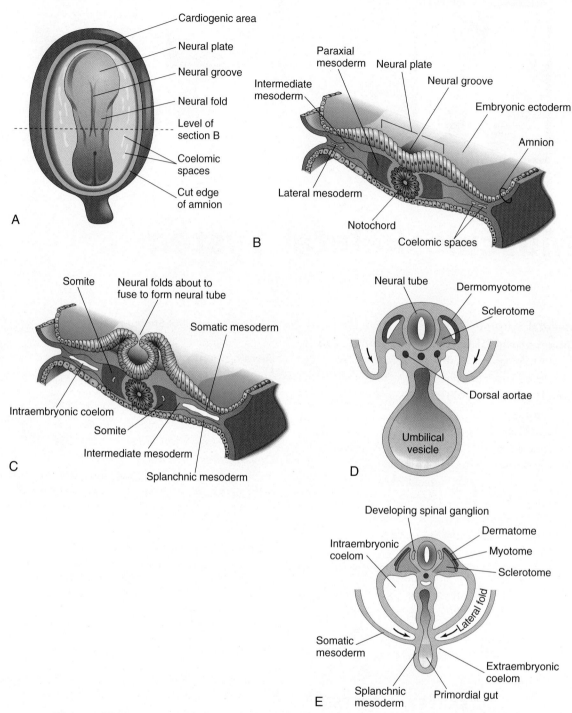

Figure 15–1 Formation and early differentiation of somites. **A,** Dorsal view of a presomite embryo (approximately 18 days). **B,** Transverse section of the embryo shown in **A,** illustrating the paraxial mesoderm from which the somites are derived. **C,** Transverse section of an embryo at approximately 22 days, at which time early somites have appeared. **D,** Transverse section of an embryo at approximately 24 days. The dermomyotome region of the somite gives rise to the dermatome and myotome. **E,** Transverse section of an embryo at approximately 26 days, showing the dermatome, myotome, and sclerotome regions of the somite. The *arrows* in **D** and **E** indicate movement of the lateral body folds.

DEVELOPMENT OF CARTILAGE AND BONE

Histogenesis of Cartilage

Cartilage develops from mesenchyme and first appears in embryos during the fifth week. In areas where cartilage is to develop, the mesenchyme condenses to form **chondrification centers**. The mesenchymal cells differentiate into **chondroblasts**, which secrete collagenous fibrils and extracellular matrix. Subsequently, collagenous or elastic fibers or both are deposited in the intercellular substance or matrix. *Three types of cartilage* are distinguishable according to the type of matrix that is formed:

- *Hyaline cartilage*, the most widely distributed type (e.g., in synovial joints)
- *Fibrocartilage* (e.g., in intervertebral discs)
- *Elastic cartilage* (e.g., in auricle of the ear)

Histogenesis of Bone

Bone develops primarily in two types of connective tissue—mesenchyme and cartilage—but it can also develop in other connective tissues. Most flat bones develop in mesenchyme within preexisting membranous sheaths; this type of osteogenesis is called **intramembranous bone formation**. Mesenchymal models of most limb bones are transformed into cartilaginous bone models, which later become ossified by **endochondral bone formation**. Like cartilage, bone consists of cells and an organic intercellular substance—**bone matrix**, which comprises collagen fibrils embedded in an amorphous component.

Studies of cellular and molecular events that occur during embryonic bone formation suggest that osteogenesis and chondrogenesis are programmed early in development and are independent processes under the influence of vascular events.

Bone morphogenetic proteins 5 and 7 and growth and differentiation factor 5, members of the tumor growth factor-b superfamily, as well as other signaling molecules, have been implicated as endogenous regulators of chondrogenesis and skeletal development.

Intramembranous Ossification

The mesenchyme condenses and becomes highly vascular; some cells differentiate into **osteoblasts** (bone-forming cells) and begin to deposit unmineralized matrix—**osteoid** (Fig. 15-2). Calcium phosphate is then deposited in the **osteoid tissue** as it is organized into bone. Osteoblasts are trapped in the matrix and become **osteocytes**. Spicules of bone soon become organized and coalesce into lamellae (layers).

Concentric lamellae develop around blood vessels, forming **osteons** (Haversian systems). Some osteoblasts remain at the periphery of the bone and continue to lay down layers, forming plates of compact bone on the surfaces. Between the surface plates, the intervening bone remains spiculated, or spongy. This spongy environment is somewhat accentuated by the action of **osteoclasts**, which reabsorb bone. In the interstices of the spongy

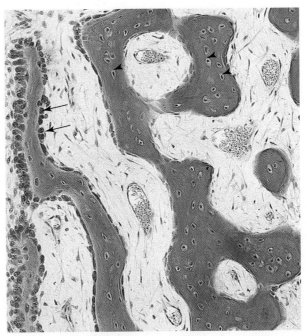

Figure 15–2 Light micrograph of intramembranous ossification (×132). The trabeculae of the bone are being formed by osteoblasts lining their surface (*arrows*). Observe that osteocytes are trapped in the lacunae (*arrowheads*) and that primordial osteons are beginning to form. The osteons (canals) contain blood capillaries. (*From Gartner LP, Hiatt JL: Color Textbook of Histology, 2nd ed. Philadelphia, WB Saunders, 2001.*)

bone, the mesenchyme differentiates into **bone marrow**. During fetal and postnatal life, continuous remodeling of bone occurs by the coordinated action of osteoclasts and osteoblasts.

Endochondral Ossification

Endochondral ossification is a type of bone formation that occurs in preexisting cartilaginous models (Fig. 15-3A to E). In a long bone, the **primary center of ossification** appears in the **diaphysis**, which forms the **shaft** of the bone (Fig. 15-3B). Here the cartilage cells hypertrophy, the matrix becomes calcified, and the cells die. Concurrently, a thin layer of bone is deposited under the **perichondrium** surrounding the diaphysis; thus, the perichondrium becomes the **periosteum** (Fig. 15-3A and B). Invasion of the vascular connective tissue by the blood vessels surrounding the periosteum breaks up the cartilage. Some invading cells differentiate into **hemopoietic cells**, which are responsible for the formation of blood cells in the bone marrow. This process continues toward the **epiphyses**, or ends of the bone. The spicules of bone are remodeled by the action of osteoclasts and osteoblasts.

Lengthening of the long bones occurs at the diaphysial-epiphysial junction. The lengthening of bone depends on the **epiphysial cartilage plates** (growth plates), whose chondrocytes proliferate and participate in endochondral bone formation (Fig. 15-3D and E). Toward the diaphysis, the cartilage cells hypertrophy and the matrix becomes calcified. Spicules are isolated from each other by vascular invasion from the marrow or **medullary cavity**. Bone

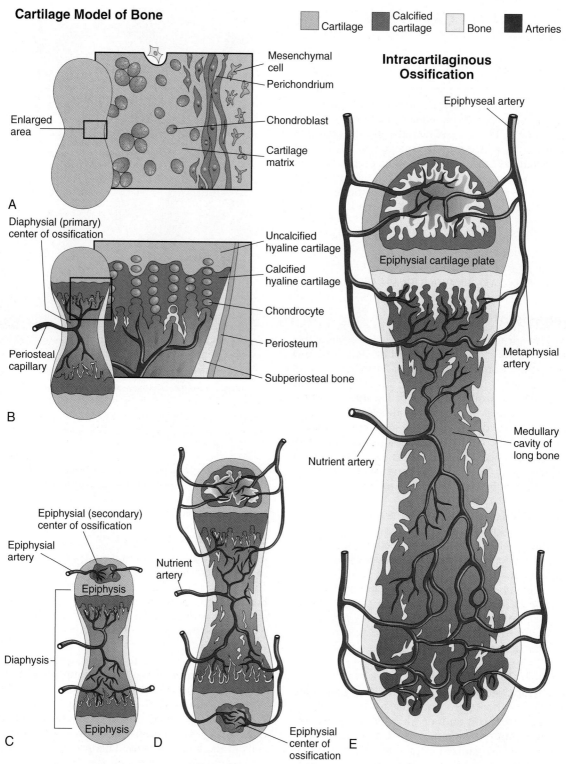

Figure 15–3 **A** to **E,** Schematic longitudinal sections, showing endochondral ossification in a developing long bone.

is deposited on these spicules by osteoblasts; resorption of this bone keeps the spongy bone masses relatively constant in length and enlarges the medullary cavity.

Ossification of the limb bones makes demands on the maternal supply of calcium and phosphorus beginning at approximately 8 weeks. At birth, the diaphyses are largely ossified but the epiphyses are still cartilaginous. **Secondary ossification centers** appear in the epiphyses during the first few years after birth. The epiphysial cartilage cells hypertrophy, and there is invasion by vascular connective tissue. Ossification spreads radially. The articular cartilage and the **epiphysial cartilage plate** remain

RICKETS

Rickets is a disease that occurs in children with vitamin D deficiency. This vitamin is required for calcium absorption by the intestine. The resulting calcium deficiency causes disturbances in ossification of the epiphysial cartilage plates and orientation of cells at the **metaphysis**. The limbs are shortened and deformed, with severe bowing of the bones.

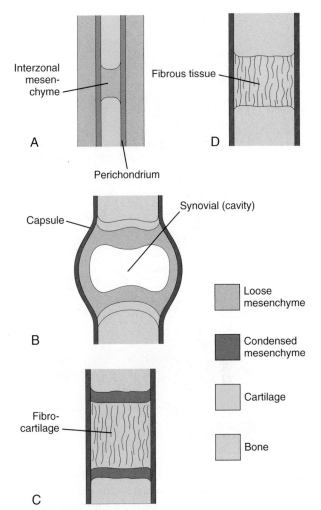

Figure 15–4 Development of joints during the sixth and seventh weeks. **A,** Condensed mesenchyme continues across the gap, or interzone, between the developing bones, enclosing some interzonal mesenchyme between them. This primordial joint may differentiate into a synovial joint **(B)**, a cartilaginous joint **(C)**, or a fibrous joint **(D)**.

cartilaginous. On completion of bone growth, this plate is replaced by spongy bone, the epiphyses and the diaphysis are united, and no further elongation of the bone occurs.

In most bones, the epiphyses have fused with the diaphysis by 20 years of age. Growth in the diameter of a bone results from deposition of bone at the periosteum and from resorption on the medullary surface. The rate of deposition and resorption is balanced to regulate the thickness of the compact bone and the size of the medullary cavity. The internal reorganization of bone continues throughout life.

DEVELOPMENT OF JOINTS

Joints begin to develop with the appearance of the **interzonal mesenchyme** during the sixth week (Fig. 15-4A), and they resemble adult joints by the end of the eighth week.

Fibrous Joints

During the development of fibrous joints, the interzonal mesenchyme between the developing bones differentiates into dense fibrous tissue (Fig. 15-4D). The sutures of the cranium are an example of fibrous joints.

Cartilaginous Joints

During the development of cartilaginous joints, the interzonal mesenchyme between the developing bones differentiates into **hyaline cartilage** (e.g., the costochondral joints) or **fibrocartilage** (Fig. 15-4C) (e.g., the pubic symphysis).

Synovial Joints

During the development of synovial joints (e.g., the knee joint), the interzonal mesenchyme between the developing bones differentiates as follows (Fig. 15-4B):

- Peripherally, it forms the capsular and other ligaments.
- Centrally it disappears and the resulting space becomes the joint cavity or synovial cavity.
- Where it lines the joint capsule and articular surfaces, it forms the synovial membrane, which secretes the synovial fluid.

DEVELOPMENT OF AXIAL SKELETON

The axial skeleton is composed of the cranium (skull), vertebral column, ribs, and sternum. During the fourth week, cells in the sclerotomes surround the neural tube (primordium of spinal cord) and the notochord, the structure around which the primordia of the vertebrae develop. This positional change of the sclerotomal cells is effected by differential growth of the surrounding structures, not by the migration of sclerotomal cells.

Development of Vertebral Column

During the precartilaginous stage, mesenchymal cells from the sclerotomes are found in three main areas (Fig. 15-5A): around the notochord, surrounding the neural tube, and in the body wall.

In a frontal section of a 4-week embryo, the **sclerotomes** appear as paired condensations of mesenchymal cells around the notochord (Fig. 15-5B). Each sclerotome

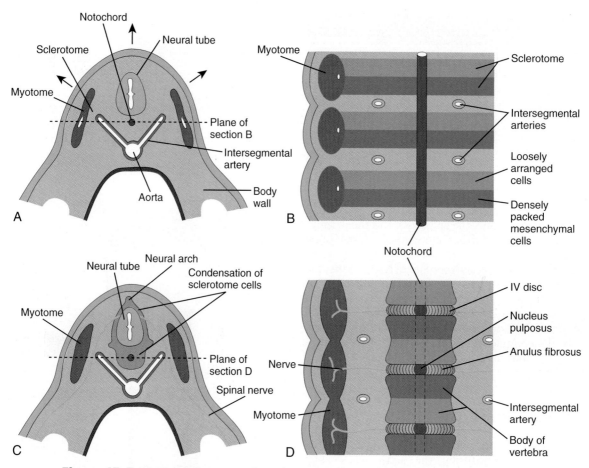

Figure 15–5 **A,** Transverse section through a 4-week embryo. The *arrows* indicate the dorsal growth of the neural tube and the simultaneous dorsolateral movement of the somite remnant, which leaves behind a trail of sclerotomal cells. **B,** Frontal section of the same embryo as in **A,** showing that the condensation of sclerotomal cells around the notochord consists of a cranial area of loosely packed cells and a caudal area of densely packed cells. **C,** Transverse section through a 5-week embryo. Note the condensation of sclerotomal cells around the notochord and the neural tube, which forms a mesenchymal vertebra. **D,** Frontal section, showing that the vertebral body forms from the cranial and caudal halves of two successive sclerotomal masses. The intersegmental arteries now cross the bodies of the vertebrae and the spinal nerves lie between the vertebrae. The notochord is degenerating, except in the region of the intervertebral disc, where it forms the nucleus pulposus.

consists of loosely arranged cells cranially and densely packed cells caudally. Some densely packed cells move cranially, opposite the center of the myotome, where they form the **intervertebral (IV) disc** (Fig. 15-5C and *D*). *These cells express Pax-1, a paired box gene.* The remaining densely packed cells fuse with the loosely arranged cells of the immediately caudal sclerotome to form the mesenchymal **centrum,** the primordium of the vertebral body. Thus, each centrum develops from two adjacent sclerotomes and becomes an intersegmental structure. The spinal nerves now lie in close relationship to the IV discs, and the intersegmental arteries lie on each side of the vertebral bodies. In the thorax, the dorsal **intersegmental arteries** become the **intercostal arteries.** *Studies indicate that the regional development of the vertebral column is regulated along the anterior-posterior axis by homeobox (Hox) and paired box (Pax) genes.*

CHORDOMA

Remnants of the notochord may persist and give rise to a chordoma. Approximately one third of these slowly growing, malignant tumors involve the base of the cranium and extend to the nasopharynx. Chordomas infiltrate bone and are difficult to remove; few patients survive longer than 5 years. Chordomas may also develop in the lumbosacral region.

Where it is surrounded by the developing vertebral bodies, the **notochord** degenerates and disappears. Between the vertebrae, the notochord expands to form the gelatinous center of the IV disc—the **nucleus pulposus** (Fig. 15-5D). This nucleus is later surrounded by

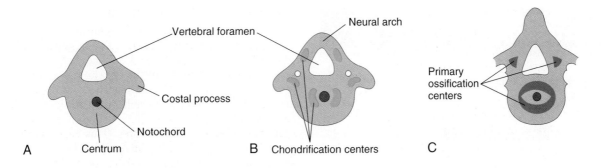

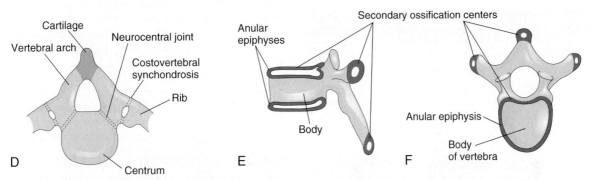

Figure 15–6 Stages of vertebral development. **A,** Mesenchymal vertebra at 5 weeks. **B,** Chondrification centers in a mesenchymal vertebra at 6 weeks. The neural arch is the primordium of the vertebral arch of the vertebra. **C,** Primary ossification centers in a cartilaginous vertebra at 7 weeks. **D,** Thoracic vertebra, consisting of three bony parts, at birth. Note the cartilage between the halves of the vertebral arch and between the arch and the centrum (neurocentral joint). **E** and **F,** Two views of a typical thoracic vertebra at puberty, showing the location of the secondary centers of ossification.

circularly arranged fibers that form the **anulus fibrosus.** The nucleus pulposus and anulus fibrosus together constitute the IV disc. The mesenchymal cells that surround the neural tube form the **neural arch,** the primordium of the vertebral arch (Figs. 15-5C and 15-6D). The mesenchymal cells in the body wall form the **costal processes,** which form the ribs in the thoracic region.

Cartilaginous Stage of Vertebral Development

During the sixth week, chondrification centers appear in each mesenchymal vertebra (Fig. 15-6A and B). At the end of the embryonic period, the two centers in each centrum fuse to form a cartilaginous centrum. Concomitantly, the centers in the neural arches fuse with each other and the centrum. The spinous and transverse processes develop from extensions of chondrification centers in the vertebral arch. Chondrification spreads until a cartilaginous vertebral column is formed.

Bony Stage of Vertebral Development

Ossification of typical vertebrae begins during the embryonic period and usually ends by the 25th year. There are **primary ossification centers** in the centrum—ventral and dorsal (Fig. 15-6C), which soon fuse to form one center.

Primary centers are also present by the end of the embryonic period in each half of the vertebral arch.

Ossification becomes evident in the neural arches during the eighth week. At birth, each vertebra consists of three bony parts connected by cartilage (Fig. 15-6D). The bony halves of the **vertebral arch** usually fuse during the first 3 to 5 years of life. The arches first unite in the lumbar region, and union progresses cranially. The vertebral arch articulates with the **centrum** at cartilaginous **neurocentral joints.** These articulations permit the vertebral arches to grow as the spinal cord enlarges. These joints disappear when the vertebral arch fuses with the centrum during the third to sixth years. Five **secondary ossification centers** appear in the vertebrae after puberty:

- One for the tip of the spinous process
- One for the tip of each transverse process
- Two *anular epiphyses,* one on the superior rim and one on the inferior rim of the vertebral body (Fig. 15-6E and F)

The **vertebral body** is a composite of the anular epiphyses and the mass of bone between them. All secondary centers unite with the rest of the vertebrae at approximately 25 years of age. Variations in the ossification of vertebrae occur in C_1 (atlas), C_2 (axis), and C_7 vertebrae, and in the lumbar vertebrae, sacrum, and coccyx.

VARIATIONS IN THE NUMBER OF VERTEBRAE

Most people have 7 cervical, 12 thoracic, 5 lumbar, and 5 sacral vertebrae. A few have one or two more vertebrae or one less. An apparent extra (or absent) vertebra in one segment of the column may be compensated for by an absent (or extra) vertebra in an adjacent segment.

KLIPPEL-FEIL SYNDROME

The main features of the *Klippel-Feil syndrome* (*Brevicollis*) are a short neck, a low hairline, and restricted neck movements. In most cases, the number of cervical vertebral bodies is fewer than normal. In some cases, there is a lack of segmentation of several elements of the cervical region of the vertebral column. The number of cervical nerve roots may be normal, but they are small, as are the intervertebral foramina. Persons with this syndrome are often otherwise normal, but the association of this anomaly with other congenital anomalies is not uncommon.

Development of Ribs

The ribs develop from the mesenchymal **costal processes** of the thoracic vertebrae (Fig. 15-6A). They become cartilaginous during the embryonic period and ossify during the fetal period. The original site of union of the costal processes with the vertebrae is replaced by **costovertebral synovial joints** (Fig. 15-6D). Seven pairs of ribs (**true ribs**) attach by their own cartilages to the sternum. Five pairs of ribs (**false ribs**) attach to the sternum through the cartilage of another rib or ribs. The last two pairs of ribs (**floating ribs**) do not attach to the sternum.

Development of Sternum

A pair of vertical mesenchymal bands—**sternal bars**—develops ventrolaterally in the body wall. Chondrification occurs in these bars as they move medially. *They fuse craniocaudally in the median plane* to form cartilaginous models of the manubrium, sternebrae (segments of the sternal body), and xiphoid process. Centers of ossification appear craniocaudally in the sternum before birth, except the ossification center for the xiphoid process, which appears during childhood.

Development of Cranium

The cranium (skull) develops from the mesenchyme around the developing brain. The cranium consists of:

- The *neurocranium*, a protective case for the brain
- The *viscerocranium*, the skeleton of the face

Cartilaginous Neurocranium

Endochondral ossification of the neurocranium forms the bones of the base of the cranium. The ossification pattern of these bones has a definite sequence, beginning with the occipital bone, the body of the sphenoid, and the ethmoid bone. The **parachordal cartilage**, or basal plate, forms around the cranial end of the notochord (Fig. 15-7A) and fuses with the cartilages derived from the sclerotome regions of the occipital somites. This cartilaginous mass contributes to the **base of the occipital bone**; later, extensions grow around the cranial end of the spinal cord and form the boundaries of the foramen magnum (Fig. 15-7C). The **hypophysial cartilage** forms around the developing pituitary gland and fuses to form the body of the sphenoid bone (Fig. 15-7B). The *trabeculae cranii* fuse to form the body of the ethmoid bone, and the ala orbitalis forms the lesser wing of the sphenoid bone.

Otic capsules develop around the otic vesicles, the primordia of the internal ears (see Chapter 17), and form the petrous and mastoid parts of the temporal bone. **Nasal capsules** develop around the nasal sacs (Chapter 10) and contribute to the formation of the ethmoid bone.

Membranous Neurocranium

Intramembranous ossification occurs in the mesenchyme at the sides and top of the brain, forming the **calvaria** (cranial vault). During fetal life, the flat bones of the calvaria are separated by dense connective tissue membranes that form fibrous joints, that is, **sutures** (Fig. 15-8). Six large fibrous areas—**fontanelles**—are present where several sutures meet. The softness of the bones and their loose connections at the sutures enable the calvaria to undergo changes of shape (**molding of fetal cranium**) during birth. The frontal bones become flat, the occipital bone is drawn out, and one parietal bone slightly overrides the other one. Within a few days after birth, the shape of the calvaria returns to normal.

Cartilaginous Viscerocranium

The cartilaginous viscerocranium is derived from the cartilaginous skeleton of the first two pairs of pharyngeal arches (see Chapter 10).

- The dorsal end of the first pharyngeal arch cartilage forms the malleus and incus.
- The dorsal end of the second pharyngeal arch cartilage forms the stapes and styloid process of the temporal bone. Its ventral end ossifies to form the lesser horn and the superior part of the body of the hyoid bone.
- The third, fourth, and sixth pharyngeal arch cartilages form only in the ventral parts of the arches. The third pharyngeal arch cartilages give rise to the greater horns and the inferior part of the body of the hyoid bone. The fourth and sixth pharyngeal arch cartilages fuse to form the laryngeal cartilages, except for the epiglottis.

Membranous Viscerocranium

Intramembranous ossification occurs in the maxillary prominence of the first pharyngeal arch (see Chapter 10) and subsequently forms the squamous temporal, maxillary, and zygomatic bones. The squamous temporal bones

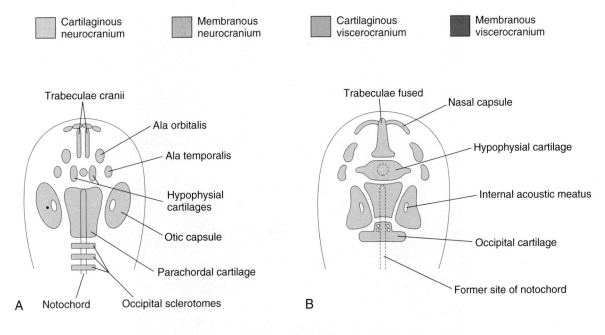

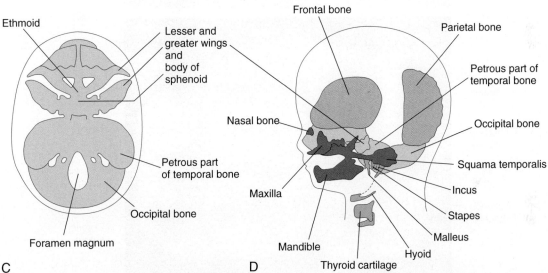

Figure 15–7 Stages in the development of the cranium. The base of the developing cranium is viewed superiorly (**A** to **C**), and laterally (**D**). **A,** At 6 weeks, showing the various cartilages that will fuse to form the chondrocranium. **B,** At 7 weeks, after fusion of some of the paired cartilages. **C,** At 12 weeks, showing the cartilaginous base of the cranium, or chondrocranium, formed by the fusion of various cartilages. **D,** At 20 weeks, indicating the derivation of the bones of the fetal cranium.

become part of the neurocranium. The mandibular prominence forms the mandible. Some endochondral ossification occurs in the median plane of the chin and in the mandibular condyle.

Newborn Cranium

The cranium of a neonate is large in proportion to the rest of the skeleton, and the face is relatively small compared with the calvaria (roof of cranium). The small facial region of the cranium results from the small size of the jaws, the virtual absence of paranasal (air) sinuses, and underdevelopment of the facial bones.

Postnatal Growth of Cranium

The fibrous sutures permit the brain and calvaria to enlarge during infancy and childhood. The increase in size is greatest during the first 2 years of life, but the calvaria continues to expand to conform to brain growth until approximately 16 years, after which its size usually increases slightly for 3 to 4 years because of thickening of its bones.

There is also rapid growth of the face and jaws, coinciding with eruption of the primary (deciduous) teeth. These facial changes are more marked after the secondary (permanent) teeth erupt (see Chapter 18).

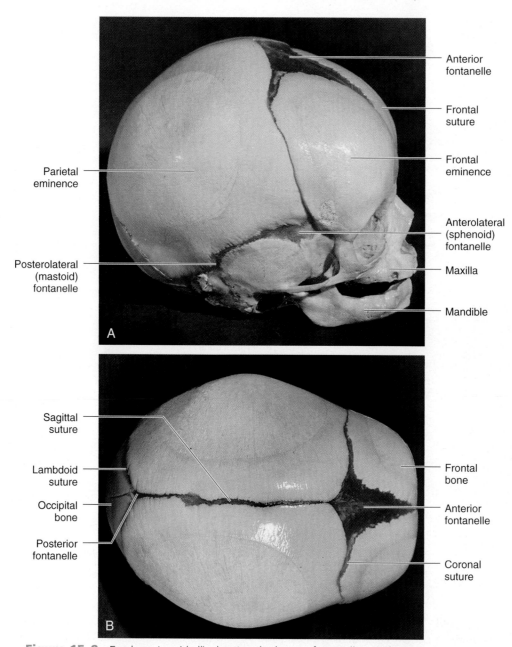

Figure 15–8   Fetal cranium (skull), showing the bones, fontanelles, and connecting sutures. **A,** Lateral view. **B,** Superior view. The posterior and anterolateral fontanelles disappear within 2 or 3 months after birth because of the growth of the surrounding bones, but they remain as sutures for several years. The posterolateral fontanelles disappear in a similar manner by the end of the first year, and the anterior fontanelle disappears by the end of the second year. The halves of the frontal bone normally begin to fuse during the second year, and the frontal suture is usually obliterated by the eighth year.

ACCESSORY RIBS

Accessory ribs, usually rudimentary, result from the development of costal processes from the cervical or lumbar vertebrae (Fig. 15-6A). The most common type of accessory rib is a **lumbar rib,** but it is clinically insignificant. **Cervical ribs** occur in 0.5% to 1% of people (Fig. 15-9A). A cervical rib is attached to the seventh cervical vertebra and may be unilateral or bilateral. Pressure of a cervical rib on the brachial plexus of nerves or the subclavian artery often produces neurovascular symptoms.

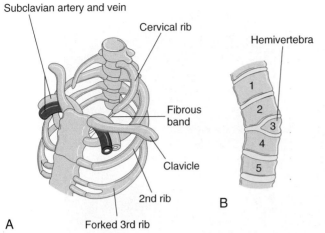

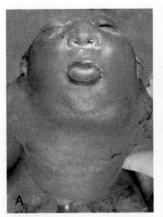 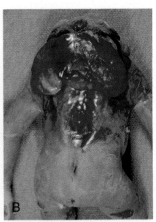

Figure 15–9 Vertebral and rib abnormalities. **A,** Cervical and forked ribs. Observe that the left cervical rib has a fibrous band that passes posterior to the subclavian vessels and attaches to the sternum. **B,** Anterior view of the vertebral column, showing a hemivertebra. The right half of the third thoracic vertebra is absent.

Figure 15–10 Anterior **(A)** and posterior **(B)** views of a 20-week fetus with severe birth defects, including acrania (absence of calvaria), cervical rachischisis (extensive clefts in the vertebral arches), cerebral regression (meroencephaly or anencephaly), and iniencephaly (defect in occiput—back of cranium). *(Courtesy of Dr. Marc Del Bigio, Department of Pathology [Neuropathology], University of Manitoba, Winnipeg, Manitoba, Canada.)*

HEMIVERTEBRA

Developing vertebral bodies have two chondrification centers that soon unite. A hemivertebra results from failure of one of the chondrification centers to appear and subsequent failure of half of the vertebra to form (see Fig. 15-9B). These vertebral defects produce **scoliosis** (lateral curvature) of the vertebral column.

RACHISCHISIS

Rachischisis (cleft vertebral column) refers to vertebral abnormalities in a complex group of anomalies (**axial dysraphic disorders**) that primarily affect axial structures (Fig. 15-10). In affected infants, the neural folds do not fuse, either because of faulty induction by the underlying notochord or because of a teratogenic agent.

ACRANIA

In acrania, the calvaria is absent, and extensive defects of the vertebral column are often present (Fig. 15-10). Acrania is associated with **meroencephaly (anencephaly)**. Partial absence of the brain occurs in approximately 1 in 1000 births and is incompatible with life. Meroencephaly occurs when the cranial end of the neural tube does not close during the fourth week of development, resulting in subsequent failure of the calvaria to form.

CRANIOSYNOSTOSIS

Several cranial deformities result from premature closure of the cranial sutures. Prenatal closure results in the most severe abnormalities. The cause of craniosynostosis is unclear, but genetic factors appear to be important. *Homeobox gene (MSX2 and ALX4) mutations have been implicated in cases of craniosynostosis* and other cranial defects. These abnormalities are much more common in males than in females, and they are often associated with other skeletal anomalies. The type of cranial deformation produced depends on which sutures close prematurely. If the sagittal suture closes early, the cranium becomes elongated and wedge-shaped, a condition known as **scaphocephaly** (Fig. 15-11A). This type of cranial deformity constitutes approximately half of the cases of craniosynostosis. Another 30% of cases involve premature closure of the coronal suture, which results in a high, tower-like cranium, a condition known as **brachycephaly** (see Fig. 15-11B). If the coronal suture closes prematurely on one side only, the cranium is twisted and asymmetrical, resulting in a condition known as **plagiocephaly**. Premature closure of the metopic suture results in a deformity of the frontal bone and other anomalies, known collectively as **trigonocephaly**.

There is concurrent enlargement of the frontal and facial regions, associated with the increase in the size of the paranasal sinuses (e.g., the maxillary sinuses). Growth of these sinuses is important in adding resonance to the voice.

DEVELOPMENT OF APPENDICULAR SKELETON

The appendicular skeleton consists of the pectoral and pelvic girdles and the limb bones. During the sixth week, the **mesenchymal bone models** undergo chondrification

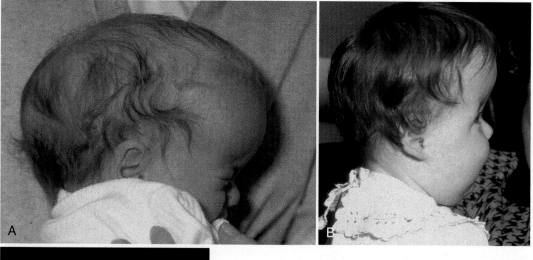

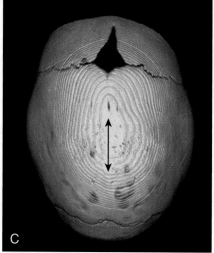

Figure 15–11 Craniosynostosis. **A,** An infant with scapho-cephaly (long narrow head) resulting from premature closure of the sagittal suture. **B,** An infant with bilateral premature closure of the coronal suture—brachycephaly—resulting in a high, tower-like forehead. **C,** Cranium of a 9-month-old infant with scaphocephaly resulting from premature closure of the sagittal suture (sagittal synostosis; *double arrow*). CT recon-structed image. (**A, B,** *Courtesy of Dr. John A. Jane, Sr., Department of Neurological Surgery, University of Virginia Health System, Charlottesville, VA.* **C,** *Courtesy of Dr. Gerald S. Smyser, Altru Health System, Grand Forks, ND.*)

to form **hyaline cartilage bone models** (Fig. 15-12). The clavicle initially develops by intramembranous ossifica-tion; later, growth cartilages form at both ends. The models of the pectoral girdle and the upper limb bones appear slightly before those of the pelvic girdle and the lower limbs; the bone models appear in a proximodistal sequence. *The molecular mechanism of limb morphogen-esis is regulated by specialized signaling centers along three axes of development (proximal/ distal, ventral/ dorsal, and anterior/posterior). Patterning in the develop-ing limbs is controlled by Hox and other complex signal-ing pathways.*

Endochondral ossification begins in the long bones by the eighth week (Fig. 15-3B and C). By 12 weeks, primary ossification centers have appeared in nearly all limb bones (Fig. 15-13). The clavicles begin to ossify before any other bones in the body, followed by the femurs. Virtually all **primary centers of ossification** (diaphysial) are present at birth.

The secondary ossification centers of the bones at the knee are the first to appear in utero. The secondary centers for the distal end of the femur and the proximal end of the tibia usually appear during the last month of intrauterine life (34–38 weeks). The secondary centers of the other bones appear after birth. The bone formed from

the primary center in the diaphysis does not fuse at the **epiphyseal plate** with that formed from the secondary centers in the epiphyses until the bone grows to its adult length. This delay enables lengthening of the bone to continue until the final size is reached.

BONE AGE

Bone age is a good index of general maturation. A radiolo-gist can determine the bone age of a person by assessing the ossification centers using two criteria:

* The time of appearance of calcified material in the diaphy-sis, epiphysis, or both is specific for each diaphysis and epiphysis and for each bone and sex.
* The disappearance of the dark line representing the epi-physial cartilage plate indicates that the epiphysis has fused with the diaphysis.

Fusion of the diaphysial–epiphysial centers, which occurs at specific times for each epiphysis, happens 1 to 2 years earlier in females than in males. In the fetus, ultrasonography is used for the evaluation and measurement of bones.

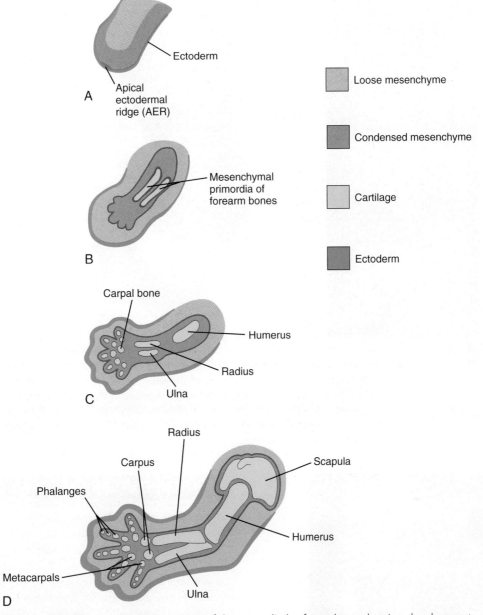

Loose mesenchyme

Condensed mesenchyme

Cartilage

Ectoderm

Figure 15–12 Longitudinal sections of the upper limb of a embryo, showing development of the cartilaginous bones. **A,** At 28 days. **B,** At 44 days. **C,** At 48 days. **D,** At 56 days.

GENERALIZED SKELETAL MALFORMATIONS

Achondroplasia is a common cause of short stature. It occurs in approximately 1 in 15,000 births. The limbs become bowed and short because of a disturbance of endochondral ossification at the epiphysial cartilage plates, particularly of the long bones, during fetal life (Fig. 15-14). The trunk is usually short, and the head is enlarged, with a bulging forehead and a "scooped-out" nose (flat nasal bone). Achondroplasia is an **autosomal dominant disorder**, and approximately 80% of cases arise from new mutations; the rate increases with paternal age. *The majority of cases are due to a point mutation (f.1,11,12) in the FGFR3 gene*, which results in magnification of the normal inhibiting effect of endochondral ossification, specifically in the zone of chondrocyte proliferation. This results in shortened bone, but does not affect growth of bone width (periosteal growth).

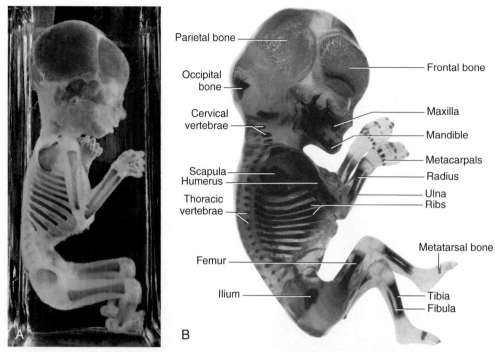

Parietal bone
Occipital bone
Cervical vertebrae
Scapula
Humerus
Thoracic vertebrae
Femur
Ilium
Frontal bone
Maxilla
Mandible
Metacarpals
Radius
Ulna
Ribs
Metatarsal bone
Tibia
Fibula

A
B

Figure 15–13 **A,** Alizarin-stained fetus, 20-week fetus. **B,** Alizarin-stained, 12-week fetus. Observe the degree of progression of ossification from the primary centers of ossification, which are endochondral in the appendicular and axial parts of the skeleton, except for most of the cranial bones. Note that the carpus and tarsus are wholly cartilaginous at this stage, as are the epiphyses of all long bones. (**A,** *Courtesy of Dr. David Bolender, Department of Cell Biology, Neurobiology, and Anatomy, Medical College of Wisconsin, Milwaukee, Wisconsin.* **B,** *Courtesy of Dr. Gary Geddes, Lake Oswego, Oregon.*)

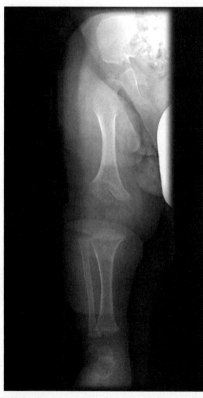

Figure 15–14 Radiograph of achondroplasia showing proximal shortening of the lower limbs. (*From Dr. Frank Gaillard, Radiopaedia.org, with permission.*)

HYPERPITUITARISM

Congenital infantile hyperpituitarism, which causes abnormally rapid growth in infancy, is rare. This condition may result in **gigantism** (excessive height and body proportions). In adults, hyperpituitarism results in **acromegaly** (enlargement of the soft tissues, visceral organs, and bones of the face, hands, and feet). In acromegaly, the epiphysial and diaphysial centers of the long bones fuse, thereby preventing elongation of the bones. Both gigantism and acromegaly result from an excessive secretion of growth hormone.

MUSCULAR SYSTEM

The muscular system develops from the **mesoderm,** except for the muscles of the iris, which develop from the **neuroectoderm.** Myoblasts—embryonic muscle cells— are derived from mesenchyme.

Development of Skeletal Muscle

The myoblasts that form the skeletal muscles of the trunk are derived from the mesenchyme in the myotome regions of the somites. The limb muscles develop from **myogenic precursor cells** in the limb buds. Studies show that these cells originate from the ventral **dermomyotome of somites** in response to molecular signals from nearby tissues

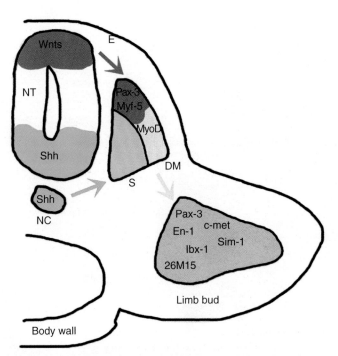

Figure 15-15 A model for molecular interactions during myogenesis. Shh and Wnt, produced by the neural tube *(NT)* and the notochord *(NC)*, induce Pax-3 and Myf-5 in the somites. Either of them can activate the initiation of MyoD transcription and myogenesis. The surface ectoderm *(E)* is also capable of inducing Myf-5 and MyoD. Pax-3 also regulates the expression of c-met, which, in turn, is necessary for the migratory ability of the myogenic precursor cells, which also express En-1, Sim-1, lbx-1, and 26M15. *DM*, dermomyotome; *S*, sclerotome. *(From Kablar B, Rudnicki MA: Skeletal muscle development in the mouse embryo. Histol Histopathol 15:649, 2000.)*

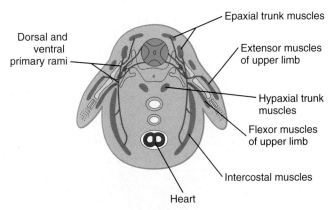

Figure 15-16 Transverse section of the embryo, showing the epaxial and hypaxial derivatives of a myotome.

Fibroblasts produce the perimysium and epimysium layers of the fibrous sheath; the endomysium is formed by the external lamina, which is derived from the muscle fiber, and by reticular fibers. Most skeletal muscle develops before birth, and almost all remaining muscles are formed by the end of the first year. The increase in the size of a muscle after the first year results from an increase in the diameter of the fibers because of the formation of more myofilaments. Muscles increase in length and width to grow with the skeleton.

Myotomes

Typically, each myotome part of a somite divides into a dorsal **epaxial division** and a ventral **hypaxial division** (Fig. 15-16). Each developing **spinal nerve** also divides and sends a branch to each division, with the **dorsal primary ramus** supplying the epaxial division and the **ventral primary ramus** supplying the hypaxial division. Some muscles—the intercostal muscles, for example—remain segmentally arranged like the somites, but most myoblasts migrate away from the myotome and form nonsegmented muscles.

Derivatives of Epaxial Divisions of Myotomes

Myoblasts from the epaxial divisions of the myotomes form the segmental muscles of the main body axis, the extensor muscles of the neck and vertebral column (Fig. 15-17). The embryonic extensor muscles that are derived from the sacral and coccygeal myotomes degenerate; their adult derivatives are the dorsal sacrococcygeal ligaments.

Derivatives of Hypaxial Divisions of Myotomes

Myoblasts from the hypaxial divisions of the cervical myotomes form the scalene, prevertebral, geniohyoid, and infrahyoid muscles (Fig. 15-17A). Those from the thoracic myotomes form the lateral and ventral flexor muscles of the vertebral column, whereas the lumbar myotomes form the quadratus lumborum muscle. The muscles of the limbs, the intercostal muscles, and the abdominal muscles are also derived from the hypaxial division of the myotomes. The sacrococcygeal myotomes form the muscles of the pelvic diaphragm and probably the striated muscles of the anus and sex organs.

(Fig. 15-15). The myogenic precursor cells migrate into the limb buds, where they undergo epitheliomesenchymal transformation. The first indication of **myogenesis** (muscle formation) is the elongation of the nuclei and cell bodies of mesenchymal cells as they differentiate into myoblasts. These **primordial muscle cells** soon fuse to form elongated, multinucleated, cylindric structures—**myotubes.** *At the molecular level, these events are preceded by gene activation and expression of the MyoD family of muscle-specific basic helix-loop-helix transcription factors (MyoD, myogenin, Myf-5, and MRF4) in the precursor myogenic cells. It has been suggested that signaling molecules from the ventral neural tube (Shh), the notochord (Shh), the dorsal neural tube (Wnt, BMP-4), and the overlying ectoderm (Wnt, BMP-4) regulate the beginning of myogenesis and the induction of the myotome.*

Muscle growth during development results from the ongoing fusion of myoblasts and myotubes. **Myofilaments** develop in the cytoplasm of the myotubes during or after fusion of the myoblasts. Soon after that, **myofibrils** and other organelles characteristic of striated muscle cells develop. Because muscle cells are long and narrow, they are called **muscle fibers.** As the myotubes differentiate, they become invested with external laminae, which segregate them from the surrounding connective tissue.

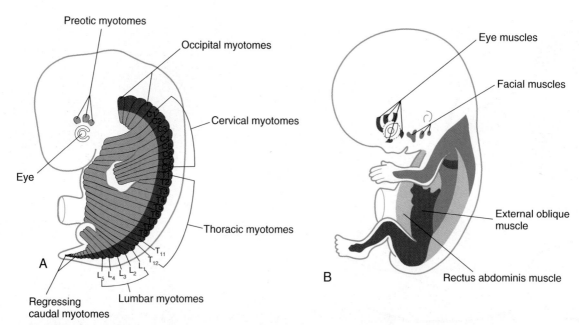

Figure 15–17   The developing muscular system. **A,** A 6-week embryo. The myotome regions of the somites give rise to most skeletal muscles. **B,** A 8-week embryo, showing the developing trunk and limb musculature.

Pharyngeal Arch Muscles

Myoblasts from the pharyngeal arches form the muscles of mastication and facial expression as well as those of the pharynx and larynx (see Chapter 10). These muscles are innervated by the pharyngeal arch nerves.

Ocular Muscles

The mesoderm in the prechordal plate area is believed to give rise to three *preotic myotomes* from which myoblasts differentiate (see Fig. 15-17*B*). Groups of myoblasts, each supplied by its own cranial nerve (CN III, CN IV, or CN VI), form the extrinsic muscles of the eye.

Tongue Muscles

Myoblasts from the *occipital (postotic) myotomes* form the tongue muscles, which are innervated by the hypoglossal nerve (CN XII).

Limb Muscles

The musculature of the limbs develops from myoblasts surrounding the developing bones (Fig. 15-16). The **precursor myogenic cells** in the limb buds originate from the somites. These cells are first located in the ventral part of the dermomyotome, and they are epithelial (see Fig. 15-1*D*). After **epitheliomesenchymal transformation,** the cells migrate into the primordium of the limb.

Development of Smooth Muscle

Some smooth muscle fibers differentiate from the splanchnic mesenchyme surrounding the endoderm of the primordial gut and its derivatives (see Fig. 15-1*E*). The smooth muscle in the walls of many blood and lymphatic vessels arises from the somatic mesoderm. The muscles of the iris (sphincter and dilator pupillae) and the

myoepithelial cells in the mammary and sweat glands are believed to be derived from mesenchymal cells that originate from ectoderm.

The first sign of differentiation of smooth muscle is the development of elongated nuclei in spindle-shaped myoblasts. During early development, new myoblasts continue to differentiate from mesenchymal cells, but do not fuse; they remain mononucleated. During later development, the division of existing myoblasts gradually replaces the differentiation of new myoblasts in the production of new smooth muscle tissue. Filamentous, but nonsarcomeric, contractile elements develop in their cytoplasm, and the external surface of each differential cell acquires a surrounding external lamina. As smooth muscle fibers develop into sheets or bundles, they receive autonomic innervation; fibroblasts and muscle cells synthesize and lay down collagenous, elastic, and reticular fibers.

Development of Cardiac Muscle

The lateral splanchnic mesoderm gives rise to the mesenchyme surrounding the developing heart tube (see Chapter 14). **Cardiac myoblasts** are derived from this mesenchyme by differentiation and growth of single cells, unlike striated skeletal muscle fibers, which develop by the fusion of cells. The myoblasts adhere to each other as in developing skeletal muscle, but the intervening cell membranes do not disintegrate; these areas of adhesion give rise to **intercalated discs.** Growth of cardiac muscle fibers results from the formation of new **myofilaments.** Late in the embryonic period, special bundles of muscle cells develop that have relatively few myofibrils and relatively larger diameters than typical cardiac muscle fibers. These atypical cardiac muscle cells—**Purkinje fibers**—form the conducting system of the heart (see Chapter 14).

ANOMALIES OF MUSCLES

Any muscle in the body may occasionally be absent; common examples are the sternocostal head of the pectoralis major, the palmaris longus, the trapezius, the serratus anterior, and the quadratus femoris. Absence of the pectoralis major, often its sternal part, is usually associated with syndactyly (fusion of digits). This anomaly is part of the **Poland syndrome**, which also includes breast and nipple aplasia or hypoplasia, deficiencies of axillary hair and subcutaneous fat, and shortened arms and fingers.

Congenital absence of the diaphragm is usually associated with pulmonary atelectasis (incomplete expansion of the lungs or part of a lung) and pneumonitis (pneumonia). The sternocleidomastoid muscle is sometimes injured at birth, resulting in **congenital torticollis**. There is fixed rotation and tilting of the head because of concomitant muscle fibrosis, as well as shortening of the sternocleidomastoid muscle on one side (Fig. 15-18). Although birth trauma is commonly considered a cause of congenital torticollis, this may also result from malpositioning in utero.

ACCESSORY MUSCLES

Accessory muscles occasionally develop. For example, an *accessory soleus muscle* is present in approximately 6% of the population. It has been suggested that the primordium of the soleus muscle may undergo early splitting to form an accessory soleus.

DEVELOPMENT OF LIMBS

Early Stages of Limb Development

The **limb buds** first appear toward the end of the fourth week as small elevations of the ventrolateral body wall (Fig. 6-9). Limb development begins with the activation of a group of mesenchymal cells in the lateral mesoderm. The upper limb buds are visible by day 26 or 27, whereas the lower limb buds appear 1 to 2 days later. Each limb bud consists of a mass of mesenchyme covered by ectoderm (Fig. 15-12A and B). The mesenchyme is derived from the somatic layer of the lateral mesoderm. The limb buds elongate by the proliferation of the mesenchyme. Although the early stages of limb development are alike for the upper and lower limbs (Figs. 6-9 and 6-10), there are distinct differences because of their form and function. The **upper limb buds** develop opposite the caudal cervical segments, whereas the **lower limb buds** form opposite the lumbar and upper sacral segments.

At the apex of each limb bud, the ectoderm thickens to form an **apical ectodermal ridge** (AER) (Fig. 15-12A). The AER, a multilayered epithelial structure, interacts with the mesenchyme in the limb bud, promoting

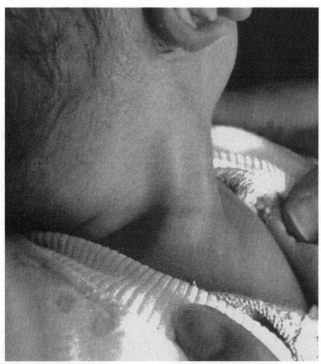

Figure 15–18 Congenital muscular torticollis (wry neck), showing extensive involvement of the left sternocleidomastoid muscle in an infant at 2 months. *(Courtesy of Professor Jack C.Y. Cheng, Department of Orthopaedics & Traumatology, The Chinese University of Hong Kong, Hong Kong, China.)*

outgrowth of the bud. Retinoic acid promotes the formation of the limb bud by inhibiting fibroblast growth factor (FGF8) signaling. The AER exerts an inductive influence on the limb mesenchyme that initiates growth and development of the limbs in a proximodistal axis. Mesenchymal cells aggregate at the posterior margin of the limb bud to form a **zone of polarizing activity**. Fibroblast growth factors from the AER activate the zone of polarizing activity, causing expression of the sonic hedgehog gene (Shh), which controls the patterning of the limb along the anteroposterior axis. *Expression of Wnt7 from the dorsal epidermis of the limb bud and engrailed-1 (En-1) from the ventral aspect is involved in specifying the dorsoventral axis. Curiously, the AER itself is maintained by inductive signals from Shh and Wnt7.* The mesenchyme adjacent to the AER consists of undifferentiated, rapidly proliferating cells, whereas the mesenchymal cells proximal to it differentiate into blood vessels and cartilage bone models. The distal ends of the limb buds eventually flatten into hand- and foot-plates (Fig. 15-19).

By the end of the sixth week of development, mesenchymal tissue in the **handplates** has condensed to form *finger buds—digital rays—*(Figs. 15-19 and 15-20A to C), which outline the pattern of the digits. During the seventh week, similar condensations of mesenchyme in foot plates form *toe buds—digital rays—*(Fig. 15-20G to I). At the tip of each digital ray, a part of the AER induces development of the mesenchyme into the

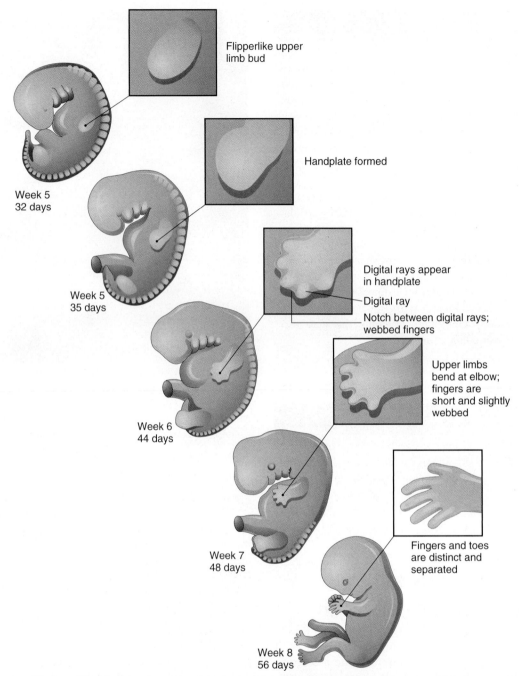

Figure 15–19   Development of the limbs (32-56 days). Note that development of the upper limbs precedes that of the lower limbs.

mesenchymal primordia of the bones (phalanges) in the digits. The intervals between the digital rays are occupied by loose mesenchyme. Soon the intervening regions of mesenchyme undergo **apoptosis** (*programmed cell death*), forming *notches between the digital rays* (see Figs. 15-19 and 15-20D and J). As this tissue breakdown progresses, separate digits are produced by the end of the eighth week of development (see Fig. 15-19). Blocking of cellular and molecular events during this process may account for webbing, or fusion, of the fingers or toes, a condition known as **syndactyly** (see Fig. 15-25C and D).

Final Stages of Limb Development

The mesenchyme in the limb bud gives rise to bones, ligaments, and blood vessels (Fig. 15-12). As the limb buds elongate during the early part of the fifth week of development, mesenchymal models of the bones are formed by cellular aggregations (see Fig. 15-12A and B). **Chondrification centers** appear later in the fifth week. By the end of the sixth week, the entire limb skeleton is cartilaginous (see Fig. 15-12C and D).

Osteogenesis of the long bones begins in the seventh week from primary ossification centers in the diaphyses of the long bones. **Primary ossification centers** are present

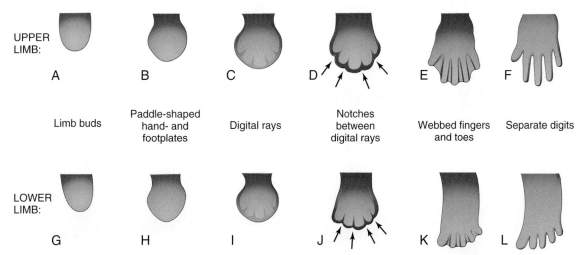

UPPER LIMB:

A — B — C — D — E — F

Limb buds | Paddle-shaped hand- and footplates | Digital rays | Notches between digital rays | Webbed fingers and toes | Separate digits

LOWER LIMB:

G — H — I — J — K — L

Figure 15–20 Development of the hands and feet between the fourth and eighth weeks. The early stages of limb development are similar, except that development of the hands precedes that of the feet by approximately 1 day. **A,** At 27 days. **B,** At 32 days. **C,** At 41 days. **D,** At 46 days. **E,** At 50 days. **F,** At 52 days. **G,** At 28 days. **H,** At 36 days. **I,** At 46 days. **J,** At 49 days. **K,** At 52 days. **L,** At 56 days. The *arrows* in **D** and **J** indicate the tissue breakdown processes that separate the fingers and toes.

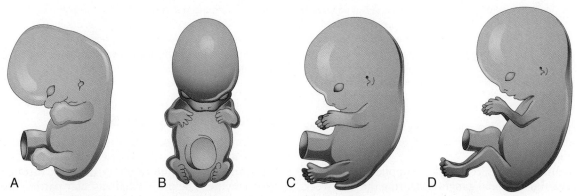

A — B — C — D

Figure 15–21 Positional changes of the developing limbs of human embryos. **A,** At approximately 48 days, showing the limbs extending ventrally and the handplates and footplates facing each other. **B,** At approximately 51 days, showing the upper limbs bent at the elbows and the hands curved over the thorax. **C,** At approximately 54 days, showing the soles of the feet facing medially. **D,** At approximately 56 days. Note that the elbows now point caudally and the knees, cranially.

in all *long* bones by the 12th week. Primary ossification of the carpal (wrist) bones begins during the first year after birth.

From the **dermomyotome regions of the somites,** myogenic precursor cells also migrate into the limb bud and later differentiate into **myoblasts,** the precursors of muscle cells. As the long bones form, myoblasts aggregate and form a large muscle mass in each limb bud (Fig. 15-16). In general, this muscle mass separates into dorsal (extensor) and ventral (flexor) components.

Early in the seventh week, the limbs extend ventrally and the preaxial and postaxial borders are cranial and caudal, respectively (see Fig. 15-22*A* and *D*). The *upper limbs rotate laterally* through 90 degrees on their longitudinal axes; thus, the future elbows point dorsally and the extensor muscles lie on the lateral and posterior aspects of the limb. The *lower limbs rotate medially*

through almost 90 degrees; thus, the future knees face ventrally and the extensor muscles lie on the anterior aspect of the lower limb (Fig. 15-21*A* to *D*).

The radius and the tibia are homologous bones, as are the ulna and the fibula, just as the thumb and the great toe are homologous digits. **Synovial joints** appear at the beginning of the fetal period, coinciding with functional differentiation of the limb muscles and their innervation.

Cutaneous Innervation of Limbs

Motor axons arising from the spinal cord enter the limb buds during the fifth week of development and grow into the dorsal and ventral muscle masses. **Sensory axons** enter the limb buds after the motor axons and use them for guidance. **Neural crest cells,** the precursors of Schwann

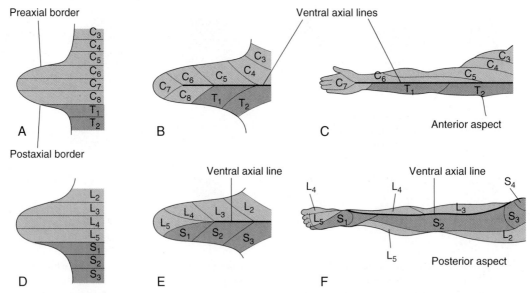

Figure 15–22   Development of the dermatomal patterns of the limbs. The axial lines indi-cate where there is no sensory overlap. **A** and **D,** Ventral aspect of the limb buds early in the fifth week. At this stage, the dermatomal patterns show the primordial segmental arrangement. **B** and **E,** Similar views later in the fifth week, showing the modified arrangement of dermatomes. **C** and **F,** The dermatomal patterns in the adult upper and lower limbs. The primordial derma-tomal pattern has disappeared, but an orderly sequence of dermatomes can still be recognized. In **F,** note that most of the original ventral surface of the lower limb lies on the back of the adult limb. This results from the medial rotation of the lower limb that occurs toward the end of the embryonic period. In the upper limb, the ventral axial line extends along the anterior surface of the arm and forearm. In the lower limb, the ventral axial line extends along the medial side of the thigh and knee, to the posteromedial aspect of the leg to the heel.

cells, surround the motor and sensory nerve fibers in the limbs and *form the neurolemmal and myelin sheaths* (see Chapter 16).

A **dermatome** is the area of skin supplied by a single spinal nerve and its spinal ganglion. During the fifth week of development, the peripheral nerves grow from the developing **limb** (brachial and lumbosacral) **plexuses** into the mesenchyme of the limb buds (Fig. 15-22A and B). The spinal nerves are distributed in segmental bands, supplying both the dorsal and the ventral surfaces of the limb buds. As the limbs elongate, the cutaneous distribu-tion of the spinal nerves migrates along the limbs and no longer reaches the surface in the distal part of the limbs. Although the original **dermatomal pattern** changes during growth of the limbs, an orderly sequence of distribution can still be recognized in the adult (Fig. 15-22C and F). In the upper limb, the areas supplied by C_5 and C_6 adjoin the areas supplied by T_2, T_1, and C_8, but the overlap between them is minimal at the ventral axial line.

Because there is overlapping of **dermatomes**, a particu-lar area of skin is not exclusively innervated by a single segmental nerve. The limb dermatomes may be traced progressively down the lateral aspect of the upper limb and back up its medial aspect. A comparable distribution of dermatomes occurs in the lower limbs and may be traced down the ventral aspect and then up the dorsal aspect of the lower limb. When the limbs extend and rotate, they carry their nerves with them; this explains the oblique course of the nerves arising from the brachial and lumbosacral plexuses.

Blood Supply to Limbs

The limb buds are supplied by branches of the **interseg-mental arteries** (Fig. 15-23A), which arise from the dorsal aorta and form a fine capillary network throughout the mesenchyme. The primordial vascular pattern consists of a **primary axial artery** and its branches (Fig. 15-23B and C), which drain into a peripheral marginal sinus. Blood in the sinus drains into a peripheral vein.

The vascular pattern changes as the limbs develop, chiefly as a result of vessels sprouting from existing vessels (**angiogenesis**). The new vessels coalesce with other sprouts to form new vessels. The primary axial artery becomes the **brachial artery** in the arm and the **ulnar and radial arteries** in the forearm, its terminal branches of the brachial artery (see Fig. 15-23B). As the digits form, the marginal sinus breaks up and the final venous pattern, represented by the basilic and cephalic veins and their tributaries, develops. In the thigh, the primary axial artery is represented by the **deep artery of the thigh** (pro-funda femoris artery). In the leg, the primary axial artery is represented by the anterior and posterior **tibial arteries** (Fig. 15-23C).

CLINICALLY ORIENTED QUESTIONS

1. Occasionally, accessory ribs are associated with the seventh cervical vertebra and the first lumbar verte-bra. Are these accessory ribs of clinical importance? What is the embryologic basis of accessory ribs?

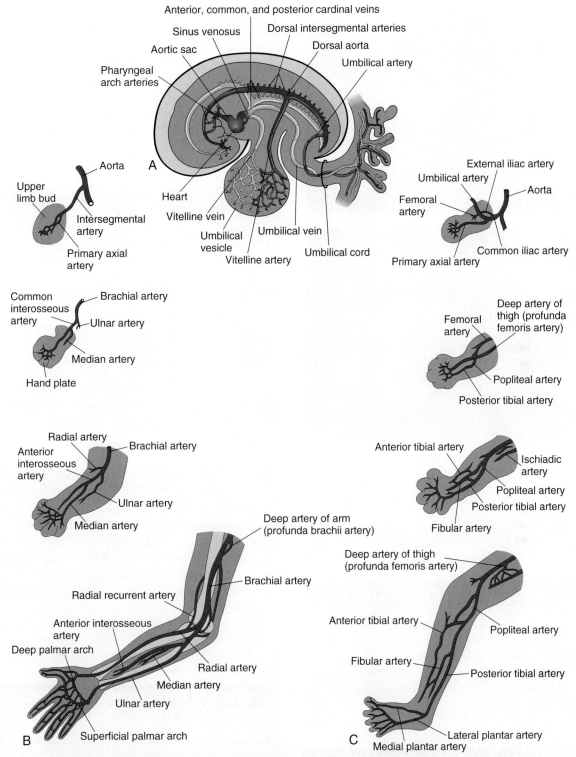

Figure 15–23 Development of the limb arteries. **A** and **B,** Development of the arteries in the upper limb. **C,** Development of the arteries in the lower limb.

2. What vertebral defect can produce scoliosis? Define this condition. What is the embryologic basis of the vertebral defect?

3. What is meant by the term *craniosynostosis*? What results from this developmental abnormality? Give a common example and describe it.

4. A child presented with characteristics of Klippel-Feil syndrome. What are the main features of this condition? What vertebral anomalies are usually present?

5. A newborn infant was born with prune-belly syndrome caused by failure of the abdominal musculature to develop normally. What do you think would

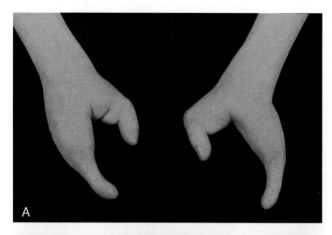

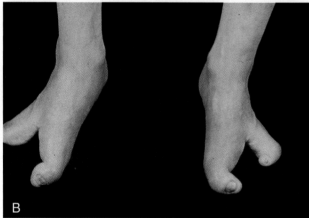

Figure 15–24 Anomalies of the hands and feet. **A,** Ectrodactyly in a child. Note the absence of the central digits of the hands, resulting in split hands. **B,** A similar type of defect involving the feet. These limb defects can be inherited in an autosomal dominant pattern. *(Courtesy of A.E. Chudley, M.D., Section of Genetics and Metabolism, Department of Pediatrics and Child Health, University of Manitoba, Children's Hospital, Winnipeg, Manitoba, Canada.)*

CLEFT HAND AND CLEFT FOOT

In the rare *cleft hand* or *cleft foot* abnormalities, one or more central digits are absent—**ectrodactylyl**—resulting from failure of one or more digital rays to develop (Fig. 15-24A and B). The hand or foot is divided into two parts that oppose each other. The remaining digits are partially or completely fused (**syndactyly**).

CONGENITAL ABSENCE OF RADIUS

In some individuals, the radius is partially or completely absent. The hand deviates laterally (radially), and the ulna bows with the concavity on the lateral side of the forearm. This anomaly results from failure of the mesenchymal primordium of the radius to form during the fifth week of development. Absence of the radius is usually caused by genetic factors.

POLYDACTYLY

Supernumerary digits are common (Fig. 15-25A and B). Often, the extra digit is incompletely formed and lacks proper muscular development, rendering it useless. If the hand is affected, the extra digit is most commonly medial or lateral rather than central. In the foot, the extra toe is usually on the lateral side. Polydactyly is inherited as a dominant trait.

SYNDACTYLY

Syndactyly occurs with a frequency of approximately 1 in 2200 births. **Cutaneous syndactyly** (simple webbing of the digits) is the most common limb anomaly (see Fig. 15-25C). It occurs more frequently in the foot than in the hand (see Fig. 15-25C and D). Syndactyly is most frequently observed between the third and fourth fingers and between the second and third toes (see Fig. 15-25D). It is inherited as a simple dominant or simple recessive trait. Cutaneous syndactyly results from failure of the webs to degenerate between two or more digits. In some cases, there is fusion of the bones (synostosis). **Osseous syndactyly** occurs when the notches between the digital rays do not develop during the seventh week; as a result, separation of the digits does not occur.

ARTHROGRYPOSIS

Arthrogryposis multiplex congenita refers to a heterogeneous group of musculoskeletal disorders characterized by multiple contractures and immobility of two or more joints from birth. The incidence of arthrogryposis multiplex congenita is 1 in 3000 live births and males are more affected in sex-linked cases. The causes may be both neurological (central and peripheral nervous system abnormalities) and nonneurological (cartilaginous abnormalities and restricted movement *in utero*).

CONGENITAL TALIPES (CLUBFOOT)

Talipes occurs at a rate of approximately 1 in 1000 births. **Talipes equinovarus**, the most common type (Fig. 15-26), occurs approximately twice as frequently in males as in females. The sole of the foot is turned medially, and the foot is inverted. There is much uncertainty about the cause of talipes. Hereditary factors are involved in some cases, and it appears that environmental factors are involved in most cases. Talipes appears to follow a **multifactorial pattern of inheritance**; hence, any intrauterine position that results in abnormal positioning of the feet may cause talipes if the fetus is genetically predisposed to this deformity.

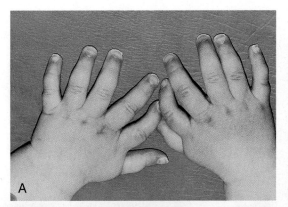
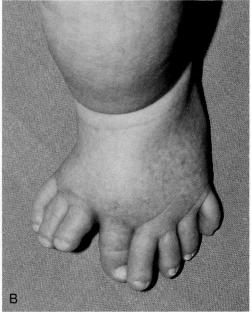
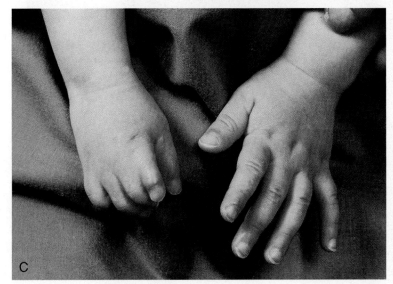
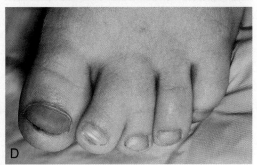

Figure 15–25 Various types of digital defects. **A,** Polydactyly of the hands. **B,** Polydactyly of the foot. This condition results from the formation of one or more extra digital rays during the embryonic period. **C** and **D,** Various forms of syndactyly involving the fingers and toes. Cutaneous syndactyly **(C)** is probably caused by incomplete apoptosis in the tissues between the digital rays during embryonic life. Syndactyly of the second and third toes is shown in **D.** In osseous syndactyly, the digital rays merge as a result of lack of apoptosis, causing fusion of the bones. *(Courtesy of A.E. Chudley, M.D., Section of Genetics and Metabolism, Department of Pediatrics and Child Health, University of Manitoba, Children's Hospital, Winnipeg, Manitoba, Canada.)*

LIMB ANOMALIES

There are two main types of limb anomalies:
* **Amelia**—complete absence of a limb
* **Meromelia**—partial absence of a limb

Terms such as hemimelia, peromelia, ectromelia, and phocomelia are also used.

Anomalies of the limbs originate at different stages of development. Suppression of limb bud development during the early part of the fourth week results in **amelia** (Fig. 15-27A). Arrest or disturbance of the differentiation or growth of the limbs during the fifth week results in **meromelia** (Fig. 15-27B and C). Some limb defects are caused by the following:

* Genetic factors, such as chromosomal abnormalities associated with trisomy 18 (Chapter 19).

* Mutant genes, as in brachydactyly (shortness of digits) or osteogenesis imperfecta (connective tissue disorders). *Molecular studies have implicated gene mutation (Hox gene, BMP, Shh, Wnt7, En-1, and others) in some cases of limb anomalies.*

* Environmental factors, such as teratogens (e.g., thalidomide).

* A combination of genetic and environmental factors (*multifactorial inheritance*), as in congenital dislocation of the hip.

* Vascular disruption and ischemia, as in limb reduction defects.

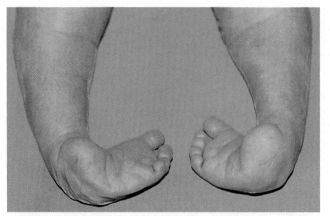

Figure 15–26 Neonate with bilateral talipes equinovarus deformities (club feet), illustrating the classic type of this anomaly, characterized by inversion and medial rotation of the soles of the feet. (*Courtesy of A.E. Chudley, M.D., Section of Genetics and Metabolism, Department of Pediatrics and Child Health, University of Manitoba, Children's Hospital, Winnipeg, Manitoba, Canada.*)

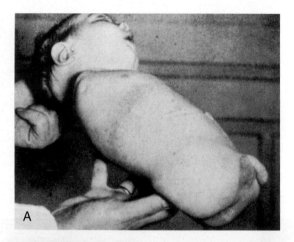

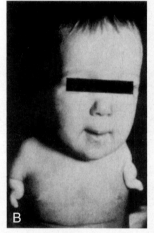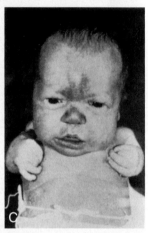

Figure 15–27 Limb anomalies due to thalidomide. **A,** Quadruple amelia (absence of the upper and lower limbs). **B,** Meromelia (partial absence) of the upper limbs. The limbs are represented by rudimentary stumps. **C,** Meromelia in which the rudimentary upper limbs are attached directly to the trunk. (*From Lenz W, Knapp K: Foetal malformations due to thalidomide. Ger Med Mon 7:253, 1962.*)

cause this congenital anomaly? What urinary anomaly results from abnormal development of the anterior abdominal wall?

6. A boy asked his mother why one of his nipples was much lower than the other one. She was unable to explain this anomaly. How would you explain the abnormally low position of the nipple?

7. An 8-year-old girl asked her doctor why the muscle on one side of her neck was so prominent. What would you tell her? What would happen if this muscle were not treated?

8. After strenuous exercise, a young athlete complained of pain on the posteromedial aspect of his ankle. He was told that he had an accessory calf muscle. Is this possible? If so, what is the embryologic basis of this anomaly?

9. An infant had short limbs. His trunk was normally proportioned, but his head was slightly larger than normal. Both parents had normal limbs, and these problems had never occurred in either of their families. Could the mother's ingestion of drugs during pregnancy have caused these abnormalities? If not, what would be the probable cause of these skeletal disorders? Could they occur again if the couple had more children?

10. A woman is interested in marrying a man who happens to have very short fingers (brachydactyly). He says that two of his relatives have short fingers, but none of his brothers or sisters has them. The woman has normal digits, and so does everyone else in her family. Clearly, heredity is involved, but what are the chances that the couple's children would have brachydactyly if they were to marry?

11. Approximately 1 year ago, a woman was reported to have given birth to a child with no right hand. She

had taken a drug that contained doxylamine and dicyclomine to alleviate nausea during the 10th week of her pregnancy (8 weeks after fertilization). The woman is instituting legal proceedings against the company that makes the drug. Does this drug cause limb defects? If it does, could it have caused failure of the child's hand to develop?

12. An infant had syndactyly of the left hand and absence of the left sternal head of the pectoralis major muscle. The infant seemed normal, except that the nipple on the left side was approximately 2 inches lower than the other one. What is the cause of these anomalies? Can they be corrected?

13. What is the most common type of clubfoot? How common is it? What is the appearance of the feet of infants born with this anomaly?

The answers to these questions are at the back of the book.

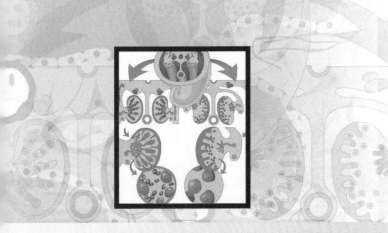

Nervous System

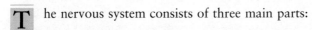

T he nervous system consists of three main parts:

- The **central nervous system** (CNS), which includes the brain and the spinal cord
- The **peripheral nervous system** (PNS), which includes neurons outside the CNS and the cranial and spinal nerves that connect the brain and spinal cord with the peripheral structures
- The **autonomic nervous system** (ANS), which has parts in both the CNS and PNS and which consists of neurons that innervate smooth muscle, cardiac muscle, glandular epithelium, or combinations of these tissues

ORIGIN OF NERVOUS SYSTEM

The nervous system develops from the **neural plate**, a thickened area of embryonic ectoderm (Fig. 16-1*A* and *B*). The notochord and paraxial mesoderm induce the overlying ectoderm to differentiate into the neural plate. Formation of the neural folds, neural tube, and neural crest from the neural plate is shown in Figure 16-1*B* to *F*. The **neural tube** differentiates into the CNS, consisting of the brain and spinal cord. The **neural crest** gives rise to the cells that form most of the PNS and ANS.

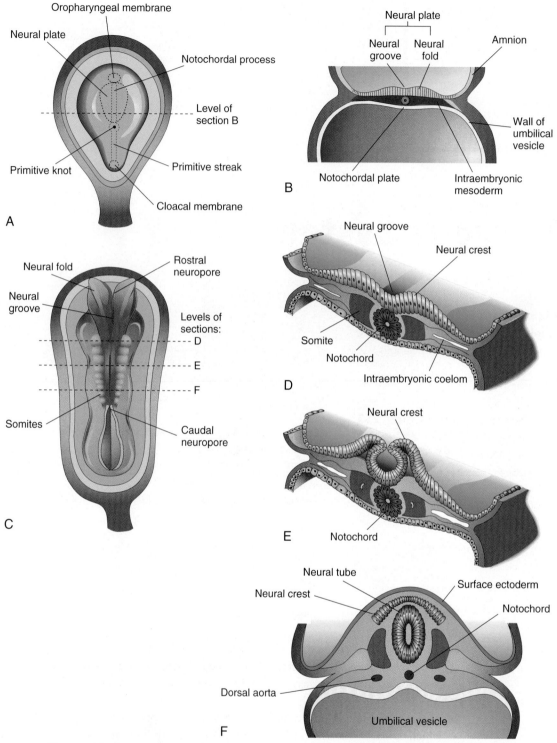

Figure 16–1 The neural plate and formation of the neural tube. **A,** Dorsal view of an embryo at approximately 18 days, exposed by removing the amnion. **B,** Transverse section of the embryo, showing the neural plate and early development of the neural groove and neural folds. **C,** Dorsal view of an embryo at approximately 22 days. The neural folds have fused opposite the fourth to sixth somites, but are open at both ends. **D to F,** Transverse sections of this embryo at the levels shown in **C,** showing the formation of the neural tube and its detachment from the surface ectoderm.

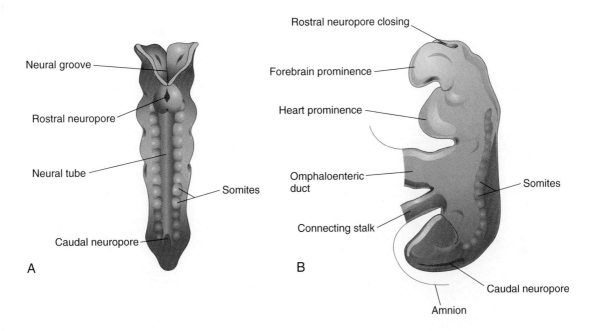

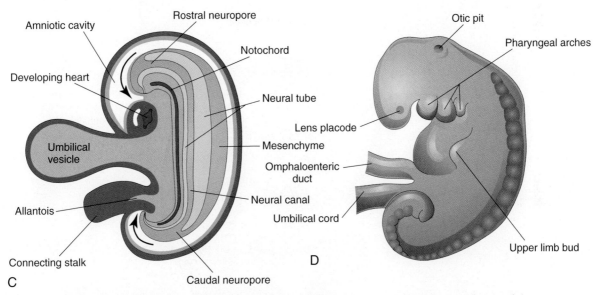

Figure 16–2 **A,** Dorsal view of an embryo at approximately 23 days, showing fusion of the neural folds, leading to formation of the neural tube. **B,** Lateral view of an embryo at approximately 24 days, showing the forebrain prominence and closing of the rostral neuropore. **C,** Sagittal section of the embryo, showing the transitory communication of the neural canal with the amniotic cavity (*arrows*). **D,** Lateral view of an embryo at approximately 27 days. Note that the neuropores shown in **B** are closed.

Formation of the neural plate and neural tube, a process known as **neurulation**, begins during the early part of the fourth week (22-23 days). Fusion of the **neural folds** proceeds in cranial and caudal directions until only small areas remain open at both ends (Fig. 16-2A and B). At these sites, the lumen of the neural tube—the **neural canal**—communicates freely with the amniotic cavity (Fig. 16-2C). The cranial opening—the *rostral neuropore*—closes on approximately the 25th day; the *caudal neuropore* closes 2 days later (Fig. 16-2D). **Closure of the neuropores** coincides with the establishment of a vascular circulation for the neural tube. The walls of the neural tube thicken to form the brain and spinal cord (Fig. 16-3). The neural canal forms the ventricular system of the brain and central canal of the spinal cord. *The dorsoventral patterning of the neural tube appears to involve the sonic hedgehog (Shh) gene, Pax genes, bone morphogenetic proteins, and dorsalin, a transforming growth factor (TGF-β).*

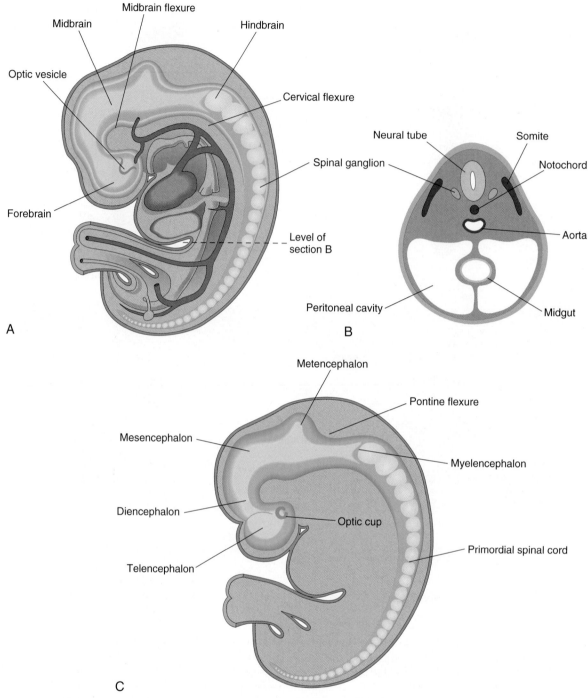

Figure 16–3 **A,** Lateral view of an embryo at approximately 28 days, showing the three primary brain vesicles: forebrain, midbrain, and hindbrain. Two flexures demarcate the primary divisions of the brain. **B,** Transverse section of the embryo, showing the neural tube that will develop into the spinal cord in this region. The spinal ganglia derived from the neural crest are also shown. **C,** Lateral view of the central nervous system of a 6-week embryo, showing the secondary brain vesicles and pontine flexure.

DEVELOPMENT OF SPINAL CORD

The neural tube caudal to the fourth pair of somites develops into the spinal cord (Fig. 16-3). The lateral walls of the neural tube thicken and gradually reduce the size of the neural canal to a minute **central canal** (Fig. 16-4A to C). Initially, the wall of the neural tube is composed

of a thick, pseudostratified, columnar neuroepithelium (Fig. 16-4D). These neuroepithelial cells constitute the **ventricular zone** (ependymal layer), which gives rise to all neurons and macroglial cells (e.g., astrocytes and oligodendrocytes) in the spinal cord (Fig. 16-5). Soon, a **marginal zone** composed of the outer parts of the neuroepithelial cells is recognizable (see Fig. 16-4E). This zone

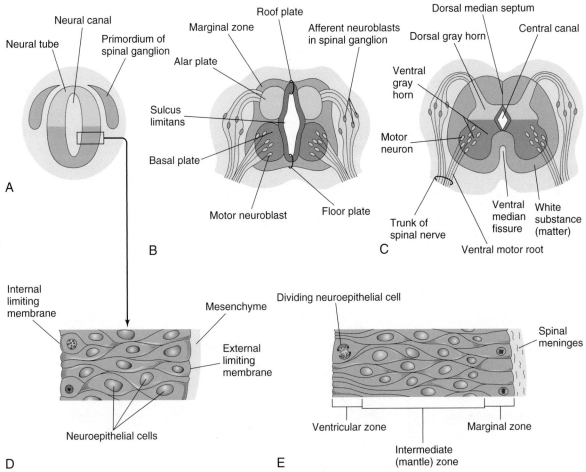

Figure 16–4 Development of the spinal cord. **A,** Transverse section of the neural tube of an embryo at approximately 23 days. **B** and **C,** Similar sections in 6- and 9-week embryos, respectively. **D,** Section of the wall of the neural tube shown in **A. E,** Section of the wall of the developing spinal cord, showing its three zones.

gradually becomes the white matter of the spinal cord as axons grow into it from nerve cell bodies in the spinal cord, spinal ganglia, and brain.

Some neuroepithelial cells in the ventricular zone differentiate into primordial neurons—**neuroblasts**. These embryonic cells form an **intermediate zone** (mantle layer) between the ventricular and marginal zones. Neuroblasts become neurons as they develop cytoplasmic processes (Fig. 16-5). The primordial supporting cells of the CNS—the **glioblasts** (spongioblasts)—differentiate from the neuroepithelial cells, mainly after neuroblast formation has ceased. The glioblasts migrate from the ventricular zone into the intermediate and marginal zones. Some glioblasts become **astroblasts** and later **astrocytes**, whereas other glioblasts become oligodendroblasts and eventually **oligodendrocytes** (Fig. 16-5). When neuroepithelial cells cease producing neuroblasts and glioblasts, they differentiate into ependymal cells, which form the **ependyma** lining the central canal of the spinal cord.

Microglial cells (**microglia**), which are scattered throughout the gray and white matter, are small cells that are derived from mesenchymal cells (Fig. 16-5). Microglial cells invade the CNS rather late in the fetal period,

after it has been penetrated by blood vessels. Microglia originate in the bone marrow and are part of the mononuclear phagocytic cell population.

Proliferation and differentiation of neuroepithelial cells in the developing spinal cord produce thick walls and a thin roof and floor plates (Fig. 16-4B). Differential thickening of the lateral walls of the spinal cord soon produces a shallow, longitudinal groove on each side, the **sulcus limitans** (Figs. 16-4B and 16-6). This groove separates the dorsal part, the **alar plate** (lamina), from the ventral part, the **basal plate** (lamina). The alar and basal plates produce longitudinal bulges extending through most of the length of the developing spinal cord. This regional separation is of fundamental importance because the alar and basal plates are later associated with afferent and efferent functions, respectively.

Cell bodies in the alar plates form the **dorsal gray columns** that extend the length of the spinal cord. In transverse sections, these columns are the **dorsal gray horns** (Fig. 16-7). Neurons in these columns constitute afferent nuclei, which form the dorsal roots of the spinal nerves. As the alar plates enlarge, the **dorsal median septum** forms. Cell bodies in the basal plates form the

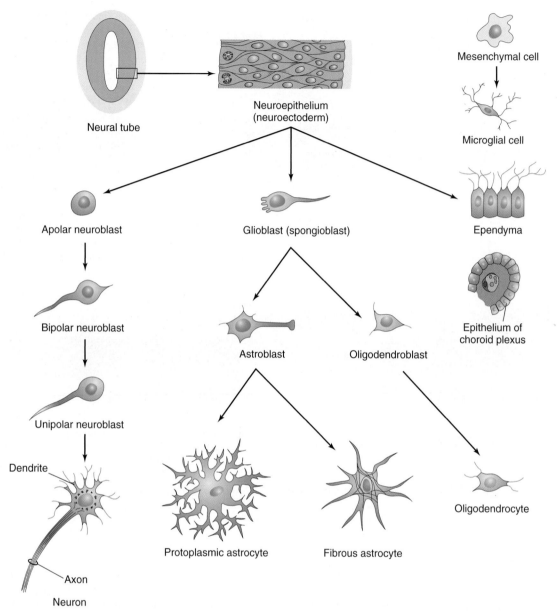

Figure 16–5   Histogenesis of cells in the central nervous system. After further development, the multipolar neuroblast *(lower left)* becomes a nerve cell or a neuron. Neuroepithelial cells give rise to all neurons and macroglial cells.

ventral and lateral gray columns. In transverse sections of the spinal cord, these columns are the **ventral gray horns** and **lateral gray horns**, respectively. Axons of the ventral horn cells grow out of the cord and form the **ventral roots of the spinal nerves** (Fig. 16-7). As the basal plates enlarge, they bulge ventrally on each side of the median plane. As this bulging occurs, the *ventral median septum* forms and a deep longitudinal groove—the ventral median fissure—develops on the ventral surface of the cord.

Development of Spinal Ganglia

The unipolar neurons in the spinal ganglia (dorsal root ganglia) are derived from **neural crest cells** (Fig. 16-7). The peripheral processes of the **spinal ganglion cells** pass in the spinal nerves to sensory endings in somatic or visceral structures. The central processes enter the spinal cord, constituting the **dorsal roots of the spinal nerves**.

Development of Spinal Meninges

The mesenchyme surrounding the neural tube condenses to form the **primordial meninx** or **meninges** (Figs. 16-2C and 16-4A, D, and E). The external layer of this membrane gives rise to the **dura mater** (Fig. 16-8A). The internal layer—the **pia mater** and **arachnoid mater**—**leptomeninges**—is derived from neural crest cells. Fluid-filled spaces appear within the leptomeninges that soon coalesce to form the **subarachnoid space** (Fig. 16-9A). Embryonic **cerebrospinal fluid** (CSF) begins to form during the fifth week.

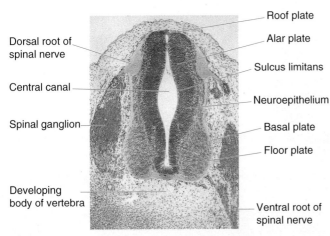

Dorsal root of spinal nerve

Central canal

Spinal ganglion

Developing body of vertebra

Roof plate

Alar plate

Sulcus limitans

Neuroepithelium

Basal plate

Floor plate

Ventral root of spinal nerve

Figure 16–6 Transverse section of an embryo (×100) at 40 days. The ventral root of the spinal nerve is composed of nerve fibers arising from neuroblasts in the basal plate, whereas the dorsal root is formed by nerve processes arising from neuroblasts in the spinal ganglion.

Positional Changes of Spinal Cord

The spinal cord in the embryo extends the entire length of the vertebral canal at 8 weeks (Fig. 16-8A). The spinal nerves pass through the intervertebral foramina opposite their levels of origin. Because the vertebral column and dura mater grow more rapidly than the spinal cord, the positional relationship to the spinal nerves does not persist. The caudal end of the spinal cord gradually comes to lie at relatively higher levels. At 24 weeks, it lies at the level of the first sacral vertebra (Fig. 16-8B). The **spinal cord in the newborn infant** terminates at the level of the second or third lumbar vertebra (Fig. 16-8C). The **spinal cord in the adult** usually terminates at the inferior border of the first lumbar vertebra (Fig. 16-8D). As a result, the spinal nerve roots, especially those of the lumbar and sacral segments, run obliquely from the spinal cord to the corresponding level of the vertebral column. The nerve roots inferior to the end of the cord— the **medullary cone** (Latin *conus medullaris*)—form a sheaf of nerve roots, the **cauda equina** (Latin horse's tail). Although in adults the dura mater and arachnoid mater usually end at the S₂ vertebra distal to the caudal end of the spinal cord, the pia mater forms a long, fibrous thread, the **terminal filum** (Latin *filum terminale*) (Fig. 16-8C and D). The filum extends from the medullary cone to the periosteum of the first coccygeal vertebra.

Myelination of Nerve Fibers

Myelin sheaths surrounding nerve fibers within the spinal cord begin to form during the late fetal period and continue to form during the first postnatal year. In general, fiber tracts become myelinated at approximately the time they become functional. Motor roots are myelinated before sensory roots. The **myelin sheaths** surrounding the nerve fibers within the spinal cord are formed by **oligodendrocytes**. The myelin sheaths surrounding

SPINA BIFIDA OCCULTA

Spina bifida occulta results from failure of the embryonic halves of the neural arch to grow normally and fuse in the median plane (Fig. 16-9A). Spina bifida occulta occurs in vertebra L₅ or S₁ in approximately 10% of otherwise normal people. In its most minor form, the only evidence of its presence may be a small dimple with a tuft of hair arising from it (Fig. 16-10). Spina bifida occulta usually produces no clinical symptoms.

SPINA BIFIDA CYSTICA

Severe types of spina bifida, involving protrusion of the spinal cord, meninges, or both through the defects in the vertebral arches, are referred to collectively as **spina bifida cystica** because of the cystlike sac that is associated with these anomalies (Figs. 16-9B to D and 16-11). Spina bifida cystica occurs in approximately 1 in 1000 births. When the sac contains meninges and CSF, the anomaly is called **spina bifida with meningocele** (Fig. 16-9B). The spinal cord and spinal roots are in their normal position, but spinal cord abnormalities may be present. If the spinal cord, nerve roots, or both are included in the sac, the anomaly is called **spina bifida with meningomyelocele** (Figs. 16-9C and 16-11). Spina bifida with meningomyelocele involving several vertebrae is often associated with partial absence of the brain— meroencephaly (anencephaly) (Fig. 16-12).

the axons of peripheral nerve fibers are formed by the plasma membranes of the **neurolemma cells (Schwann cells)**. *Myelination of the nerve fibers is regulated by β-1 integrins.* These neuroglial cells are derived from **neural crest cells** that migrate peripherally and wrap themselves around the axons of somatic motor neurons and presynaptic autonomic motor neurons as they pass out of the CNS (Fig. 16-7). These cells also wrap themselves around both the central and peripheral processes of the somatic and the visceral sensory neurons, as well as around the axons of postsynaptic autonomic motor neurons.

BIRTH DEFECTS OF SPINAL CORD

Most congenital anomalies of the spinal cord result from defective closure of the neural tube during the fourth week. These **neural tube defects** (NTDs) affect the tissues overlying the spinal cord, including the meninges, neural arches, muscles, and skin (Fig. 16-9B to D). Anomalies involving the neural arches are referred to as **spina bifida**.

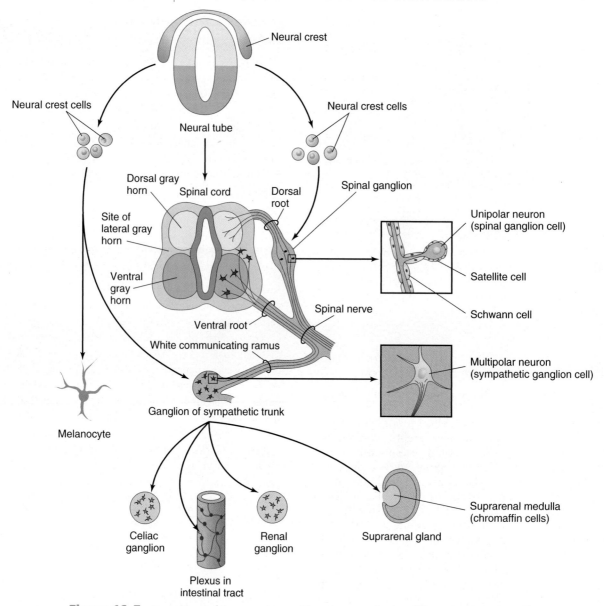

Figure 16–7 Derivatives of the neural crest. Neural crest cells also differentiate into the cells in the afferent ganglia of cranial nerves and many other structures.

CAUSES OF NEURAL TUBE DEFECTS

Genetic, nutritional, and environmental factors play a role in the production of NTDs. Epidemiologic studies have shown that folic acid supplements (400 μg daily) taken at least 1 month before conception and continuing through the first trimester reduce the incidence of NTDs. Certain drugs increase the risk of NTD. For example, valproic acid, an anticonvulsant, causes NTDs in 1% to 2% of pregnant women if given during the fourth week of development, when the neural folds are fusing.

DEVELOPMENT OF BRAIN

The **neural tube** cranial to the fourth pair of somites develops into the brain. Even before the neural folds are completely fused, three distinct vesicles are recognizable in the rostral end of the developing neural tube. From rostral to caudal, these **primary brain vesicles** (Fig. 16-13) form the *forebrain* (prosencephalon), *midbrain* (mesencephalon), and *hindbrain* (rhombencephalon). During the fifth week, the forebrain partially divides into two **secondary brain vesicles**, the *telencephalon* and *diencephalon*; the midbrain does not divide. The hindbrain divides into the metencephalon and myelencephalon; consequently, there are five secondary brain vesicles.

Brain Flexures

The embryonic brain grows rapidly during the fourth week and bends ventrally with the head fold. This bending produces the **midbrain flexure** in the midbrain region and the **cervical flexure** at the junction of the hindbrain and the spinal cord (Fig. 16-14A). Later, unequal growth of the developing brain between these flexures produces the **pontine flexure** in the opposite direction. This flexure

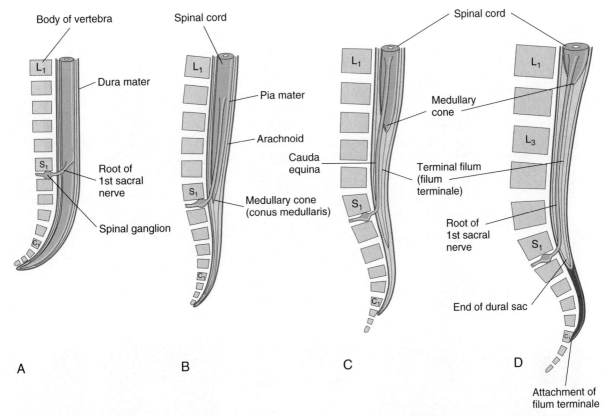

Figure 16–8 The position of the caudal end of the spinal cord in relation to the vertebral column and the meninges at various stages of development are shown. The increasing inclination of the root of the first sacral nerve is also shown. **A,** At 8 weeks. **B,** At 24 weeks. **C,** Newborn infant. **D,** Adult.

results in thinning of the roof of the hindbrain. The **sulcus limitans** extends cranially to the junction of the midbrain and forebrain, and the alar and basal plates are recognizable only in the midbrain and the hindbrain (Figs. 16-4*B* and 16-14*C*).

Hindbrain

The *cervical flexure* demarcates the hindbrain from the spinal cord (Fig. 16-14*A*). The *pontine flexure* divides the hindbrain into caudal (myelencephalon) and rostral (metencephalon) parts. The *myelencephalon* becomes the **medulla oblongata** (often called the medulla), whereas the *metencephalon* becomes the **pons** and **cerebellum**. The cavity of the hindbrain becomes the fourth ventricle and the central canal in the caudal part of the medulla (Fig. 16-14*B* and *C*).

Myelencephalon

Neuroblasts from the alar plates in the myelencephalon migrate into the marginal zone and form isolated areas of gray matter: the **gracile nuclei** medially and the **cuneate nuclei** laterally (Fig. 16-14*B*). These nuclei are associated with correspondingly named nerve tracts that enter the medulla from the spinal cord. The ventral area of the medulla contains a pair of fiber bundles—**pyramids**—that consist of corticospinal fibers descending from the developing cerebral cortex.

The rostral part of the myelencephalon is wide and rather flat, especially opposite the pontine flexure (Fig. 16-14*C* and *D*). As the pontine flexure forms, the walls of the medulla move laterally and the alar plates come to lie lateral to the basal plates (Fig. 16-14*C*). As the positions of the plates change, the motor nuclei generally develop medial to the sensory nuclei.

Neuroblasts in the basal plates of the medulla, like those in the spinal cord, develop into motor neurons. In the medulla, the neuroblasts form nuclei (groups of nerve cells) and organize into three cell columns on each side (Fig. 16-14*D*). From medial to lateral, they are:

- The *general somatic efferent*, represented by neurons of the hypoglossal nerve
- The *special visceral efferent*, represented by neurons innervating muscles derived from the pharyngeal arches (see Chapter 10)
- The *general visceral efferent*, represented by some neurons of the vagus and the glossopharyngeal nerves

Neuroblasts from the alar plates of the medulla form neurons that are arranged in four columns on each side (Fig. 16-14*D*). From medial to lateral, they are:

- The *general visceral afferent*, receiving impulses from the viscera
- The *special visceral afferent*, receiving taste fibers

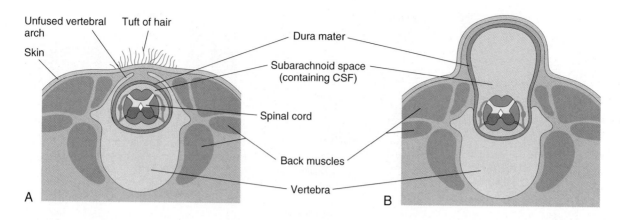

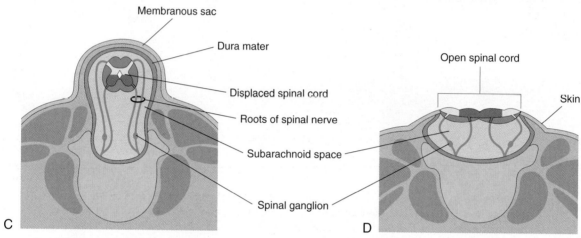

Figure 16–9 Various types of spina bifida. **A,** Spina bifida occulta. Observe the unfused vertebral arch. **B,** Spina bifida with meningocele. **C,** Spina bifida with meningomyelocele. **D,** Spina bifida with myeloschisis. The types shown in **B** to **D** are referred to collectively as *spina bifida cystica* because of the cystlike sac that is associated with them.

- The *general somatic afferent,* receiving impulses from the surface of the head
- The *special somatic afferent,* receiving impulses from the ear

Some neuroblasts from the alar plates migrate ventrally and form the neurons in the **olivary nuclei** (Fig. 16-14C and D).

Metencephalon

The walls of the metencephalon form the **pons** and **cerebellum**; its cavity forms the *superior part of the fourth ventricle* (Fig. 16-15). As in the rostral part of the myelencephalon, the pontine flexure causes divergence of the lateral walls of the pons, which spreads the gray matter in the floor of the fourth ventricle.

The **cerebellum** develops from the dorsal parts of the alar plates (Fig. 16-15A and B). Initially, the **cerebellar swellings** project into the fourth ventricle (Fig. 16-15C). As the swellings enlarge and fuse in the median plane, they overgrow the rostral half of the fourth ventricle and overlap the pons and the medulla (Fig. 16-15D). Some neuroblasts in the intermediate zone of the alar plates migrate to the marginal zone and differentiate into the

neurons of the **cerebellar cortex.** Other neuroblasts from these plates give rise to the central nuclei, the largest of which is the **dentate nucleus** (Fig 16-15D). Cells from the alar plates also give rise to the **pontine nuclei,** the cochlear and vestibular nuclei, and the sensory nuclei of the trigeminal nerve.

Nerve fibers connecting the cerebral and cerebellar cortices with the spinal cord pass through the marginal layer of the ventral region of the metencephalon—**the pons** (Fig. 16-15C and D).

Choroid Plexuses and Cerebrospinal Fluid

The thin ependymal roof of the fourth ventricle is covered externally by *pia mater* (Fig. 16-15C and D). This vascular membrane, together with the ependymal roof, forms the **tela choroidea** of the fourth ventrical. Because of the active proliferation of the pia mater, the tela choroidea invaginates the fourth ventricle, where it differentiates into the **choroid plexus** (infoldings of choroidial arteries of the pia mater). Similar choroid plexuses develop in the roof of the third ventricle and in the medial walls of the lateral ventricles.

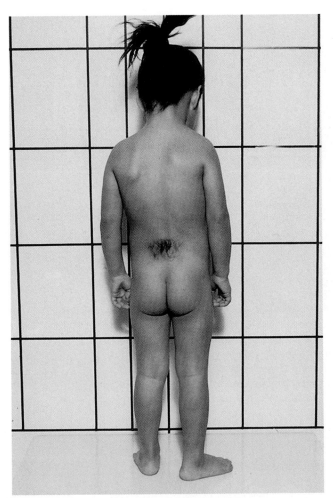

Figure 16–10 A female child with a hairy patch in the lumbosacral region, indicating the site of a spina bifida occulta. *(Courtesy of A.E. Chudley, M.D., Section of Genetics and Metabolism, Department of Pediatrics and Child Health, Children's Hospital and University of Manitoba, Winnipeg, Manitoba, Canada.)*

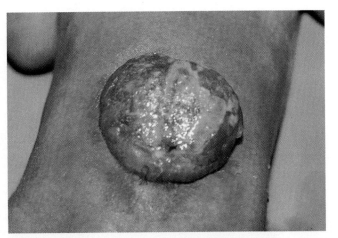

Figure 16–11 The back of a newborn infant with a large lumbar meningomyelocele. The neural tube defect is covered with a thin membrane. *(Courtesy of A.E. Chudley, M.D., Section of Genetics and Metabolism, Department of Pediatrics and Child Health, Children's Hospital and University of Manitoba, Winnipeg, Manitoba, Canada.)*

The choroid plexuses secrete ventricular fluid, which becomes CSF. The thin roof of the fourth ventricle evaginates in three locations. These outpouchings rupture to form openings, the **median and lateral apertures.** These apertures permit CSF to enter the **subarachnoid space** from the fourth ventricle.

Midbrain

The midbrain (mesencephalon) undergoes very little change. The neural canal narrows and becomes the **cerebral aqueduct** (see Fig. 16-15D), a canal that connects the third and fourth ventricles. Neuroblasts migrate from the alar plates of the midbrain into the **tectum** (roof), where they aggregate to form four large groups of neurons—the paired **superior and inferior colliculi** (Fig. 16-16B), which are concerned with visual and auditory reflexes, respectively. Neuroblasts from the basal plates appear to give rise to groups of neurons in the **tegmentum** (red nuclei, nuclei of the third and fourth cranial nerves, and reticular nuclei). The **substantia nigra,** a broad layer of gray matter adjacent to the cerebral peduncle

(Fig. 16-16D and E), may also differentiate from the basal plate, but some authorities believe that it is derived from cells in the alar plate that migrate ventrally. Fibers growing from the cerebrum form the **cerebral peduncles** anteriorly (Fig. 16-16B). These peduncles become progressively more prominent as additional descending fiber groups (corticopontine, corticobulbar, and corticospinal) pass through the developing midbrain on their way to the brainstem and spinal cord.

Forebrain

As closure of the rostral neuropore occurs, two lateral outgrowths—**optic vesicles**—appear (Fig. 16-3A), one on each side of the forebrain. The optic vesicles are the primordia of the retinas and optic nerves. A second pair of diverticula soon arises more dorsally and rostrally, representing the **telencephalic vesicles** (Fig. 16-16C). They are the primordia of the **cerebral hemispheres** and their cavities become the **lateral ventricles.** The rostral, or anterior, part of the forebrain, including the primordia of the cerebral hemispheres, is known as the **telencephalon,** whereas the caudal, or posterior, part of the forebrain is called the **diencephalon.** The cavities of the telencephalon and diencephalon contribute to the formation of the **third ventricle** (Fig. 16-17D and E).

Diencephalon

Three swellings develop in the lateral walls of the third ventricle, which later become the thalamus, hypothalamus, and epithalamus (Fig. 16-17C to E). The **thalamus** develops rapidly on each side and bulges into the cavity of the third ventricle, eventually reducing it to a narrow cleft. The **hypothalamus** arises by the proliferation of neuroblasts in the intermediate zone of the diencephalic walls. A pair of nuclei, the **mammillary bodies,** form pea-sized swellings on the ventral surface of the hypothalamus (Fig. 16-17C). The **epithalamus** develops from the

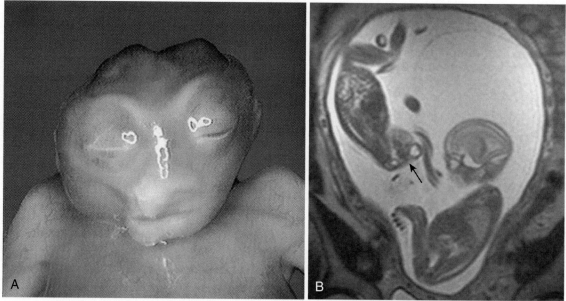

Figure 16–12 **A,** A fetus with meroencephaly (anencephaly). **B,** Magnetic resonance image (MRI) of diamniotic-monochorionic twins, one with meroencephaly. Note the absent calvarium of the abnormal twin and the amnion of the normal twin. (**A,** *Courtesy of Wesley Lee, M.D., Division of Fetal Imaging, Department of Obstetrics and Gynecology, William Beaumont Hospital, Royal Oak, MI.* **B,** *Courtesy of Deborah Levine, MD, Director of Obstetric and Gynecologic Ultrasound, Beth Israel Deaconess Medical Center, Boston, Massachusetts.*)

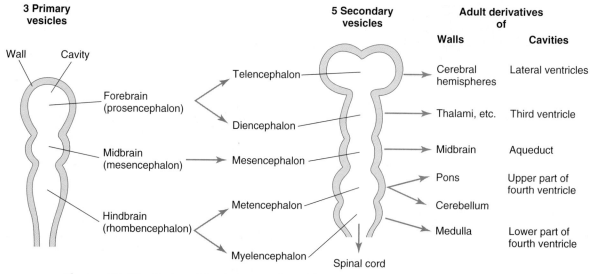

Figure 16–13 Brain vesicles, indicating the adult derivatives of their walls and cavities. The rostral part of the third ventricle forms from the cavity of the telencephalon; most of this ventricle is derived from the cavity of the diencephalon.

roof and dorsal part of the lateral wall of the diencephalon. Initially, the epithalamic swellings are large, but later they become relatively small.

The **pineal gland** (pineal body) develops as a median diverticulum of the caudal part of the roof of the diencephalon (Fig. 16-17D). Proliferation of the cells in its walls soon converts it into a solid, cone-shaped gland.

The **pituitary gland** (Fig. 16-18 and Table 16-1) is ectodermal in origin. It develops from two sources:

- An upgrowth from the ectodermal roof of the stomodeum—the **hypophysial diverticulum (Rathke pouch)**
- A downgrowth from the neuroectoderm of the diencephalon—the **neurohypophysial diverticulum**

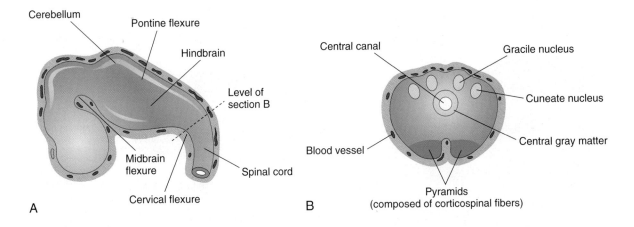

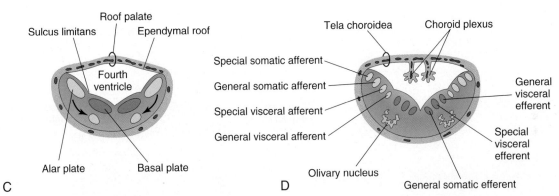

Figure 16–14 **A**, The developing brain at the end of the fifth week, showing the three primary divisions of the brain and the brain flexures. **B**, Transverse section of the caudal part of the myelencephalon. **C** and **D**, Similar sections of the rostral part of the myelencephalon, showing the position and successive stages of differentiation of the alar and basal plates. The *arrows* in **C** show the pathway taken by the neuroblasts from the alar plates to form the olivary nuclei.

Table 16–1   Derivation and Terminology of Pituitary Gland

Oral Ectoderm			
(Hypophysial diverticulum from roof of stomodeum)	⟶	Adenohypophysis (glandular portion)	{ Pars anterior Pars tuberalis Pars intermedia	Anterior lobe
	⟶		
Neuroectoderm			
(Neurohypophysial diverticulum from floor of diencephalon)		Neurohypophysis (nervous portion)	{ Pars nervosa Infundibular stem Median eminence	Posterior lobe

This double embryonic origin of the pituitary gland explains why it is composed of two different types of tissue.

- The **adenohypophysis** (glandular part), or anterior lobe, arises from the oral ectoderm.
- The **neurohypophysis** (nervous part), or posterior lobe, originates from the neuroectoderm.

During the third week, a **hypophysial diverticulum** projects from the roof of the stomodeum and lies adjacent to the floor (ventral wall) of the diencephalon (Fig. 16-18*A* and *B*). By the fifth week, this diverticulum has elongated and constricted at its attachment to the

oral epithelium, giving it a nipple-like appearance (Fig. 16-18*C*). By this stage, it has come into contact with the **infundibulum** (derived from the neurohypophysial diverticulum), a ventral downgrowth of the diencephalon. The stalk of the hypophysial diverticulum gradually regresses (Fig. 16-18*C* to *E*). The parts of the pituitary gland that develop from the ectoderm of the stomodeum—pars anterior, pars intermedia, and pars tuberalis—form the **adenohypophysis** (Table 16-1).

Cells of the anterior wall of the hypophysial diverticulum proliferate and give rise to the **pars anterior** of the pituitary gland. Later, an extension, the **pars tuberalis**, grows around the *infundibular stem* (Fig. 16-18*F*). The extensive proliferation of the anterior wall of the

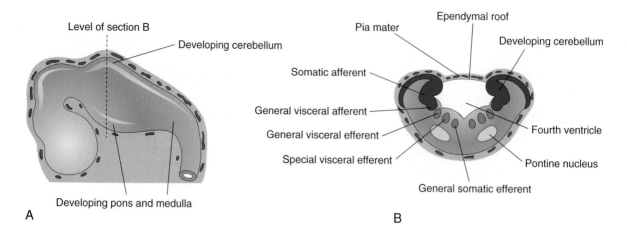

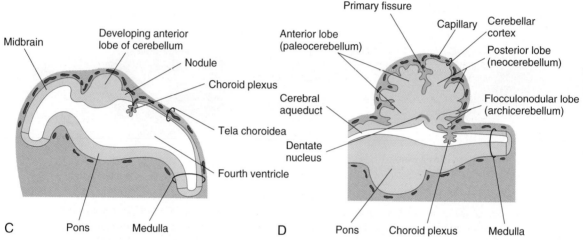

Figure 16–15 **A,** The developing brain at the end of the fifth week. **B,** Transverse section of the metencephalon (developing pons and cerebellum), showing the derivatives of the alar and basal plates. **C** and **D,** Sagittal sections of the hindbrain at 6 and 17 weeks, respectively, showing successive stages in the development of the pons and cerebellum.

hypophysial diverticulum reduces its lumen to a narrow cleft (Fig. 16-18E). Cells in the posterior wall of the hypophysial diverticulum do not proliferate; they give rise to the thin, poorly defined **pars intermedia** (Fig. 16-18F). The part of the pituitary gland that develops from the neuroectoderm of the brain (infundibulum) is the **neurohypophysis** (Table 16-1). The infundibulum gives rise to the *median eminence, infundibular stem,* and *pars nervosa.*

Telencephalon

The telencephalon consists of a median part and two lateral diverticula, the cerebral vesicles (Fig. 16-18A). These vesicles are the primordial of the cerebral hemispheres, which are identifiable at 7 weeks (Fig. 16-19A). The cavity of the median part of the telencephalon forms the extreme anterior part of the third ventricle. At first, the cerebral hemispheres are in wide communication with the cavity of the third ventricle through the interventricular foramina (Fig. 16-19B). As the cerebral hemispheres expand, they cover successively the diencephalon, midbrain, and hindbrain. The hemispheres eventually meet each other in the midline, flattening their medial surfaces.

The **corpus striatum** appears during the sixth week as a prominent swelling in the floor of each cerebral hemisphere (Fig. 16-20B). As a result, the floor of each hemisphere expands more slowly than its thin cortical wall, and the cerebral hemispheres become C-shaped (Fig. 16-21). The growth and curvature of the hemispheres also affect the shape of the lateral ventricles. They become roughly C-shaped cavities filled with CSF. The caudal end of each cerebral hemisphere turns ventrally and then rostrally, forming the temporal lobe; in so doing, it carries with it the ventricle (forming the **temporal horn**) and the **choroid fissure** (Fig. 16-21). Here, the thin medial wall of the hemisphere is invaginated along the **choroid fissure** by the vascular pia mater to form the *choroid plexus of the temporal horn* of the lateral ventricle (Figs. 16-20B and 16-21B).

As the cerebral cortex differentiates, fibers passing to and from it pass through the **corpus striatum** and divide it into the *caudate and lentiform nuclei.* This fiber pathway—the **internal capsule** (Fig. 16-20C)—becomes C-shaped as the hemisphere assumes this form. The **caudate nucleus** becomes elongated and C-shaped, conforming to the outline of the lateral ventricle (Fig. 16-21A to C). Its pear-shaped head and elongated body lie in the

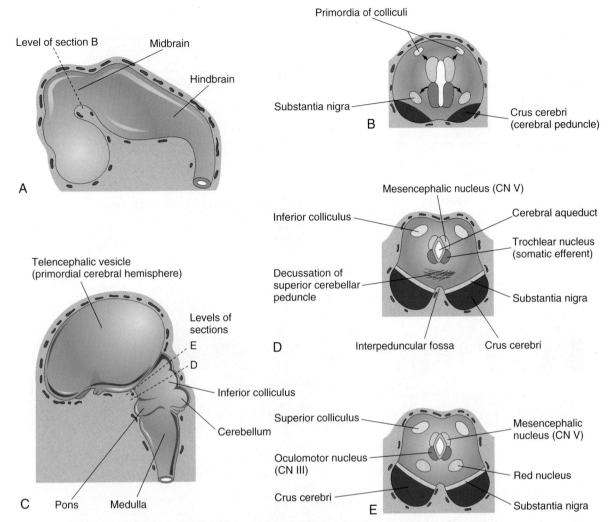

Figure 16–16 **A,** The developing brain at the end of the fifth week. **B,** Transverse section of the developing midbrain, showing the early migration of cells from the basal and alar plates. **C,** The developing brain at 11 weeks. **D** and **E,** Transverse sections of the developing midbrain at the level of the inferior and superior colliculi, respectively.

floor of the frontal horn and the body of the lateral ventricle; its tail makes a U-shaped turn to gain the roof of the temporal horn.

Cerebral Commissures

As the cerebral cortex develops, groups of fibers—**commissures**—connect corresponding areas of the cerebral hemispheres with one another (Fig. 16-20). The most important commissures cross in the **lamina terminalis**, the rostral end of the forebrain. This lamina extends from the roof plate of the diencephalon to the optic chiasm. The **anterior commissure** connects the olfactory bulb and related brain areas of one hemisphere with those of the opposite side. The **hippocampal commissure** connects the hippocampal formations. The **corpus callosum**, the largest cerebral commissure, connects the neocortical areas (Fig. 16-20*A*). The rest of the lamina terminalis becomes stretched to form the **septum pellucidum**, a thin plate of brain tissue. By birth, the corpus callosum extends over the roof of the diencephalon.

The **optic chiasm**, which develops in the ventral part of the lamina terminalis (Fig. 16-20*A*), consists of fibers from the medial halves of the retinas that cross to join the optic tract of the opposite side.

Initially, the surface of the hemispheres is smooth (Fig. 16-22); however, as growth proceeds, **sulci** (grooves) and **gyri** (convolutions) develop (Fig. 16-22). The sulci and gyri permit a considerable increase in the surface area of the cerebral cortex without requiring an extensive increase in cranial size. As each cerebral hemisphere grows, the cortex covering the external surface of the corpus striatum grows relatively slowly and is soon overgrown. This buried cortex, hidden from view in the depths of the lateral sulcus (fissure) of the cerebral hemisphere, is the **insula**.

CONGENITAL ANOMALIES OF BRAIN

Most major congenital anomalies of the brain result from defective closure of the rostral neuropore during the fourth week of development (Fig. 16-23*A*) and involve the overlying tissues (meninges and calvaria). MRI is often used for evaluation of the fetal brain in pregnancies at risk for fetal defects. The factors causing neural tube defects (NTDs) are genetic, nutritional, or environmental.

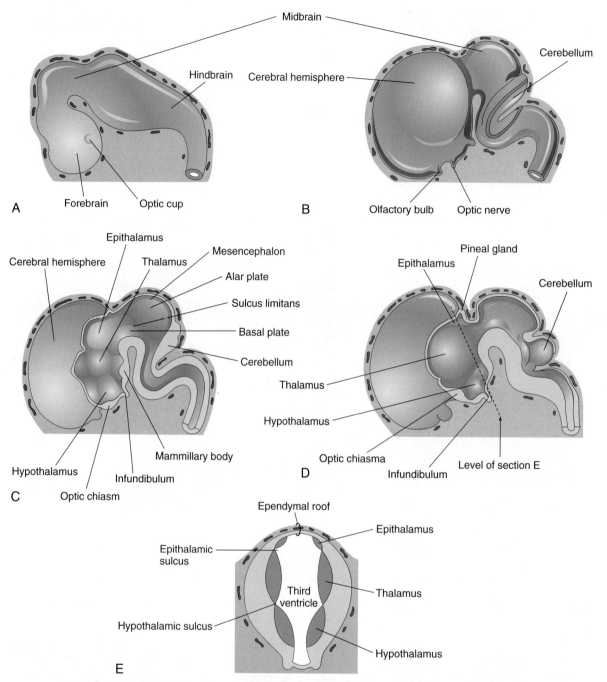

Figure 16–17 **A,** External view of the brain at the end of the fifth week. **B,** Similar view at 7 weeks. **C,** Median section of the brain, showing the medial surface of the forebrain and midbrain. **D,** Similar section at 8 weeks. **E,** Transverse section of the diencephalon, showing the epithalamus dorsally, the thalamus laterally, and the hypothalamus ventrally.

PHARYNGEAL HYPOPHYSIS AND CRANIOPHARYNGIOMA

A remnant of the stalk of the hypophysial diverticulum may persist and form a pharyngeal hypophysis in the roof of the oropharynx (Fig. 16-18E and F). Occasionally, craniopharyngiomas from remnants of the stalk of the hypophysial diverticulum develop in the pharynx or in the basisphenoid (posterior part of the sphenoid bone), but most often, they form in or superior to the sella turcica of the cranium (Fig. 16-24).

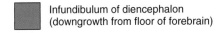

Hypophysial pouch of stomodeum
(upgrowth from roof of primitive mouth)

Infundibulum of diencephalon
(downgrowth from floor of forebrain)

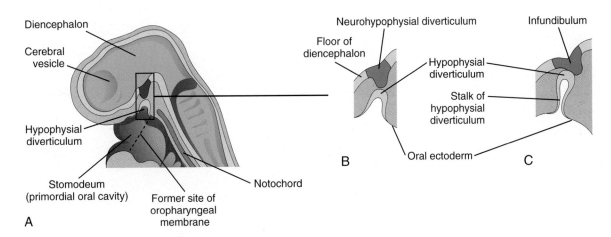

Diencephalon

Cerebral vesicle

Hypophysial diverticulum

Stomodeum (primordial oral cavity)

Former site of oropharyngeal membrane

Notochord

A

Neurohypophysial diverticulum

Floor of diencephalon

Hypophysial diverticulum

Stalk of hypophysial diverticulum

Oral ectoderm

Infundibulum

B

C

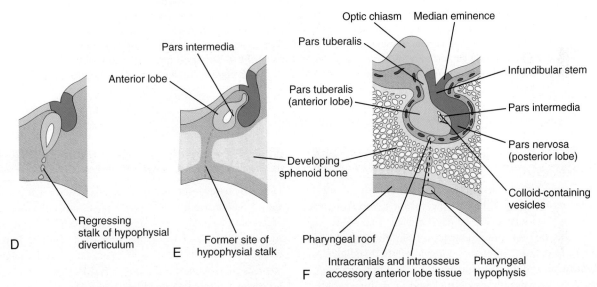

Pars intermedia

Anterior lobe

Regressing stalk of hypophysial diverticulum

D

Former site of hypophysial stalk

E

Optic chiasm   Median eminence

Pars tuberalis

Pars tuberalis (anterior lobe)

Developing sphenoid bone

Pharyngeal roof

Intracranials and intraosseus accessory anterior lobe tissue

F

Infundibular stem

Pars intermedia

Pars nervosa (posterior lobe)

Colloid-containing vesicles

Pharyngeal hypophysis

Figure 16–18 Development of the pituitary gland. **A**, Sagittal section of the cranial end of an embryo at approximately 36 days, showing the hypophysial diverticulum, an upgrowth from the stomodeum, and the neurohypophysial diverticulum, a downgrowth from the forebrain. **B** to **D**, Successive stages of the developing pituitary gland. By 8 weeks, the diverticulum loses its connection with the oral cavity and is in close contact with the infundibulum and posterior lobe (neurohypophysis) of the pituitary gland. **E** and **F**, Later stages, showing proliferation of the anterior wall of the hypophysial diverticulum to form the anterior lobe (adenohypophysis) of the pituitary gland.

CRANIUM BIFIDUM

Defects in the formation of the cranium (cranium bifidum) are often associated with congenital anomalies of the brain, meninges, or both. Defects of the cranium (skull) usually involve the median plane of the calvaria. The defect is often in the squamous part of the occipital bone and may include the posterior part of the foramen magnum. When the defect is small, usually only the meninges herniate, and the anomaly is called a *cranial meningocele*. Cranium bifidum associated with herniation of the brain, the meninges, or both occurs in approximately 1 in 2000 births. When the cranial defect is large, the meninges and part of the brain herniate, forming a meningoencephalocele (Fig. 16-23A and B). If the protruding brain contains part of the ventricular system, the anomaly is called a *meningohydroencephalocele* (Fig. 16-23).

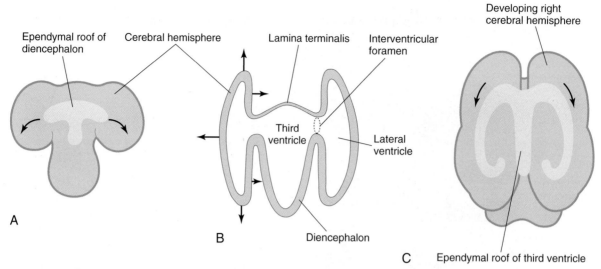

Figure 16–19 **A,** Dorsal surface of the forebrain, showing how the ependymal roof of the diencephalon is carried out to the dorsomedial surface of the cerebral hemispheres. **B,** The forebrain, showing how the developing cerebral hemispheres grow from the lateral walls of the forebrain and expand in all directions until they cover the diencephalon. The rostral wall of the forebrain, the lamina terminalis, is very thin. **C,** The forebrain, showing how the ependymal roof is finally carried into the temporal lobes as a result of the C-shaped growth pattern of the cerebral hemispheres. The *arrows* indicate some of the directions in which the hemispheres expand.

MEROENCEPHALY (ANENCEPHALY)

Meroencephaly (anencephaly) is a severe anomaly of the brain that results from failure of the rostral neuropore to close during the fourth week of development (Fig. 16-12). Most of the infant's brain extrudes from the cranium. Although this defect is often called *anencephaly*, a rudimentary brainstem and functioning neural tissue are present. Meroencephaly is usually associated with a multifactorial pattern of inheritance.

MICROCEPHALY

In microcephaly, the calvaria and brain are small, but the face is of normal size. Affected infants are usually severely mentally challenged (IQ below 35-40) because the cranium and brain are underdeveloped. Some cases of microcephaly appear to be genetic (autosomal recessive); others are caused by environmental factors such as cytomegalovirus infection in utero (see Chapter 19). Exposure during the fetal period to large amounts of ionizing radiation, infectious agents, and certain drugs is a contributing factor in some cases.

HYDROCEPHALUS

Hydrocephalus results from impaired circulation and absorption of cerebrospinal fluid (CSF) or, in unusual cases, from increased production of CSF. An excess of CSF is present in the ventricular system of the brain (Fig. 16-25). Impaired circulation of CSF often results from congenital aqueductal stenosis (narrow cerebral aqueduct). Blockage of CSF circulation results in dilation of the ventricles proximal to the obstruction and increased pressure on the cerebral hemispheres. This squeezes the brain between the ventricular fluid and the calvaria. In infants, the internal pressure results in an accelerated rate of expansion of the brain and calvaria because the fibrous sutures of the calvaria are not fused.

ARNOLD-CHIARI MALFORMATION

Arnold-Chiari malformation is the most common congenital anomaly involving the cerebellum (Fig. 16-26). A tongue-like projection of the medulla and inferior displacement of the vermis of the cerebellum herniate through the foramen magnum into the vertebral canal. The condition results in a type of communicating hydrocephalus in which there is interference with the absorption of CSF; as a result, the entire ventricular system is distended.

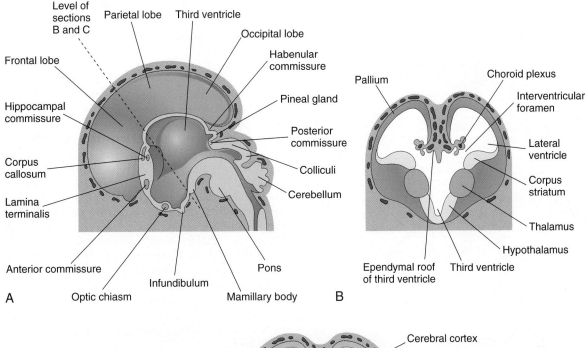

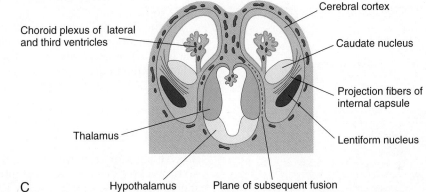

Figure 16–20 **A,** Medial surface of the forebrain of a 10-week embryo, showing the diencephalic derivatives, the main commissures, and expanding cerebral hemispheres. **B,** Transverse section of the forebrain at the level of the interventricular foramina, showing the corpus striatum and choroid plexuses of the lateral ventricles. **C,** Similar section at approximately 11 weeks, showing division of the corpus striatum into the caudate and lentiform nuclei by the internal capsule.

DEVELOPMENT OF PERIPHERAL NERVOUS SYSTEM

The peripheral nervous system (PNS) consists of cranial, spinal, and visceral nerves and cranial, spinal, and autonomic ganglia. All sensory cells (somatic and visceral) of the PNS are derived from **neural crest cells**. The cell bodies of these sensory cells are located outside the CNS. The cell body of each afferent neuron is closely invested by a capsule of modified Schwann cells, known as *satellite cells* (Fig. 16-7), which are derived from neural crest cells. This capsule is continuous with the **neurolemmal sheath** of Schwann cells that surrounds the axons of afferent neurons.

Neural crest cells in the developing brain migrate to form sensory ganglia only in relation to the trigeminal (CN V), facial (CN VII), vestibulocochlear (CN VIII), glossopharyngeal (CN IX), and vagus (CN X) nerves. Neural crest cells also differentiate into multipolar neurons of the *autonomic ganglia* (Fig. 16-7), including ganglia of the sympathetic trunks that lie along the sides of the vertebral bodies; collateral or prevertebral, ganglia in the plexuses of the thorax and abdomen (e.g., cardiac, celiac, and mesenteric plexuses); and parasympathetic, or terminal, ganglia in or near the viscera (e.g., the submucosal, or Meissner, plexus). Paraganglia—**chromaffin cells**—are also derived from the neural crest. The term *paraganglia* includes several widely scattered groups of cells that are similar in many ways to the medullary cells of the suprarenal glands. The cell groups largely lie retroperitoneally, often in association with sympathetic ganglia. The carotid and aortic bodies also have small

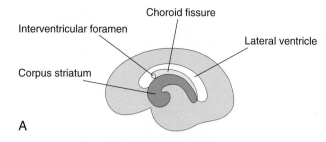

A

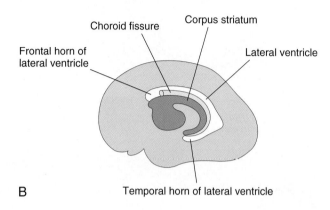

B

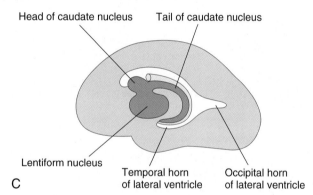

C

Figure 16–21 Medial surface of the developing right cerebral hemisphere, showing the development of the lateral ventricle, choroid fissure, and corpus striatum. **A,** At 13 weeks. **B,** At 21 weeks. **C,** At 32 weeks.

islands of chromaffin cells associated with them. These widely scattered groups of chromaffin cells constitute the **chromaffin system.**

Spinal Nerves

Motor nerve fibers arising from the spinal cord begin to appear at the end of the fourth week (Fig. 16-4). The nerve fibers arise from cells in the *basal plates* of the developing spinal cord and emerge as a continuous series of rootlets along its ventrolateral surface. The fibers destined for a particular developing muscle group become arranged in a bundle, forming a **ventral nerve root** (Figs. 16-6 and 16-7). The nerve fibers of the **dorsal nerve root** are formed by axons derived from neural crest cells that migrate to the dorsolateral aspect of the spinal cord, where they differentiate into the cells of the **spinal ganglion** (Fig. 16-7). The central processes of the neurons in the spinal ganglion form a single bundle that grows into the spinal cord, opposite the apex of the dorsal horn of gray matter (Fig. 16-4*B* and *C*). The distal processes of the spinal ganglion cells grow toward the ventral nerve root and eventually join it to form a **spinal nerve** (Fig. 16-7).

As the limb buds develop, the nerves from the spinal cord segments opposite to them elongate and grow into the limbs. The nerve fibers are distributed to its muscles, which differentiate from myogenic cells that originate from the somites (see Chapter 15). The skin of the developing limbs is also innervated in a segmental manner.

Cranial Nerves

Twelve pairs of cranial nerves form during the fifth and sixth weeks. They are classified into three groups according to their embryologic origins.

Somatic Efferent Cranial Nerves

The trochlear (CN IV), abducent (CN VI), hypoglossal (CN XII), and the greater part of the oculomotor (CN III) nerves, are homologous with the ventral roots of the spinal nerves (Fig. 16-27A). The cells of origin of these nerves are located in the *somatic efferent column* (derived

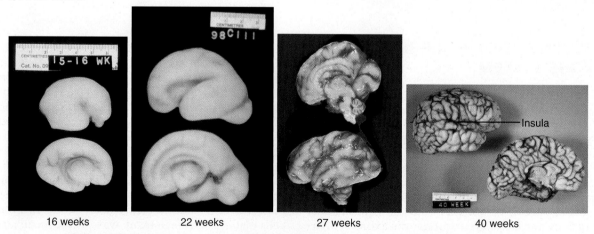

Figure 16–22 Lateral and medial surfaces of human fetal brains at 16, 22, 27, and 40 weeks gestation. *(Courtesy of Dr. Marc R. Del Bigio, Department of Pathology [Neuropathology], University of Manitoba and Health Sciences Centre, Winnipeg, Manitoba, Canada.)*

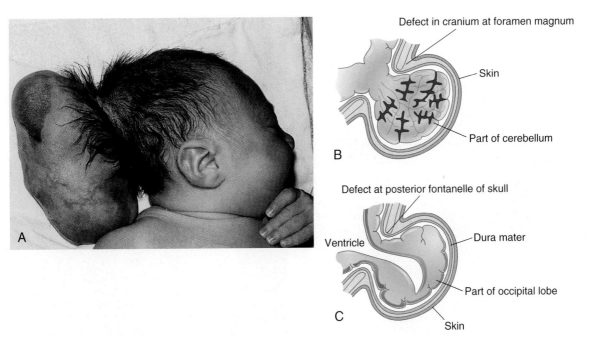

Figure 16–23 Cranium bifidum (bony defect of the cranium) and herniation of the brain and meninges. **A,** Infant with a large meningoencephalocele in the occipital area. **B,** Meningoencephalocele consisting of a protrusion of part of the cerebellum that is covered by meninges and skin. **C,** Meningohydroencephalocele consisting of a protrusion of part of the occipital lobe that contains part of the posterior horn of a lateral ventricle. (**A,** *Courtesy of A.E. Chudley, M.D., Section of Genetics and Metabolism, Department of Pediatrics and Child Health, Children's Hospital and University of Manitoba, Winnipeg, Manitoba, Canada.*)

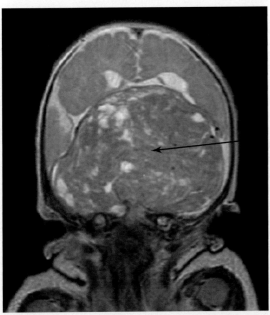

Figure 16–24 Magnetic resonance image (MRI) of a large craniopharyngioma *(arrow)*. *(Courtesy of Dr. R. Shane Tubbs and Dr. W. Jerry Oakes, Children's Hospital, Birmingham, Alabama.)*

from the basal plates) of the brainstem. Their axons are distributed to the muscles derived from the head myotomes (preotic and occipital) (see Fig. 15-17*A*).

The **trochlear nerve** (CN IV) arises from nerve cells in the somatic efferent column in the posterior part of the midbrain. Although a motor nerve, it emerges from the brainstem dorsally and passes ventrally to supply the superior oblique muscle of the eye.

The **abducent nerve** (CN VI) arises from nerve cells in the basal plates of the metencephalon. It passes from its ventral surface to the posterior of the three preotic myotomes from which the lateral rectus muscle of the eye is thought to originate.

The **hypoglossal nerve** (CN XII) develops by fusion of the ventral root fibers of three or four occipital nerves (Fig. 16-27*A*). Sensory roots, corresponding to the dorsal roots of the spinal nerves, are absent. The somatic motor fibers originate from the *hypoglossal nucleus*. These fibers leave the ventrolateral wall of the medulla in several groups—the *hypoglossal nerve roots*—which converge to form the common trunk of CN XII (Fig. 16-27*B*). They grow rostrally and eventually innervate the muscles of the tongue, which are derived from the occipital myotomes (see Fig. 15-17*A*).

The **oculomotor nerve** (CN III) supplies the superior, inferior, and medial recti and inferior oblique muscles of the eye.

Nerves of Pharyngeal Arches

Cranial nerves V, VII, IX, and X supply the embryonic pharyngeal arches; thus, the structures that develop from these arches are innervated by these cranial nerves (Fig. 16-27*A* and Table 10-1).

The **trigeminal nerve** (CN V) is the nerve of the first pharyngeal arch, but it has an ophthalmic division that is not a pharyngeal arch component. *CN V is the*

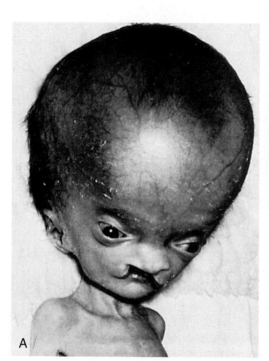
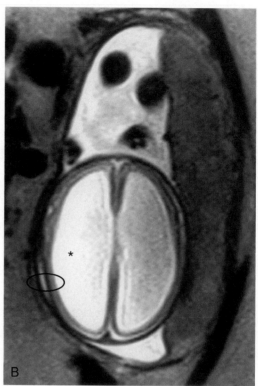

Figure 16–25 **A,** An infant with hydrocephalus and a bilateral cleft palate. Hydrocephalus often produces thinning of the bones of the calvaria, prominence of the forehead, and atrophy of the cerebral cortex and white substance. **B,** Axial magnetic resonance imaging scan (transverse section through the brain) of a fetus with X-linked hydrocephalus at approximately 29 weeks gestation, showing the massively enlarged ventricles (*) and thinned cortex *(oval)*. *(Courtesy of Dr. E.H. Whitby, Magnetic Resonance Imaging Unit, University of Sheffield, United Kingdom.)*

principal sensory nerve for the head. The cells of the large **trigeminal ganglion** are derived from the most anterior part of the neural crest. The central processes of the cells in this ganglion form the large sensory root of CN V, which enters the lateral part of the pons. The peripheral processes of cells in this ganglion separate into three large divisions (ophthalmic, maxillary, and mandibular nerves). Their sensory fibers supply the skin of the face as well as the lining of the mouth and nose. The *motor fibers of CN V* arise from cells in the most anterior part of the *special visceral efferent* column in the metencephalon. These fibers pass to the muscles of mastication and to other muscles that develop in the mandibular prominence of the first pharyngeal arch (see Table 10-1). The mesencephalic nucleus of CN V differentiates from cells in the midbrain.

The **facial nerve** (CN VII) is the nerve of the second pharyngeal arch. It consists mostly of motor fibers that arise principally from a nuclear group in the *special visceral efferent column* in the caudal part of the pons. These fibers are distributed to the *muscles of facial expression* and to other muscles that develop in the mesenchyme of the second pharyngeal arch (see Table 10-1). The small general visceral efferent component of CN VII terminates in the peripheral autonomic ganglia of the head. The sensory fibers of CN VII arise from the cells of the

geniculate ganglion. The central processes of these cells enter the pons, and the peripheral processes pass to the greater superficial petrosal nerve and, via the chorda tympani nerve, to the taste buds in the anterior two thirds of the tongue.

The **glossopharyngeal nerve** (CN IX) is the nerve of the third pharyngeal arch. Its motor fibers arise from the special and, to a lesser extent, the general visceral efferent columns of the anterior part of the myelencephalon. CN IX forms from several rootlets that arise from the medulla just caudal to the developing internal ear. All the fibers from the special visceral efferent column are distributed to the stylopharyngeus muscle, which is derived from the mesenchyme in the third pharyngeal arch (see Table 10-1). The general efferent fibers are distributed to the otic ganglion from which postsynaptic fibers pass to the parotid and posterior lingual glands. The *sensory fibers of CN IX* are distributed as general sensory and special visceral afferent fibers (taste fibers) to the posterior part of the tongue.

The **vagus nerve** (CN X) is formed by fusion of the nerves of the fourth and sixth pharyngeal arches (see Table 10-1). The nerve of the fourth pharyngeal arch becomes the superior laryngeal nerve, which supplies the cricothyroid muscle and the constrictor muscles of the pharynx. The nerve of the sixth pharyngeal arch becomes

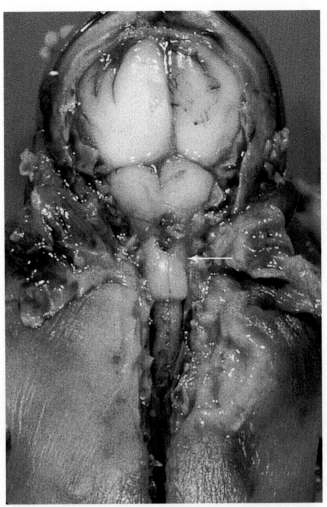

Figure 16–26 Arnold-Chiari type II malformation in a 23-week fetus. In situ exposure of the hindbrain shows cerebellar tissue well below the foramen magnum *(arrow)*. *(Courtesy of Dr. Marc R. Del Bigio, Department of Pathology [Neuropathology], University of Manitoba and Health Sciences Centre, Winnipeg, Manitoba, Canada.)*

the recurrent laryngeal nerve, which supplies various laryngeal muscles.

The **spinal accessory nerve** (CN XI) arises from the cranial five or six cervical segments of the spinal cord (Fig. 16-26). The spinal accessory nerve supplies the sternocleidomastoid and trapezius muscles.

Special Sensory Nerves

The **olfactory nerve** (CN I) arises from the olfactory bulb. The olfactory cells are bipolar neurons that differentiate from cells in the epithelial lining of the primordial nasal sac. The axons of the olfactory cells are collected into 18 to 20 bundles around which the cribriform plate of the ethmoid bone develops. These unmyelinated nerve fibers end in the olfactory bulb.

The **optic nerve** (CN II) is formed by more than a million nerve fibers that grow into the brain from neuroblasts in the primordial retina. Because the optic nerve develops from the evaginated wall of the forebrain, it actually represents a fiber tract of the brain. Development of the optic nerve is described in Chapter 17.

The **vestibulocochlear nerve** (CN VIII) consists of two kinds of sensory fiber in two bundles; these fibers are known as *the vestibular and cochlear nerves*. The **vestibular nerve** originates in the semicircular ducts, whereas the **cochlear nerve** proceeds from the cochlear duct, in which the **spiral organ** (of Corti) develops (see Chapter 17). The bipolar neurons of the vestibular nerve have their cell bodies in the **vestibular ganglion**. The central processes of these cells terminate in the vestibular nuclei in the floor of the fourth ventricle. The bipolar neurons of the cochlear nerve have their cell bodies in the **spiral ganglion**. The central processes of these cells end in the ventral and dorsal *cochlear nuclei* in the medulla.

DEVELOPMENT OF AUTONOMIC NERVOUS SYSTEM

Functionally, the autonomic system can be divided into sympathetic (thoracolumbar) and parasympathetic (craniosacral) parts.

Sympathetic Nervous System

During the fifth week, neural crest cells in the thoracic region migrate along each side of the spinal cord, where they form paired cellular masses (ganglia) dorsolateral to the aorta (Fig. 16-7). All these segmentally arranged **sympathetic ganglia** are connected in a bilateral chain by longitudinal nerve fibers. These ganglionated cords—**sympathetic trunks**—are located on each side of the vertebral bodies. Some neural crest cells migrate ventral to the aorta and form neurons in the **preaortic ganglia**, such as the celiac and mesenteric ganglia (Fig. 16-7). Other neural crest cells migrate to the area of the heart, lungs, and gastrointestinal tract, where they form terminal ganglia in **sympathetic organ plexuses**, located near or within these organs.

After the sympathetic trunks have formed, axons of sympathetic neurons located in the **intermediolateral cell column** (lateral horn) of the thoracolumbar segments of the spinal cord, pass through the ventral root of a spinal nerve and a **white communicating ramus** to a paravertebral ganglion (Fig. 16-7). Here they may synapse with neurons or ascend or descend in the sympathetic trunk to synapse at other levels. Other presynaptic fibers pass through the **paravertebral ganglia** without synapsing, forming splanchnic nerves to the viscera. The postsynaptic fibers course through a **gray communicating ramus**, passing from a sympathetic ganglion into a spinal nerve; hence, the sympathetic trunks are composed of ascending and descending fibers.

Parasympathetic Nervous System

The presynaptic parasympathetic fibers arise from neurons in the nuclei of the brainstem and in the sacral region of the spinal cord. The fibers from the brainstem leave through the oculomotor (CN III), facial (CN VII), glossopharyngeal (CN IX), and vagus (CN X) nerves. The

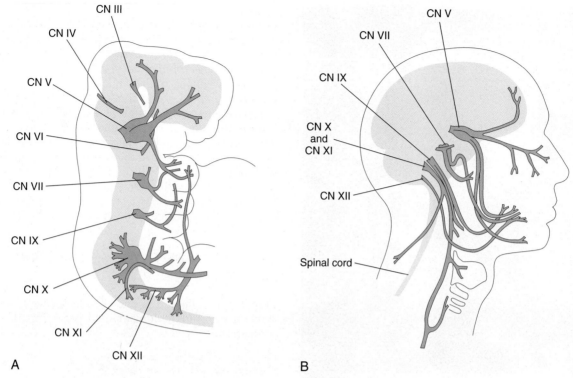

Figure 16–27 **A,** A 5-week embryo, showing the distribution of most of the cranial nerves, especially those supplying the pharyngeal arches. **B,** The head and neck of an adult, showing the general distribution of most of the cranial nerves.

postsynaptic neurons are located in the peripheral ganglia or in plexuses near or within the structure being innervated (e.g., pupil of the eye, salivary glands).

CLINICALLY ORIENTED QUESTIONS

1. Are neural tube defects hereditary? A woman had an infant with spina bifida cystica, and her daughter had an infant with meroencephaly. Is the daughter likely to have another child with a neural tube defect? Can meroencephaly and spina bifida be detected early in fetal life?

2. Some say that pregnant women who are heavy drinkers may have infants who exhibit mental and growth retardation. Is this true? There are reports of women who get drunk during pregnancy, yet have infants who seem to be normal. Is there a safe threshold for alcohol consumption during pregnancy?

3. A woman was told that cigarette smoking during pregnancy probably caused the slight mental retardation of her infant. She is not a heavy smoker. Was the woman correctly informed?

4. Do all types of spina bifida cause loss of motor function in the lower limbs? What treatments are there for infants with spina bifida cystica?

The answers to these questions are at the back of the book.

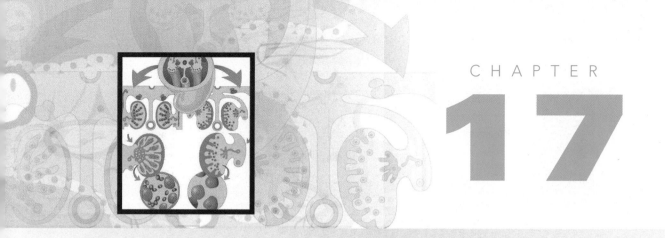

Eyes and Ears

DEVELOPMENT OF EYES AND RELATED STRUCTURES

Early eye development results from a series of inductive signals and is first evident at the beginning of the fourth week, when **optic grooves** appear in the cranial neural folds (Fig. 17-1*A* and *B*). As the neural folds fuse, the optic grooves evaginate to form hollow diverticula—**optic vesicles**—which project from the wall of the forebrain into the adjacent mesenchyme (Fig. 17-1*C*). Formation of the optic vesicles is induced by the mesenchyme adjacent to the developing brain. As the optic vesicles enlarge, their connections with the forebrain constrict to form hollow **optic stalks** (Fig. 17-1*D*).

An inductive signal passes from the optic vesicles and stimulates the surface ectoderm to thicken and form **lens placodes,** the primordia of the lenses (Fig. 17-1*C*). These placodes invaginate and sink deep to the surface ectoderm, forming **lens pits** (Figs. 17-1*D* and 17-2). The edges of each lens pit approach and fuse to form spherical **lens vesicles** (Fig. 17-1*F* and *H*), which soon lose their connection with the surface ectoderm. As the lens vesicles develop, the optic vesicles invaginate to form double-walled **optic cups** (Figs. 17-1*H* and 17-2), with the lens becoming infolded by the rim of the optic cup (Fig. 17-3*A*). By this stage, the lens vesicles have entered the cavities of the optic cups (Fig. 17-4). Linear grooves—**retinal (optic) fissures**—develop on the ventral surface of the optic cups and along the optic stalks (Figs. 17-1*E* to *H* and 17-3*A* to *D*). The retinal fissures contain vascular mesenchyme from which the hyaloid blood vessels develop. The **hyaloid artery** supplies the inner layer of the optic cup, the lens vesicle, and the mesenchyme in the optic cup (Figs. 17-1*H* and 17-3). As the edges of the retinal fissure fuse, the hyaloid vessels are enclosed within the **primordial optic nerve** (Fig. 17-3*C* to *F*). Distal parts of the hyaloid vessels eventually degenerate, but proximal parts persist as the **central artery** and **vein of the retina** (Fig. 17-5*D*).

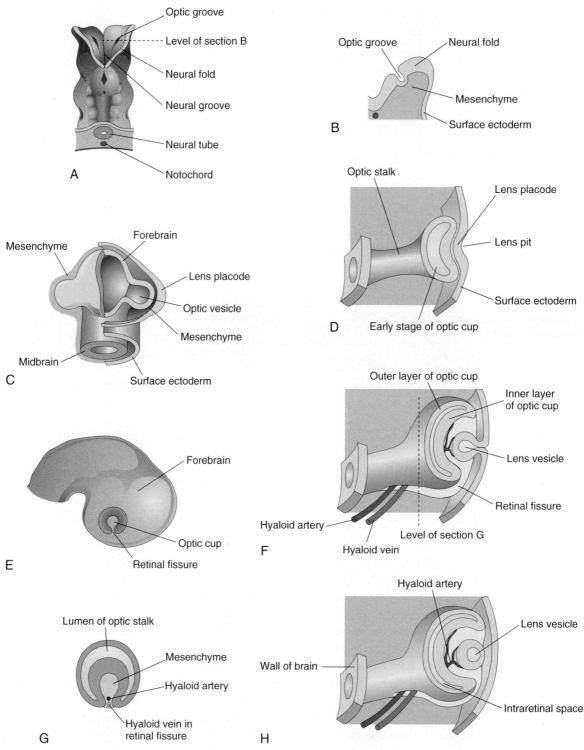

Figure 17–1 **A,** Dorsal view of the cranial end of an embryo at approximately 22 days, showing the optic grooves, the first indication of eye development. **B,** Transverse section of a neural fold, showing the optic groove. **C,** Forebrain of an embryo (approximately 28 days). **D, F,** and **H,** The developing eye, showing successive stages in the development of the optic cup and the lens vesicle. **E,** Lateral view of an embryo (approximately 32 days), showing the external appearance of the optic cup. **G,** Transverse section of the optic stalk, showing the retinal fissure and its contents.

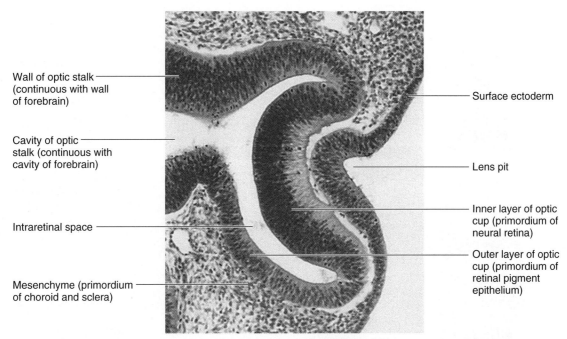

Figure 17–2 Photomicrograph of a sagittal section of the eye of an embryo at approximately 32 days. Observe the primordium of the lens (invaginated lens placode), the walls of the optic cup (primordium of the retina), and the optic stalk (primordium of the optic nerve). *(From Moore KL, Persaud TVN, Shiota K: Color Atlas of Clinical Embryology, 2nd ed. Philadelphia, WB Saunders, 2000.)*

Labels on figure:
- Wall of optic stalk (continuous with wall of forebrain)
- Cavity of optic stalk (continuous with cavity of forebrain)
- Intraretinal space
- Mesenchyme (primordium of choroid and sclera)
- Surface ectoderm
- Lens pit
- Inner layer of optic cup (primordium of neural retina)
- Outer layer of optic cup (primordium of retinal pigment epithelium)

Development of Retina

The retina develops from the walls of the **optic cup** (Figs. 17-1 and 17-2). In the invaginated optic cup, the deeper, thinner layer becomes the **retinal pigment epithelium**, whereas the more superficial, thicker layer differentiates into the **neural retina**. The two retinal layers are separated by an **intraretinal space** (Figs. 17-1H and 17-4), which is the original cavity of the optic cup. Before birth, this space gradually disappears as the two layers of the retina fuse (Fig. 17-5D). Because the optic cup is an outgrowth of the forebrain, the layers of the optic cup are continuous with the wall of the brain (Fig. 17-1H). Under the influence of the developing lens, the inner layer of the optic cup proliferates to form a thick **neuroepithelium** (Fig. 17-4). Subsequently, the cells of the inner layer closest to the retinal pigment epithelium differentiate into the **neural retina**, the light-sensitive region of the retina (Fig. 17-4). This region contains **photoreceptors** (rods and cones) and the cell bodies of neurons (e.g., ganglion cells). Because the optic vesicle invaginates as it forms the optic cup, the neural retina is "inverted"; that is, light-sensitive parts of the photoreceptor cells are adjacent to the retinal pigment epithelium. As a result, light must pass through the thickest part of the retina before reaching the receptors; however, because the retina is transparent, it does not form a barrier to light.

The axons of the ganglion cells in the superficial layer of the neural retina grow proximally in the wall of the optic stalk to the brain (Fig. 17-3A). The cavity of the **optic stalk** is gradually obliterated as the axons of the ganglion cells form the **optic nerve** (Fig. 17-3F).

RETINAL DETACHMENT

Congenital detachment of the retina occurs when the inner and outer layers of the optic cup do not fuse during the fetal period to form the retina and obliterate the intraretinal space (Figs. 17-3 and 17-5). The separation of the neural and pigmented layers may be partial or complete. Retinal detachment may result from unequal rates of growth of the two retinal layers; as a result, the layers of the optic cup are not in perfect apposition. Although separated from the retinal pigment epithelium, the neural retina retains its blood supply (central artery of retina). Normally, the retinal pigment epithelium becomes firmly fixed to the choroid, but its attachment to the neural retina is not firm; hence, retinal detachment is not uncommon.

COLOBOMA OF RETINA

Retinal coloboma is a defect that is characterized by a localized gap in the retina, usually inferior to the optic disc. The defect is bilateral in most cases. A typical coloboma results from defective closure of the retinal fissure.

Myelination of the optic nerve fibers begins late in the fetal period and is completed by the 10th week after birth. Molecular studies have shown that the homeobox genes PAX6 and OTX2 regulate retinal differentiation and pigment formation, respectively.

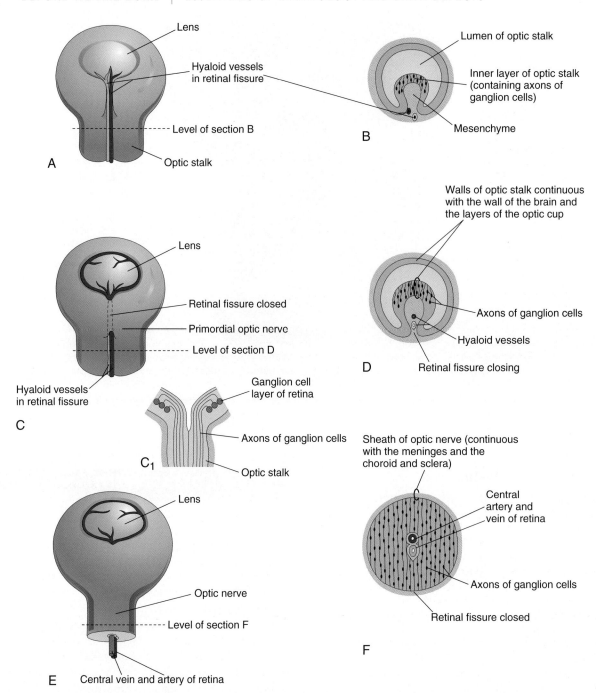

Figure 17–3 Closure of the retinal fissure and formation of the optic nerve. **A, C,** and **E,** Views of the inferior surface of the optic cup and optic stalk, showing progressive stages in the closure of the retinal fissure. **C₁,** Longitudinal section of a part of the optic cup and optic stalk, showing the axons of the ganglion cells of the retina growing through the optic stalk to the brain. **B, D,** and **F,** Transverse sections of the optic stalk, showing successive stages in the closure of the retinal fissure and formation of the optic nerve.

COLOBOMA OF IRIS

In infants with coloboma of the iris, a defect in the inferior sector of the iris or the pupillary margin gives the pupil a keyhole appearance (Fig. 17-6). The coloboma may be limited to the iris, or it may extend deeper and involve the ciliary body and retina. A typical coloboma *results from failure of closure of the retinal fissure* during the sixth week. The defect may be genetically determined, or it may be caused by environmental factors. A simple coloboma of the iris is frequently hereditary and is transmitted as an autosomal dominant characteristic.

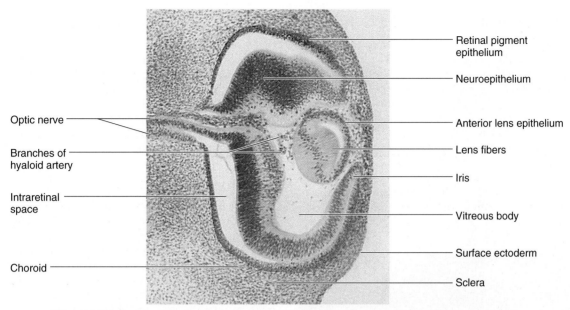

Optic nerve

Branches of
hyaloid artery

Intraretinal
space

Choroid

Retinal pigment
epithelium

Neuroepithelium

Anterior lens epithelium

Lens fibers

Iris

Vitreous body

Surface ectoderm

Sclera

Figure 17–4 Photomicrograph of a sagittal section of the eye of an embryo at approximately 44 days. Observe that the posterior wall of the lens vesicle forms the lens fibers. The anterior wall does not change appreciably as it becomes the anterior lens epithelium. *(From Nishimura H [ed]: Atlas of Human Prenatal Histology. Tokyo, Igaku-Shoin, 1983.)*

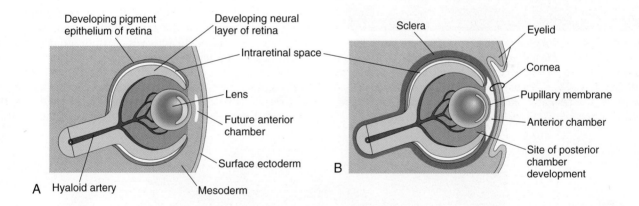

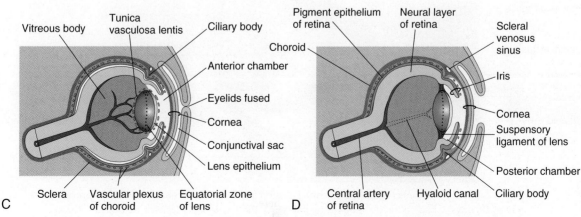

Figure 17–5 Sagittal sections of the eye, showing successive developmental stages of the lens, retina, iris, and cornea. **A,** At 5 weeks. **B,** At 6 weeks. **C,** At 20 weeks. **D,** Newborn infant.

Development of Choroid and Sclera

The mesenchyme surrounding the optic cup differentiates into an inner, vascular layer—the **choroid**—and an outer, fibrous layer—the **sclera** (see Figs. 17-5C and 17-7). At the rim of the optic cup, the choroid forms the cores of the **ciliary processes,** consisting chiefly of capillaries supported by delicate connective tissue.

Development of Ciliary Body

The ciliary body is a wedge-shaped extension of the **choroid** (Fig. 17-5C and D). Its medial surface projects toward the lens, forming the **ciliary processes.** The

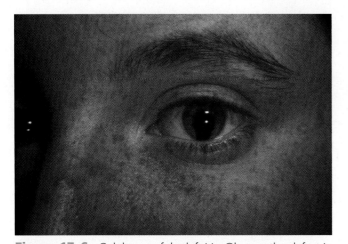

Figure 17–6   Coloboma of the left iris. Observe the defect in the inferior part of the iris (at the 6 o'clock position). The defect represents failure of fusion of the retinal fissure. *(Reprinted from Otolaryngologic Clinics of North America 40(1), Guercio J, Martyn L, Congenital malformations of the eye and orbit, 113-140, Copyright 2007, with permission from Elsevier.)*

pigmented part of the ciliary epithelium is derived from the outer layer of the optic cup and is continuous with the retinal pigment epithelium. The nonpigmented part of the ciliary epithelium represents the anterior prolongation of the neural retina, in which no neural elements develop. The smooth **ciliary muscle,** responsible for focusing the lens and the connective tissue in the ciliary body, develop from mesenchyme at the edge of the optic cup between the anterior scleral condensation and the ciliary pigment epithelium.

Development of Iris

The iris develops from the rim of the optic cup, which grows inward and partially covers the lens (Fig. 17-5D). The epithelium of the iris represents both layers of the optic cup; it is continuous with the double-layered epithelium of the ciliary body and with the retinal pigment epithelium and neural retina. The connective tissue framework of the iris is derived from neural crest cells that migrate into the iris. The **dilator pupillae** and **sphincter pupillae muscles** of the iris are derived from the *neuroectoderm of the optic cup.* These smooth muscles result from a transformation of epithelial cells into smooth muscle cells.

Development of Lens

The lens develops from the **lens vesicle,** a derivative of the surface ectoderm (Fig. 17-1). The anterior wall of the lens vesicle becomes the subcapsular **lens epithelium** (Fig. 17-5C). The nuclei of the tall columnar cells that form the posterior wall of the lens vesicle undergo dissolution. These cells lengthen considerably to form highly transparent epithelial cells, the **primary lens fibers.** As these fibers grow, they gradually obliterate the cavity of the lens vesicle (Figs. 17-5A to C). The rim of the lens—the **equatorial zone**—is located midway between the anterior

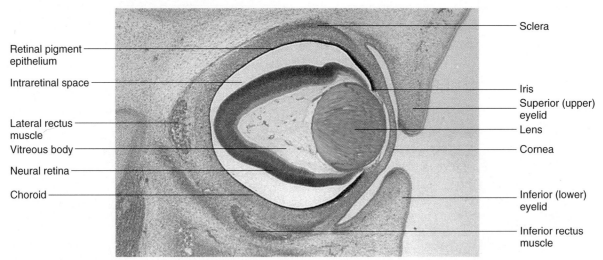

Figure 17–7   Photomicrograph of a sagittal section of the eye of an embryo (x50) at approximately 56 days. Observe the developing neural retina and the retinal pigment epithelium. Note the large intraretinal space between the two layers of the retina. *(From Moore KL, Persaud TVN, Shiota K: Color Atlas of Clinical Embryology, 2nd ed. Philadelphia, WB Saunders, 2000.)*

and the posterior poles of the lens. The cells in the equatorial zone are cuboidal; as they elongate, they lose their nuclei and become **secondary lens fibers** (Fig. 17-8). These fibers are added to the external sides of the primary lens fibers. *Lens formation involves the expression of L-Maf (lens-specific Maf) and other transcription factors in the lens placode and vesicle. The transcription factors Pitx3 and GAT-3 are also essential for the formation of the lens.*

Although secondary lens fibers continue to form during adulthood and the lens increases in diameter as a result, the primary lens fibers must last a lifetime. The developing lens is supplied with blood by the distal part of the **hyaloid artery** (Figs. 17-4 and 17-5); however, it becomes avascular in the fetal period when this part of the artery degenerates (Fig. 17-5D). After this, the lens depends on diffusion from the aqueous humor in the anterior chamber of the eye, which bathes its anterior surface, and from the vitreous humor in other parts. The lens capsule is produced by the anterior lens epithelium. The **lens capsule** represents a greatly thickened basement membrane and has a lamellar structure. The former site of the hyaloid artery is indicated by the **hyaloid canal** in the vitreous body (Fig. 17-5D); this canal is usually inconspicuous in the living eye.

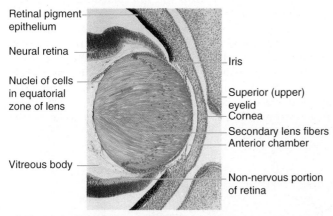

Retinal pigment epithelium
Neural retina
Nuclei of cells in equatorial zone of lens
Vitreous body
Iris
Superior (upper) eyelid
Cornea
Secondary lens fibers
Anterior chamber
Non-nervous portion of retina

Figure 17–8 Photomicrograph of a sagittal section of a portion of the developing eye of an embryo at approximately 56 days. Observe that the lens fibers have elongated and obliterated the cavity of the lens vesicle. *(From Moore KL, Persaud TVN, Shiota K: Color Atlas of Clinical Embryology, 2nd ed. Philadelphia, WB Saunders, 2000.)*

PERSISTENCE OF HYALOID ARTERY

The distal part of the hyaloid artery normally degenerates as its proximal part becomes the central artery of the retina. If part of the hyaloid artery persists distally, it may appear as a freely moving, nonfunctional vessel, a wormlike structure projecting from the optic disc, or as a fine strand traversing the vitreous body. In other cases, the hyaloids artery remnant may form a cyst.

The **vitreous body** forms within the optic cup (Fig. 17-5C). It is composed of **vitreous humor**, an avascular mass of transparent, gel-like, intercellular substance.

Development of Aqueous Chambers

The **anterior chamber of the eye** develops from a cleft-like space that forms in the mesenchyme located between the developing lens and the cornea (Fig. 17-5A and B). The **posterior chamber of the eye** develops from a space that forms in the mesenchyme posterior to the developing iris and anterior to the developing lens (Fig. 17-5D). After the lens is established, it induces the surface ectoderm to develop into the epithelium of the cornea and conjunctiva. When the pupillary membrane disappears and the pupil forms, the anterior and posterior chambers of the eye communicate with each other through the **scleral venous sinus**. This sinus encircles the anterior chamber and allows aqueous humor to flow from the anterior chamber of the eye to the venous system.

Development of Cornea

The cornea, induced by the lens vesicle, is formed from three sources:

- The external corneal epithelium, derived from the **surface ectoderm**
- The **mesenchyme**, derived from the mesoderm
- **Neural crest cells** that migrate from the lip of the optic cup and become transformed into the corneal endothelium

CONGENITAL GLAUCOMA

Intraocular tension (abnormal elevation of intraocular pressure) occurs because of an imbalance between the production of aqueous humor and its outflow. This imbalance may result from abnormal development of the scleral venous sinus (Fig. 17-5D). Congenital glaucoma is usually genetically heterogeneous, but the condition may result from rubella infection during early pregnancy (see Fig. 19-16B). It has been shown that the gene CYP1B1 is responsible for the majority of primary congenital glaucomas.

CONGENITAL CATARACTS

In congenital cataracts, the lens is opaque and frequently appears grayish white. Blindness results. Many lens opacities are inherited, with dominant transmission being more common than recessive, or sex-linked, transmission. Some congenital cataracts are caused by teratogenic agents—particularly the **rubella virus** (see Fig. 19-16A)—that affect the early development of the lenses. The lenses are vulnerable to the rubella virus between the fourth and seventh weeks, when primary lens fibers are forming. Physical agents, such as **radiation**, can also damage the lens and produce cataracts (see Chapter 19).

Development of Eyelids

The eyelids develop during the sixth week from the neural crest–derived mesenchyme and from two folds of skin that grow over the cornea (Fig. 17-5B). The eyelids adhere to one another at approximately the 10th week and remain fused until the 26th to 28th weeks (Fig. 17-5C). The **palpebral conjunctiva** lines the inner surface of the eyelids. The **eyelashes** and **glands** in the eyelids are derived from the surface ectoderm (Chapter 18). The connective tissue and **tarsal plates** develop from mesenchyme in the developing eyelids. The *orbicularis oculi muscle* is derived from the mesenchyme in the second pharyngeal arch (see Chapter 10).

CONGENITAL PTOSIS OF EYELID

Drooping of the superior (upper) eyelids at birth is relatively common. Congenital ptosis may result from dystrophy of the levator palpebrae superioris muscle. Ptosis occurs more rarely as a result of prenatal injury or dystrophy of the superior division of the **oculomotor nerve** (CN III) that supplies this muscle. Congenital ptosis may be transmitted as an autosomal dominant trait.

COLOBOMA OF EYELID

Most palpebral colobomas are characterized by a small notch in the superior eyelid. Coloboma of the inferior (lower) eyelid is rare. **Palpebral colobomas** appear to result from developmental disturbances in the formation of the eyelids.

Development of Lacrimal Glands

The lacrimal glands are derived from a number of solid buds from the surface ectoderm. The buds branch and canalize to form lacrimal excretory ducts and the alveoli of the glands. The lacrimal glands are small at birth and do not function fully until approximately 6 weeks; hence, the newborn infant does not produce tears when crying.

DEVELOPMENT OF EARS

The ears are composed of external, middle, and internal anatomical parts. The external and middle parts of the ears regulate the transference of sound waves from the exterior to the internal ears; this process converts the sound waves into nerve impulses. The internal ears are concerned with both hearing and balance.

Development of Internal Ears

The internal ears are the first of the three parts of the ear to develop. Early in the fourth week, a thickening of the surface ectoderm—the **otic placodes**—appears on each side of the embryo at the level of the caudal part of the hindbrain (Fig. 17-9A and B). Inductive influences from the notochord and paraxial mesoderm stimulate the surface ectoderm to form the otic placodes. *Fibroblast growth factor 3 (FGF-3) may play a role in this process.* Each otic placode soon invaginates and sinks deep to the surface ectoderm into the underlying mesenchyme, forming an **otic pit** (Fig. 17-9C and D). The edges of the otic pit come together and fuse to form an **otic vesicle** (Fig. 17-9E to G). The otic vesicle then loses its connection with the surface ectoderm, and a diverticulum grows from the otic vesicle and elongates to form the

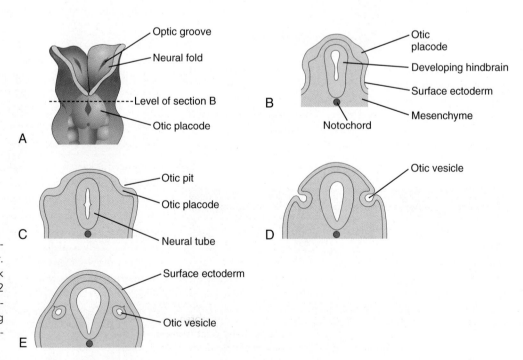

Figure 17–9 Early development of the internal ear. **A,** Dorsal view of a 4-week embryo (at approximately 22 days). **B, C, D,** and **E,** Schematic coronal sections, showing successive stages in the development of the otic vesicles.

endolymphatic duct and **sac** (Fig. 17-10*A* to *E*). As the otic vesicle grows, two regions become visible:

- A dorsal utricular part from which the endolymphatic duct, utricle, and semicircular ducts arise
- A ventral saccular part, which gives rise to the saccule and cochlear duct, in which the spiral organ (of Corti) is located

Three disc-like diverticula grow out from the utricular part of the **primordial membranous labyrinth**. The central parts of these diverticula fuse and disappear (Fig. 17-10*B* to *E*). The peripheral unfused parts of the diverticula become the **semicircular ducts**, which are attached to the utricle and are later enclosed in the **semicircular canals** of the **bony labyrinth**. Localized dilatations, the **ampullae**, develop at one end of each semicircular duct (Fig. 17-10*E*). Specialized receptor areas—**cristae ampullares**—differentiate in these ampullae as well as in the utricle and saccule.

From the ventral saccular part of the otic vesicle, a tubular diverticulum—the **cochlear duct**—grows and coils to form the **membranous cochlea** (Fig. 17-10*C* to *E*). A connection of the cochlea with the saccule, the **ductus reuniens**, soon forms. The **spiral organ** differentiates from cells in the wall of the cochlear duct (Fig. 17-10*F* to *I*). Ganglion cells of the vestibulocochlear nerve (CN VIII) migrate along the coils of the membranous cochlea and form the **spiral ganglion**. Nerve processes extend from this ganglion to the spiral organ, where they terminate on **hair cells**. The cells in the spiral ganglion retain their embryonic bipolar condition.

Inductive influences from the otic vesicle stimulate the mesenchyme around the otic vesicle to differentiate into a **cartilaginous otic capsule** (Fig. 17-10*F*). The cartilaginous otic capsule later ossifies to form the **bony labyrinth** of the internal ear. *Transforming growth factor β₁ may play a role in modulating epithelial–mesenchymal interaction in the internal ear and directing the formation of the otic capsule.* As the membranous labyrinth enlarges, vacuoles appear in the cartilaginous otic capsule that soon coalesce to form the **perilymphatic space**. As a result, the membranous labyrinth becomes suspended in perilymph (fluid in the perilymphatic space). The perilymphatic space related to the cochlear duct develops two divisions, the **scala tympani** and **scala vestibuli** (Fig. 17-10*H* and *I*). The internal ear reaches its adult size and shape by the middle of the fetal period (20-22 weeks).

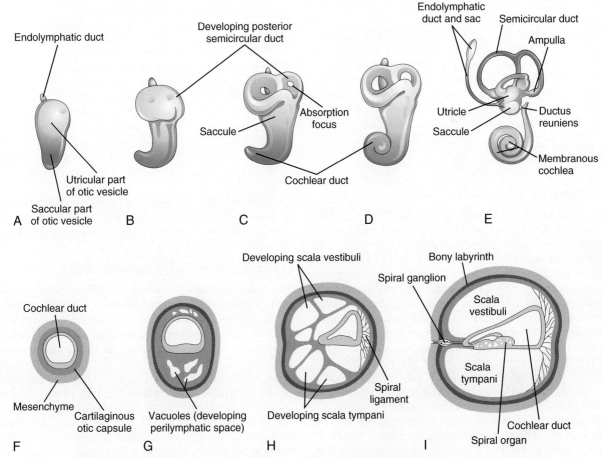

Figure 17–10 The otic vesicle, showing the development of the membranous and bony labyrinths of the internal ear. **A** to **E,** Lateral views, showing successive stages in the development of the otic vesicle into the membranous labyrinth from the fifth to eighth weeks. **F** to **I,** Sections through the cochlear duct, showing successive stages in the development of the spiral organ and the perilymphatic space from the eighth to 20th weeks.

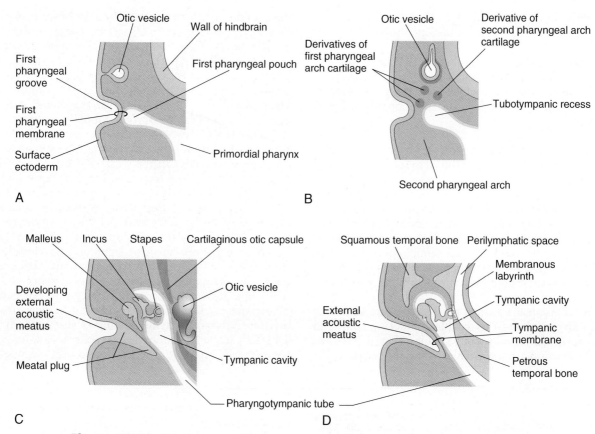

Figure 17–11 Development of the external and middle parts of the ear. **A,** At 4 weeks, showing the relation of the otic vesicle to the pharyngeal apparatus. **B,** At 5 weeks, showing the tubotympanic recess and pharyngeal arch cartilages. **C,** At a later stage, showing the tubotympanic recess (primordium of the tympanic cavity and mastoid antrum) beginning to envelop the ossicles. **D,** Final stage of ear development, showing the relation of the middle ear to the perilymphatic space and the external acoustic meatus.

Development of Middle Ears

Development of the **tubotympanic recess** (Fig. 17-11*B*) from the first pharyngeal pouch is described in Chapter 10. The proximal part of the tubotympanic recess forms the **pharyngotympanic tube** (auditory tube). The distal part of the tubotympanic recess expands and becomes the **tympanic cavity** (Fig. 17-11*C*), which gradually envelops the **auditory ossicles** (malleus, incus, and stapes), their tendons and ligaments, and the chorda tympani nerve. All these structures receive a virtually complete epithelial investment. An epithelial-type organizer, located at the tip of the tubotympanic recess, probably plays a role in the early development of the middle ear cavity by inducing programmed cell death—apoptosis. The malleus and the incus develop from the cartilage of the first pharyngeal arch, whereas the stapes develops from the cartilage of the second arch. The **tensor tympani**, the muscle attached to the malleus, is derived from the mesenchyme in the first pharyngeal arch, and the **stapedius muscle** is derived from the second pharyngeal arch. During the late fetal period, expansion of the tympanic cavity gives rise to the **mastoid antrum**, located in the temporal bone. The mastoid antrum is almost adult size at birth; however, *no mastoid cells are present in newborn infants*. By 2 years,

the mastoid cells are well developed and produce conic projections of the temporal bones, the mastoid processes. The middle ear continues to grow through puberty.

Development of External Ears

The **external acoustic meatus** develops from the dorsal part of the first pharyngeal groove. The ectodermal cells at the bottom of this tube proliferate to form a solid epithelial plate, the **meatal plug** (Fig. 17-11*C*). Late in the fetal period, the central cells of this plug degenerate, forming a cavity that becomes the internal part of the external acoustic meatus (Fig. 17-11*D*). The primordium of the **tympanic membrane** is the first pharyngeal membrane, which separates the first pharyngeal groove from the first pharyngeal pouch (Fig. 17-11*A*). The external covering of the tympanic membrane is derived from the surface ectoderm, whereas its internal lining is derived from the endoderm of the tubotympanic recess.

The **auricle** develops from the mesenchymal proliferations in the first and second pharyngeal arches. Prominences—**auricular hillocks**—surround the first pharyngeal groove (Fig. 17-12*A*). As the auricle grows, the contribution of the first arch is reduced (Fig. 17-12*B* to *D*). The

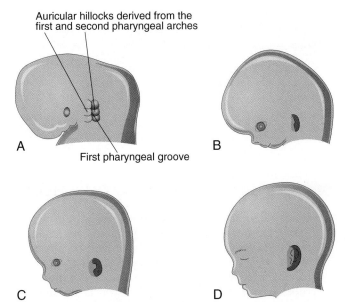

Figure 17–12   Development of the auricle of the external ear. **A,** At 6 weeks. Note that three auricular hillocks are located on the first pharyngeal arch and three are on the second arch. **B,** At 8 weeks. **C,** At 10 weeks. **D,** At 32 weeks.

CONGENITAL DEAFNESS

Approximately 1 in 1000 newborn infants have significant hearing loss. Congenital deafness may be the result of maldevelopment of the sound-conducting apparatus of the middle and external ears, or of the neurosensory structures in the internal ear. *Enlargement of the vestibular aqueduct and endolymphatic duct* is the most common congenital ear defect in children with hearing loss (Fig. 17-13). This defect is typically bilateral and is an autosomal recessive condition. *Rubella infection* during the critical period of development of the internal ear can cause maldevelopment of the spiral organ and deafness. Congenital fixation of the stapes results in conductive deafness in an otherwise normal ear. Failure of differentiation of the anular ligament, which attaches the base of the stapes to the oval window, results in fixation of the stapes to the bony labyrinth and loss of sound conduction.

AURICULAR ANOMALIES

Minor auricular deformities are common and may serve as indicators of a specific pattern of congenital anomalies. For example, the auricles are often low-set and abnormal in shape in infants with chromosomal syndromes, such as trisomy 18 (see Chapter 19), and in infants affected by maternal ingestion of certain drugs (e.g., trimethadione).

lobule (earlobe) is the last part to develop. The auricle is initially located at the base of the neck (Fig. 17-12*A* and *B*). As the mandible develops, the auricle assumes its normal position at the side of the head (Fig. 17-12*C* and *D*).

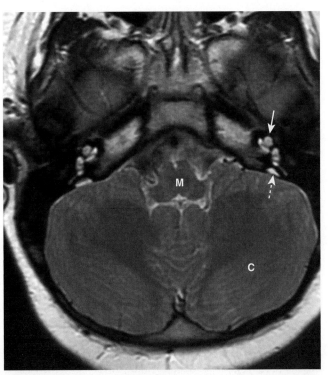

Figure 17–13   MRI of a 5-year-old child demonstrating bilateral enlargement of vestibular aqueduct and endolymphatic duct *(dashed arrow).* Also note the cochlea *(solid arrow),* the medulla *(M),* and the cerebellum *(C). (Courtesy of Dr. G. Smyser, Altru Health System, Grand Forks, North Dakota.)*

AURICULAR APPENDAGES

Auricular appendages (skin tags) are common and result from the development of accessory auricular hillocks (Fig. 17-14). The appendages usually appear anterior to the auricle, more often unilaterally than bilaterally. The appendages, often with narrow pedicles, consist of skin but they may also contain some cartilage.

MICROTIA

Microtia (small auricle) results from suppressed development of the auricular hillocks (Fig. 17-14). This anomaly often serves as an indicator of associated anomalies, such as atresia of the external acoustic meatus and abnormalities of the middle ear.

PREAURICULAR SINUSES

Shallow, pitlike cutaneous sinuses are occasionally located anterior to the auricle. These sinuses usually have pinpoint external openings. Some sinuses contain a vestigial cartilaginous mass. These defects are probably related to abnormal development of the auricular hillocks and defective closure of the dorsal part of the first pharyngeal groove. *Preauricular sinuses* are familial and are frequently bilateral.

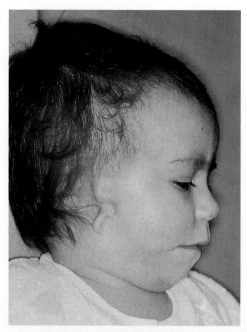

Figure 17–14 Child with a rudimentary auricle (microtia) and a preauricular tag. The external acoustic meatus is also absent. *(Courtesy of A.E. Chudley, M.D., Section of Genetics and Metabolism, Department of Pediatrics and Child Health, Children's Hospital, University of Manitoba, Winnipeg, Manitoba, Canada.)*

ATRESIA OF EXTERNAL ACOUSTIC MEATUS

Atresia (blockage) of the external acoustic meatus results from failure of the meatal plug to canalize (Fig. 17-11C). Usually the deep part of the canal is open but the superficial part is blocked by bone or fibrous tissue. Most cases are associated with the *first arch syndrome* (see Chapter 10). Often the auricle is also severely affected, and anomalies of the middle ear, internal ear, or both may be present. Atresia of the external acoustic meatus can occur bilaterally or unilaterally and usually results from autosomal dominant inheritance.

ABSENCE OF EXTERNAL ACOUSTIC MEATUS

Absence of the external acoustic meatus is rare (Fig. 17-14). This anomaly results from failure of inward expansion of the first pharyngeal groove and failure of the meatal plug to disappear.

CLINICALLY ORIENTED QUESTIONS

1. If a woman has rubella (German measles) during the first trimester of pregnancy, what are the chances that the eyes and ears of the fetus will be affected? What is the most common manifestation of late fetal rubella infection? If a pregnant woman is exposed to rubella, can it be determined if she is immune to the infection?

2. Some believe that a good way of preventing the congenital anomalies caused by rubella is by the purposeful exposure of young girls to rubella. Is this the best way for a woman to avoid rubella infection during pregnancy? If not, what can be done to provide immunization against rubella infection?

3. It has been reported that deafness and tooth defects occurring during childhood may result from a condition called fetal syphilis. Is this true? If so, how could this happen? Can these congenital defects be prevented?

4. There are reports that blindness and deafness can result from herpes virus infections. Is this true? If so, which herpes virus is involved? What are the affected infant's chances of normal development?

5. An article in the newspaper reported that methyl mercury exposure in utero can cause mental deficiency, deafness, and blindness. The article cited the eating of contaminated fish as the cause of the abnormalities. How might these anomalies be caused by methyl mercury?

The answers to these questions are at the back of the book.

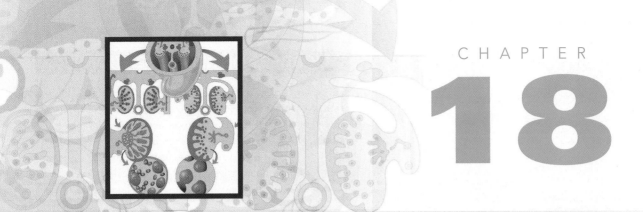

CHAPTER

18

Integumentary System

T he integumentary system consists of the skin and its appendages: sweat glands, nails, hairs, sebaceous glands, and arrector muscles of hairs. The system also includes the mammary glands and teeth.

DEVELOPMENT OF SKIN

The integument or skin consists of two layers (epidermis and dermis) that are derived from two different germ layers (Fig. 18-1): the ectoderm and mesoderm.

● The **epidermis** is a superficial epithelial tissue that is derived from surface ectoderm.
● The **dermis** is a deep layer composed of dense connective tissue that is derived from primordial connective tissue (mesenchyme).

Ectodermal (epidermal) and mesenchymal (dermal) interactions involve mutual inductive mechanisms. The embryonic skin at 4 to 5 weeks consists of a single layer of surface ecto-derm overlying the mesoderm (Fig. 18-1A).

Epidermis

The primordium of the epidermis is the surface ectoderm (Fig. 18-1A). The cells in this layer proliferate and form a layer of squamous epithelium, the **periderm**, and a basal layer (Fig. 18-1B). The cells of the periderm continually undergo keratinization and desquamation and are replaced by cells arising from the **basal layer**. The exfoliated peridermal cells form part of a white, greasy substance—**vernix caseosa**—that covers the fetal skin. Later, the vernix contains **sebum**, the secretion from the sebaceous glands in the skin (Fig. 18-2). The vernix protects the developing skin from constant exposure to amniotic fluid containing urine.

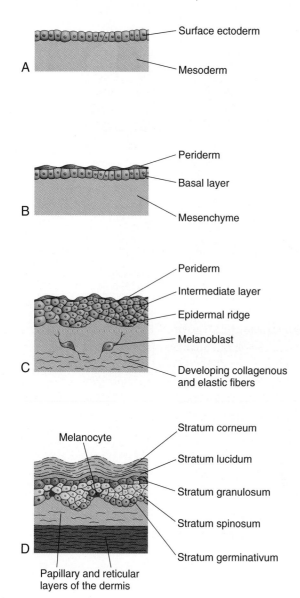

Figure 18–1 Successive stages of skin development. **A,** At 4 weeks. **B,** At 7 weeks. **C,** At 11 weeks. The cells of the periderm continually undergo keratinization and desquamation. Exfoliated peridermal cells form part of the vernix caseosa. **D,** Newborn infant. Note the position of the melanocytes in the basal layer of the epidermis. Their processes extend between the epidermal cells to supply them with melanin.

The basal layer of the epidermis becomes the **stratum germinativum** (Fig. 18-1D), which produces new cells that are displaced into the more superficial layers. By 11 weeks, cells from the stratum germinativum have formed an **intermediate layer** (Fig. 18-1C). Replacement of the peridermal cells continues until approximately the 21st week; thereafter, the periderm disappears and the **stratum corneum** forms from the **stratum lucidum** (Fig. 18-1D). Proliferation of the cells in the stratum germinativum also produces **epidermal ridges**, which extend into the developing dermis. These ridges begin to appear in embryos of 10 weeks and are permanently established by the 17th week. The pattern of epidermal ridges that develops on

DISORDERS OF KERATINIZATION

Ichthyosis is a general term for a group of skin disorders resulting from **excessive keratinization (keratin formation)**. The skin is characterized by dryness and fish-skin–like scaling, which may involve the entire body surface (Fig. 18-3). A **harlequin fetus** results from a rare keratinizing disorder that is inherited as an autosomal recessive trait. The skin is markedly thickened, ridged, and cracked. Most of the affected infants die during the first week of life. A **collodion infant** is covered at birth by a thick, taut membrane that resembles collodion or parchment. This membrane cracks with the first respiratory efforts and begins to fall off in large sheets. Complete shedding of membranes may take several weeks, occasionally leaving normal-appearing skin.

the surface of the palms of the hands and the soles of the feet is determined genetically and constitutes the basis for examining fingerprints (**dermatoglyphics**) in criminal investigations and medical genetics. Abnormal chromosome complements affect the development of ridge patterns; for example, infants with Down syndrome have distinctive ridge patterns on their hands and feet that are of diagnostic value.

Late in the embryonic period, **neural crest cells** migrate into the mesenchyme in the developing dermis and differentiate into **melanoblasts** (Fig. 18-1B and C). Later, these cells migrate to the **dermoepidermal junction** and differentiate into melanocytes (Fig. 18-1D). The **melanocytes** begin producing **melanin** before birth and distribute it to the epidermal cells. After birth, increased amounts of melanin are produced in response to ultraviolet light. The relative content of melanin in the melanocytes accounts for the different colors of skin. *Molecular studies indicate that melanocyte-stimulating hormone cell surface receptor and melanosomal P-protein determine the degree of pigmentation by regulating tyrosinase levels and activity.*

Dermis

The dermis develops from the mesenchyme underlying the surface ectoderm (Fig. 18-1A and B). The mesenchyme that differentiates into the connective tissue of the dermis originates from the somatic layer of the lateral mesoderm and from the dermatomes of the somites. By 11 weeks, the mesenchymal cells have begun to produce collagenous and elastic connective tissue fibers (Fig. 18-1C). As the **epidermal ridges** form, the dermis projects into the epidermis, forming **dermal papillae.** Capillary loops develop in some of the **dermal ridges** and provide nourishment for the epidermis. Sensory nerve endings form in other ridges.

The developing afferent nerve fibers apparently play an important role in the spatial and temporal sequence of dermal ridge formation. The blood vessels in the dermis differentiate from the mesenchyme. As the skin grows, new capillaries grow out from the primordial vessels (**angiogenesis**). Some capillaries acquire muscular

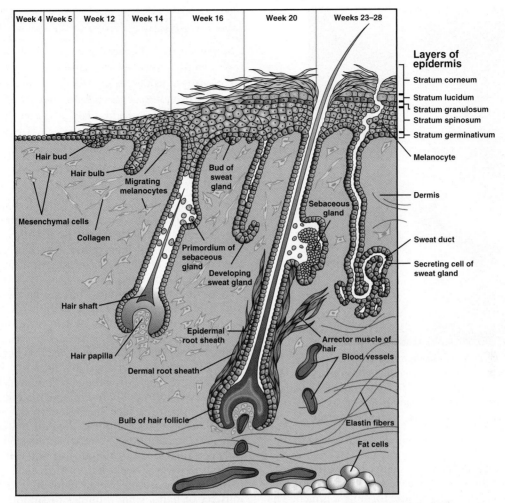

| Week 4 | Week 5 | Week 12 | Week 14 | Week 16 | Week 20 | Weeks 23–28 |

Layers of epidermis
- Stratum corneum
- Stratum lucidum
- Stratum granulosum
- Stratum spinosum
- Stratum germinativum
- Melanocyte
- Dermis
- Sweat duct
- Secreting cell of sweat gland

Hair bud
Hair bulb
Migrating melanocytes
Bud of sweat gland
Sebaceous gland
Mesenchymal cells
Collagen
Primordium of sebaceous gland
Developing sweat gland
Hair shaft
Epidermal root sheath
Arrector muscle of hair
Blood vessels
Hair papilla
Dermal root sheath
Bulb of hair follicle
Elastin fibers
Fat cells

Figure 18–2 Successive stages in the development of a hair and its associated sebaceous gland and arrector muscle. Note also the successive stages in the development of a sweat gland.

ANGIOMAS OF SKIN

Angiomas of the skin are vascular anomalies in which some transitory primordial blood vessels persist. Similar lesions that are composed of lymphatics are called **cystic lymphangiomas,** or cystic hygromas (see Chapter 14). True **angiomas** are benign tumors of endothelial cells, usually composed of solid or hollow cords; the hollow cords contain blood. Various terms are used to describe angiomatous anomalies ("birthmarks"). **Nevus flammeus** denotes a flat, pink or red, flame-like blotch that often appears on the posterior surface of the neck. A **port wine stain**, or **hemangioma**, is a larger, darker angioma than a nevus flammeus and is nearly always anterior or lateral on the face, neck, or both.

coats through the differentiation of myoblasts developing in the surrounding mesenchyme, and they become arterioles, arteries, venules, and veins. By the end of the first trimester, the blood supply of the fetal dermis is well established.

Glands of Skin

Two kinds of glands, sebaceous glands and sweat glands, are derived from the epidermis and grow into the dermis.

Sebaceous Glands

Most sebaceous glands develop as buds from the sides of the developing **epidermal root sheaths** of the hair follicles (Fig. 18-2). The glandular buds grow into the surrounding connective tissue and branch to form the primordia of the alveoli and their associated ducts. The central cells of the alveoli break down, forming an oily secretion called **sebum;** this is released into the hair follicle and passes to the surface of the skin, where it mixes with desquamated peridermal cells to form **vernix caseosa.** Sebaceous glands, independent of the hair follicles (e.g., in the glans penis and labia minora), develop in a similar manner as buds from the epidermis.

Sweat Glands

Eccrine sweat glands develop as epidermal downgrowths—**cellular buds**—into the underlying mesenchyme (Fig. 18-2). As a bud elongates, its end coils to form the primordium of the secretory part of the gland. The epithelial

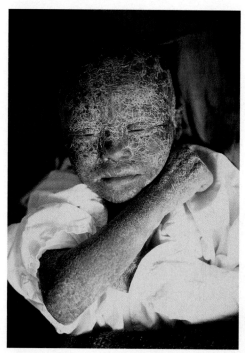

Figure 18–3 A child with epidermolytic hyperkeratosis. This condition is characterized by severe hyperkeratosis from the time of birth. It has an autosomal dominant inheritance pattern. *(Courtesy of Dr. Joao Carlos Fernandes Rodrigues, Servico de Dermatologia, Hospital de Desterro, Lisbon, Portugal.)*

ALBINISM

In *generalized albinism*, an autosomal recessive trait, the skin, hairs, and retina lack pigment; however, the iris usually shows some pigmentation. Albinism occurs when the melanocytes do not produce melanin because of a lack of the enzyme tyrosinase. In *localized albinism*—piebaldism—an autosomal dominant trait, there is a lack of melanin in patches of skin, hair, or both.

attachment of the developing gland to the epidermis forms the primordium of the sweat duct. The central cells of the primordial ducts degenerate, forming a lumen. The peripheral cells of the secretory part of the gland differentiate into *myoepithelial* and *secretory* cells (Fig. 18-2). The myoepithelial cells are believed to be specialized smooth muscle cells that assist in expelling sweat from the glands. Eccrine sweat glands begin to function shortly after birth.

Apocrine sweat glands develop from downgrowths of the stratum germinativum of the epidermis that give rise to the hair follicles. As a result, the ducts of these glands open into the upper part of the hair follicles, superficial to the openings of the sebaceous glands. They begin to secrete sweat during puberty.

DEVELOPMENT OF HAIRS

Hairs begin to develop during the 9th to 12th weeks, but they do not become easily recognizable until approximately the 20th week (Fig. 18-2). Hairs are first recognizable on the eyebrows, upper lip, and chin. A hair follicle begins as a proliferation of the stratum germinativum of the epidermis and extends into the underlying dermis. The **hair bud** soon becomes a club-shaped hair bulb. The epithelial cells of the hair bulb constitute the **germinal matrix**, which later produces the hair. The **hair bulb** is soon invaginated by a small mesenchymal **hair papilla** (Fig. 18-2). The peripheral cells of the developing hair follicle form the epidermal root sheath, and the

surrounding mesenchymal cells differentiate into the **dermal root sheath**. As cells in the germinal matrix proliferate, they are pushed toward the surface, where they keratinize to form **hair shafts**. The hair grows through the epidermis on the eyebrows and the upper lip by the end of the 12th week.

The first hairs—**lanugo** (downy hair)—are fine, soft, and lightly pigmented. Lanugo begins to appear toward the end of the 12th week and is plentiful by 17 to 20 weeks. These hairs help to hold the vernix on the skin. Lanugo is replaced during the perinatal period by coarser hairs that persist over most of the body. In the axillary and pubic regions, the lanugo is replaced at puberty by even coarser **terminal hairs**. In males, similar coarse hairs also appear on the face and often on the chest.

Melanoblasts migrate into the hair bulbs and differentiate into **melanocytes**. The melanin produced by these cells is transferred to the hair-forming cells in the germinal matrix several weeks before birth. The relative content of melanin accounts for different hair colors. **Arrector muscles of hairs**, small bundles of smooth muscle fibers, differentiate from the mesenchyme surrounding the hair follicle and attach to the dermal root sheath and the papillary layer of the dermis (Fig. 18-2). The arrector muscles are poorly developed in the hairs of the axilla and in certain parts of the face. The hairs forming the eyebrows and the cilia forming the eyelashes have no arrector muscles.

DEVELOPMENT OF NAILS

Toenails and fingernails begin to develop at the tips of the digits at approximately 10 weeks (Fig. 18-4). Development of the **fingernails** precedes that of the **toenails** by approximately 4 weeks. The primordia of the nails appear as thickened areas, or fields, of epidermis at the tip of each digit. Later, these **nail fields** migrate onto the dorsal surface (Fig. 18-4A), carrying their innervation from the ventral surface. The nail fields are surrounded laterally and proximally by folds of epidermis—**nail folds**. Cells from the proximal nail fold grow over the nail field and keratinize to form the **nail plate** (Fig. 18-4B). At first, the developing nail is covered by superficial layers of epidermis called **eponychium** (Fig. 18-4C). These layers degenerate, exposing the nail, except at its base, where it persists as the **cuticle**. The fingernails reach the fingertips at approximately 32 weeks; the toenails reach the toe tips at approximately 36 weeks.

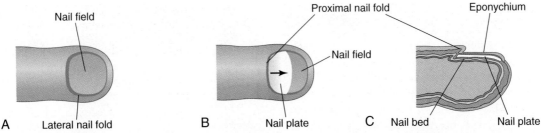

Figure 18–4 Successive stages in the development of a fingernail. **A,** The first indication of a nail is a thickening of the epidermis, the nail field, at the tip of the finger. **B,** As the nail plate develops, it slowly grows toward the tip of the finger. **C,** The fingernail normally reaches the end of the digit by 32 weeks.

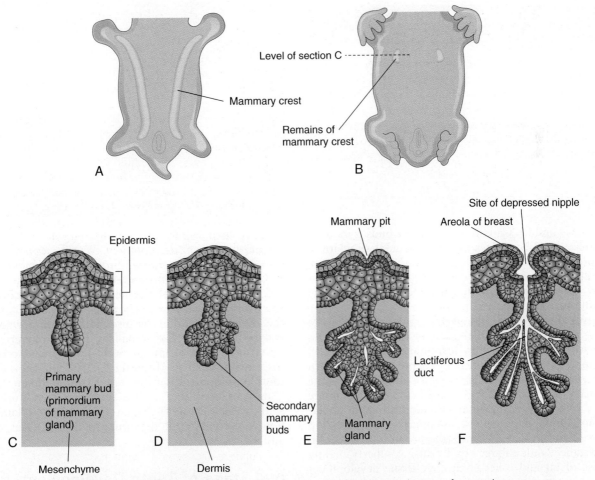

Figure 18–5 Development of the mammary glands. **A,** Ventral view of an embryo at approximately 28 days, showing mammary crests. **B,** Similar view at 6 weeks, showing the remains of these crests. **C,** Transverse section of a mammary crest at the site of a developing mammary gland. **D to F,** Similar sections, showing successive stages of breast development between the 12th week and birth.

DEVELOPMENT OF MAMMARY GLANDS

Mammary glands are modified and highly specialized types of sweat glands. **Mammary buds** begin to develop during the sixth week as solid downgrowths of the epidermis into the underlying mesenchyme (Fig. 18-5C). These changes occur in response to an inductive influence from the mesenchyme. The mammary buds develop from **mammary crests**, which are thickened strips of ectoderm extending from the axillary to the inguinal regions (Fig. 18-5A). The **mammary crests** appear during the fourth week but normally persist only in the pectoral area where the breasts develop (Fig. 18-5B). Each primary mammary bud soon gives rise to several secondary mammary buds that develop into the **lactiferous ducts** and their branches

GYNECOMASTIA

The rudimentary mammary glands in males normally undergo no postnatal development. **Gynecomastia** refers to excessive development of male mammary tissue. It occurs in most newborn males because of stimulation of the mammary glands by maternal sex hormones. This effect disappears in a few weeks. During mid-puberty, approximately two thirds of boys have varying degrees of hyperplasia of the breasts. Approximately 80% of males with Klinefelter syndrome have gynecomastia (see Chapter 19).

SUPERNUMERARY BREASTS AND NIPPLES

An extra breast (**polymastia**) or nipple (**polythelia**), an inheritable condition, occurs in approximately 1% of the female population. **Supernumerary nipples** are also relatively common in males; they are often mistaken for moles. Less commonly, **supernumerary breasts** or nipples appear in the axillary or abdominal regions of females. In these positions, the nipples or breasts arise from extra mammary buds that develop along the mammary crests.

Table 18–1 The Order and Usual Time of Eruption of Teeth and the Time of Shedding of Deciduous Teeth

TOOTH	USUAL ERUPTION TIME	SHEDDING TIME
Deciduous		
Medial incisor	6-8 mo	6-7 yr
Lateral incisor	8-10 mo	7-8 yr
Canine	16-20 mo	10-12 yr
First molar	12-16 mo	9-11 yr
Second molar	20-24 mo	10-12 yr
Permanent		
Medial incisor	7-8 yr	
Lateral incisor	8-9 yr	
Canine	10-12 yr	
First premolar	10-11 yr	
Second premolar	11-12 yr	
First molar	6-7 yr	
Second molar	12 yr	
Third molar	13-25 yr	

Data from Moore KL, Dalley AF, Agur AMR: Clinically Oriented Anatomy, 6th ed. Baltimore, Williams & Wilkins, 2010.

(Fig. 18-5D and E). Canalization of these buds is induced by maternal sex hormones entering the fetal circulation. This process continues until late gestation and by term, 15 to 20 lactiferous ducts have formed. The fibrous connective tissue and fat of the mammary gland develop from the surrounding mesenchyme.

During the late fetal period, the epidermis at the site of origin of the primordial mammary gland becomes depressed, forming a shallow **mammary pit** (Fig. 18-5E). The nipples are poorly formed and depressed in newborn infants. After birth, the nipples usually rise from the mammary pits. At birth, the main lactiferous ducts are formed (Fig. 18-5F); the mammary glands remain underdeveloped until puberty. The mammary glands develop similarly and are of the same structure in both sexes. In females, the glands enlarge rapidly during puberty, mainly because of fat and other connective tissue development in the breasts. Growth of the duct system also occurs because of the increased levels of circulating estrogens.

DEVELOPMENT OF TEETH

Two sets of teeth normally develop: the primary dentition, or **deciduous teeth**, and the secondary dentition, or **permanent teeth**. Teeth develop from the oral ectoderm, mesenchyme, and neural crest cells. The **enamel** is derived from the ectoderm of the oral cavity; all other tissues differentiate from the surrounding mesenchyme and neural crest cells. *Expression of homeobox MSX and Dlx genes and BMP in the migrating neural crest cells, as well as in the ectoderm and mesenchyme, is essential for the initiation of tooth development. Wnt/β-catenin signaling also regulates many stages of tooth development.*

Odontogenesis (tooth development) is initiated by the inductive influence of the **neural crest mesenchyme** on the overlying ectoderm. The first tooth buds appear in the anterior mandibular region; later tooth development occurs in the anterior maxillary region and progresses posteriorly in both jaws. Tooth development continues for years after birth (Table 18-1). The first indication of tooth development is a thickening of the oral epithelium, a derivative of the surface ectoderm seen during the sixth week. These U-shaped bands—**dental laminae**—follow the curves of the primordial jaws (Figs. 18-6A and 18-7A).

Bud Stage of Tooth Development

Each dental lamina develops 10 centers of proliferation from which **tooth buds** grow into the underlying mesenchyme (Figs. 18-6B and 18-7B). These buds develop into the **deciduous teeth**, which are shed during childhood (Table 18-1). There are 10 tooth buds in each jaw, one for each deciduous tooth. The tooth buds for the **permanent teeth** begin to appear at approximately 10 weeks from deep continuations of the dental laminae (Fig. 18-7D). The permanent molars have no deciduous predecessors; they develop as buds from posterior extensions of the **dental laminae.** The tooth buds for the permanent teeth appear at different times, mostly during the fetal period. The buds for the second and third permanent molars develop after birth.

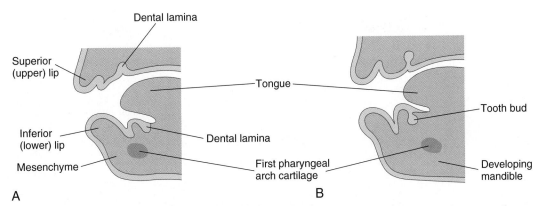

Figure 18–6 Sagittal sections through the developing jaws, showing early development of the teeth. **A,** Early in the sixth week, the dental laminae are evident. **B,** Later in the sixth week, tooth buds arise from the laminae.

Cap Stage of Tooth Development

As each tooth bud is invaginated by the mesenchyme—the **primordium of the dental papilla** and dental follicle—the bud becomes cap-shaped (Fig. 18-7C). The ectodermal part of the developing tooth, the **enamel organ**, eventually produces **enamel**. The internal part of each cap-shaped tooth, the **dental papilla**, is the primordium of the dental pulp. Together, the dental papilla and enamel organ form the **tooth germ** (primordial tooth). The outer cell layer of the enamel organ is the **outer enamel epithelium**, whereas the inner cell layer lining the "cap" is the **inner enamel epithelium** (see Fig. 18-7D).

The central core of loosely arranged cells between the layers of enamel epithelium is the **enamel reticulum or stellate reticulum** (Fig. 18-7E). As the enamel organ and dental papilla of the tooth develop, the mesenchyme surrounding the developing tooth condenses to form the **dental sac**, a vascularized capsular structure (Fig. 18-7E). The dental sac is the primordium of the **cement** and **periodontal ligament**. The cement is the bone-like, rigid connective tissue covering the root of the tooth. The **periodontal ligament** is derived from neural crest cells. It is a specialized vascular connective tissue that surrounds the root of the tooth, separating it from and attaching it to the alveolar bone (Fig. 18-7G).

Bell Stage of Tooth Development

As the enamel organ differentiates, the developing tooth becomes bell-shaped (Figs. 18-7D and 18-8). The mesenchymal cells in the dental papilla adjacent to the inner enamel epithelium differentiate into **odontoblasts**, which produce **predentine** and deposit it adjacent to the epithelium. Later, the predentine calcifies and becomes **dentin**. As the dentin thickens, the odontoblasts regress toward the center of the dental papilla; however, their cytoplasmic processes—**odontoblastic processes**—remain embedded in the dentin (Fig. 18-7F and I). Enamel is the hardest tissue in the body. It overlies the yellowish dentin, the second hardest tissue in the body, and protects it from being fractured.

Cells of the inner enamel epithelium differentiate into **ameloblasts**, which produce enamel in the form of prisms (rods) over the dentin. As the enamel increases, the ameloblasts regress toward the *outer enamel epithelium*. The **root of the tooth** begins to develop after dentin and enamel formation is well advanced. The inner and outer enamel epithelia come together in the neck region of the tooth, where they form a fold, the **epithelial root sheath** (Fig. 18-7F). This sheath grows into the mesenchyme and initiates root formation. The odontoblasts adjacent to the epithelial root sheath form dentin that is continuous with that of the crown. As the dentin increases, it reduces the pulp cavity to a narrow **root canal** through which the vessels and nerves pass. The inner cells of the dental sac differentiate into **cementoblasts**, which produce cement that is restricted to the root. Cement is deposited over the dentin of the root and meets the enamel at the neck of the tooth.

As the teeth develop and the jaws ossify, the outer cells of the dental sac also become active in bone formation. Each tooth soon becomes surrounded by bone, except over its crown. The tooth is held in its **alveolus** (bony socket) by the strong **periodontal ligament**, a derivative of the dental sac (Fig. 18-7G and H). Some fibers of this ligament are embedded in the cement; other fibers are embedded in the bony wall of the alveolus. The periodontal ligament is located between the cement of the root and the bony alveolus.

Tooth Eruption

As the **deciduous teeth** develop, they begin a continuous slow movement toward the oral cavity (Fig. 18-7F and G). The mandibular teeth usually erupt before the maxillary teeth, and girls' teeth usually erupt sooner. A child's dentition contains **20 deciduous teeth**. As the root of the tooth grows, its crown gradually erupts through the oral epithelium. The part of the oral mucosa around the erupted crown becomes the **gingiva** (gum). Usually, eruption of the deciduous teeth occurs between 6 and 24 months after birth (see Table 18-1). The mandibular

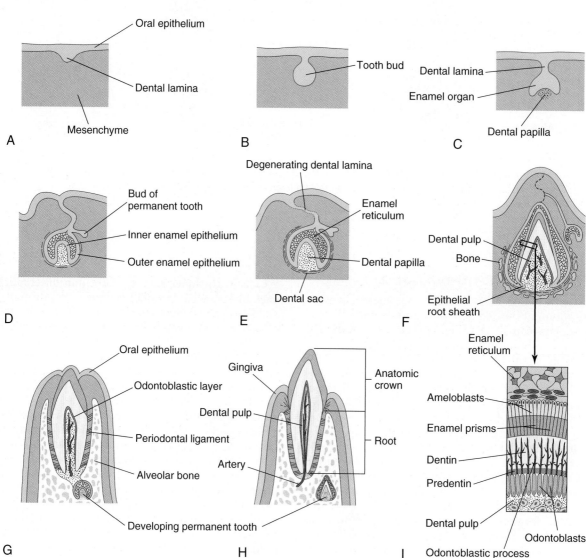

Figure 18–7 Sagittal sections, showing successive stages in the development and eruption of an incisor tooth. **A,** At 6 weeks, showing the dental lamina. **B,** At 7 weeks, showing the tooth bud developing from the dental lamina. **C,** At 8 weeks, showing the cap stage of tooth development. **D,** At 10 weeks, showing the early bell stage of a deciduous tooth and the bud stage of a permanent tooth. **E,** At 14 weeks, showing the advanced bell stage of tooth development. Note that the connection (dental lamina) of the tooth to the oral epithelium is degenerating. **F,** At 28 weeks, showing the enamel and dentin layers. **G,** At 6 months postnatally, showing early tooth eruption. **H,** At 18 months postnatally, showing a fully erupted deciduous incisor tooth. The permanent incisor tooth now has a well-developed crown. **I,** Section through a developing tooth, showing ameloblasts (enamel producers) and odontoblasts (dentin producers).

medial incisors—or **central incisors**—usually erupt 6 to 8 months after birth, but this process may not begin until 12 or 13 months in some children. Despite this, all 20 deciduous teeth are usually present by the end of the second year in healthy children

The **permanent teeth** develop in a manner similar to that described for deciduous teeth. As a permanent tooth grows, the root of the corresponding deciduous tooth is gradually resorbed by **osteoclasts**. Consequently, when the deciduous tooth is shed, it consists only of the crown and the cervical, or uppermost, part of the root. The permanent teeth usually begin to erupt during the sixth year and continue to appear until early adulthood (Fig. 18-9; see also Table 18-1).

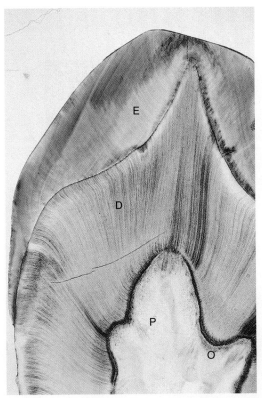

Figure 18–8 Photomicrograph (×17) of a section of the crown and neck of a tooth. Observe the enamel *(E)*, dentin *(D)*, dental pulp *(P)*, and odontoblasts *(O)*. *(From Gartner LP, Hiatt JL: Color Textbook of Histology, 2nd ed. Philadelphia, WB Saunders, 2001.)*

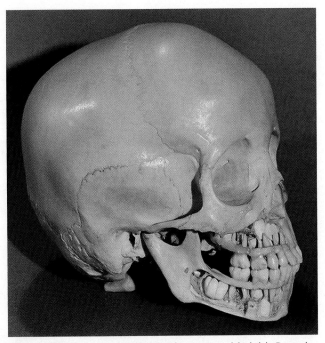

Figure 18–9 Cranium (skull) of a 4-year-old child. Bone has been removed from the jaws to show the relation of the developing permanent teeth to the erupted deciduous teeth.

ENAMEL HYPOPLASIA

Defective enamel formation causes pits, fissures, or both in the enamel. These defects result from temporary disturbances of enamel formation. Various factors may injure ameloblasts (source of enamel), such as nutritional deficiency, tetracycline therapy, and infectious diseases. **Rickets** arising during the critical period of permanent tooth development (6-12 weeks) is the most common known cause of enamel hypoplasia. Rickets is a disease affecting children who are deficient in vitamin D.

NUMERIC ABNORMALITIES OF TEETH

One or more **supernumerary teeth** may develop, or the normal number of teeth may not form (Fig. 18-10*D*). Supernumerary teeth usually develop in the area of the maxillary incisors and may disrupt the position and eruption of normal teeth. The extra teeth commonly erupt posterior to the normal teeth. In **partial anodontia**, one or more teeth are absent. Congenital absence of one or more teeth is often a familial trait. In **total anodontia**, no teeth develop; this very rare condition is usually associated with congenital ectodermal dysplasia (disorders involving tissues that are ectodermal in origin).

VARIATIONS OF TOOTH SHAPE

Abnormally shaped teeth are relatively common. Occasionally there are spherical masses of enamel—**enamel pearls**—attached to the tooth (Fig. 18-10*E*). They are formed by **aberrant groups of ameloblasts.** In other cases, the maxillary lateral incisor teeth may have a slender, tapered shape (pegshaped incisors). **Congenital syphilis** affects the differentiation of the permanent teeth, resulting in incisors with central notches.

MACRODONTIA

Macrodontia (a single large tooth) is a condition caused by the union of two adjacent tooth germs. The crowns of the two teeth can be partially or completely fused. The same applies to roots. Occasionally, a tooth bud divides or two buds partially fuse to form fused teeth. This condition is commonly observed in the mandibular incisors of the primary dentition, but can also occur in the permanent dentition.

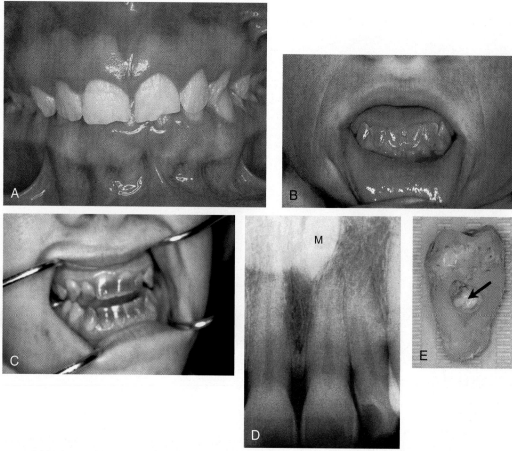

Figure 18–10   Common tooth anomalies. **A,** Amelogenesis imperfecta. **B,** Dentinogenesis imperfecta. **C,** Tetracycline-stained teeth. **D,** Midline supernumerary tooth (*M, mesiodens*), located near the root apex of the central incisor. **E,** Molar tooth with an enamel pearl (*arrow*). (**A,** *Courtesy of Dr. Blaine Cleghorn, Faculty of Dentistry, Dalhousie University, Halifax, Nova Scotia, Canada;* **B** to **D,** *Courtesy of Dr. Steve Ahing, Faculty of Dentistry, University of Manitoba, Winnipeg, Manitoba, Canada.*)

AMELOGENESIS IMPERFECTA

In amelogenesis imperfecta, the tooth enamel is soft and friable because of hypocalcification, and the teeth are yellow to brown color (Fig. 18-10*A*). The teeth are covered with only a thin layer of abnormally formed enamel through which the color of the underlying dentin is visible, giving the teeth a darkened appearance. This autosomal dominant condition affects approximately 1 in 7000 newborn infants.

DENTINOGENESIS IMPERFECTA

Dentinogenesis imperfecta is relatively common in white children (Fig. 18-10*B*). In affected children, the teeth are brown to gray-blue, with an opalescent sheen. This is caused by failure of the odontoblasts to differentiate normally, producing poorly calcified dentin. Both deciduous and permanent teeth are usually involved. The enamel tends to wear down rapidly, exposing the dentin. This anomaly is inherited as an autosomal dominant trait.

DISCOLORED TEETH

Foreign substances incorporated into the developing enamel and dentin discolor the teeth. The hemolysis (liberation of hemoglobin) associated with hemolytic disease of the newborn (Chapter 8) may produce blue to black discoloration of the teeth. *All tetracyclines are extensively incorporated into the teeth.* The critical period of risk is from approximately 14 weeks of fetal life to the 10th postnatal month for deciduous teeth, and from approximately 14 weeks of fetal life to the 16th postnatal year for permanent teeth. Tetracyclines produce brownish-yellow discoloration (mottling) and enamel hypoplasia because they interfere with the metabolic processes of the ameloblasts (Fig. 18–10*C*). The enamel is completely formed on all but the third molars by approximately 8 years of age. For this reason, *tetracyclines should not be administered to pregnant women or to children younger than 8 years.*

CLINICALLY ORIENTED QUESTIONS

1. An infant was reportedly born without skin. Is this possible? If so, could such an infant survive?

2. A dark-skinned person presented with patches of white skin on the face, chest, and limbs. He even had a white forelock. What is this condition called, and what is its developmental basis? Is there any treatment for these skin defects?

3. Some boys have enlarged breasts at birth. Is this an indication of abnormal sex development? Some boys develop breasts during puberty. Why might this occur?

4. A girl developed a breast in the axilla during puberty. She also had extra nipples on her chest. What is the embryologic basis for these anomalies?

5. An infant was born with two teeth. Would these be normal teeth? Is this a common occurrence? Are they usually extracted?

The answers to these questions are at the back of the book.

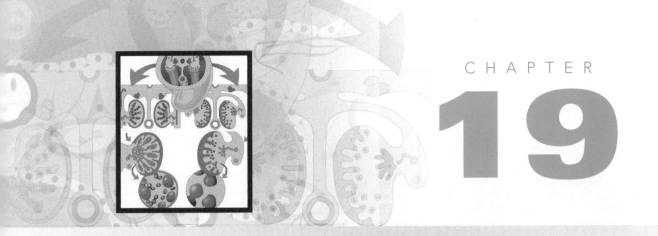

Human Birth Defects

C *ongenital birth defects*, *developmental anomalies*, and *malformations* are terms currently used to describe disorders that were established during intrauterine life. **Birth defects** are the leading cause of infant mortality and may be structural, functional, metabolic, behavioral, or hereditary. A **birth defect** is a structural abnormality of any type; however, *not all variations are anomalies*. There are four clinically significant types of birth defects: malformation, disruption, deformation, and dysplasia.

TERATOLOGY: STUDY OF ABNORMAL DEVELOPMENT

Teratology is the branch of science that studies the causes, mechanisms, and patterns of abnormal development. A fundamental concept in teratology is that certain stages of embryonic development are more vulnerable to disruption than others (see Fig. 19-11).

More than 20% of infant deaths in North America are attributable to birth defects. Major structural anomalies are observed in approximately 3% of newborn infants. Additional defects may only be detected after birth; thus, the incidence of birth defects approaches 6% in 2-year-old infants and 8% in 5-year-old children.

Birth defects may be caused by *genetic factors*, such as chromosomal abnormalities, as well as *environmental factors*, such as drugs. However, many common defects are the result of **multifactorial inheritance**; that is, they are caused by genetic and environmental factors acting together. For 50% to 60% of defects, the causes are unknown (Fig. 19-1). Birth defects may be single or multiple and of major or minor clinical significance.

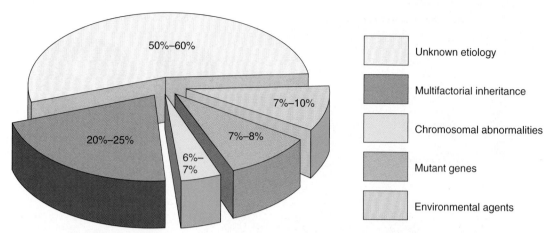

Figure 19–1 Causes of birth defects. Note that the causes of most defects are of unknown etiology and that 20% to 25% of them are caused by a combination of genetic and environmental factors (multifactorial inheritance).

Minor defects are present in approximately 14% of neonates. Anomalies of the external ear, for example, are of no serious medical significance, but they indicate the possible presence of associated major anomalies. **Major defects** are much more common in early embryos (10%-15%), but most of them abort spontaneously during the first 6 weeks. Chromosomal abnormalities are present in more than 50% to 60% of spontaneously aborted embryos.

BIRTH DEFECTS CAUSED BY GENETIC FACTORS*

In terms of the sheer number of cases, genetic factors are the most important cause of birth defects. It has been estimated that they cause approximately one third of all defects (see Fig. 19-1). Any mechanism as complex as mitosis or meiosis may occasionally malfunction; thus, *chromosomal aberrations are common and are present in 6% to 7% of zygotes.* Many of these early embryos never undergo normal cleavage to become blastocysts. The changes may affect the sex chromosomes, the autosomes, or both. Persons with chromosomal abnormalities usually have characteristic phenotypes, such as the physical characteristics of infants with Down syndrome.

Numerical Chromosomal Abnormalities

Numerical aberrations of chromosomes usually result from **nondisjunction**, an error in cell division in which a chromosome pair or two chromatids of a chromosome do not disjoin during mitosis or meiosis. As a result, the chromosome pair or chromatids pass to one daughter cell, while the other cell receives neither (Fig. 19-2).

*The authors are grateful to Dr. A.E. Chudley, MD, FRCPC, FCCMG, Professor of Pediatrics and Child Health, and Head, Section of Genetics and Metabolism, Children's Hospital, Health Sciences Centre, University of Manitoba, Winnipeg, Manitoba, Canada, for his assistance with the preparation of this section on genetic disorders.

INACTIVATION OF GENES

During embryogenesis, one of the two X chromosomes in female somatic cells is randomly inactivated and appears as a mass of **sex chromatin**. Inactivation of the genes on one X chromosome in the somatic cells of female embryos occurs during implantation.

X-inactivation is important clinically because it means that each cell from a carrier of an X-linked disease has the mutant gene causing the disease, either on the active X chromosome or on the inactivated X chromosome that is represented by sex chromatin. Uneven X-inactivation in monozygotic twins is one reason given for discordance in a variety of birth defects. The genetic basis for discordance is that one twin preferentially expresses the paternal X and the other, the maternal X.

Nondisjunction may occur during maternal or paternal gametogenesis (see Chapter 2). The chromosomes in somatic (body) cells are normally paired; the *homologous chromosomes* making up a pair are homologs. Normal human females have 22 pairs of autosomes plus two X chromosomes, whereas normal males have 22 pairs of autosomes plus one X and one Y chromosome.

Turner Syndrome

Approximately 1% of female embryos with monosomy X survive (chromosome count 45 and only one X chromosome). The incidence of 45, X—or Turner syndrome—in newborn females is approximately 1 in 8000 live births. Half of the affected individuals have 45, X; the other half have a variety of abnormalities affecting a sex chromosome. *The phenotype of Turner syndrome is female* (Figure 19-3). **Phenotype** refers to the morphologic characteristics of an individual, as determined by the genotype and environment in which it is expressed.

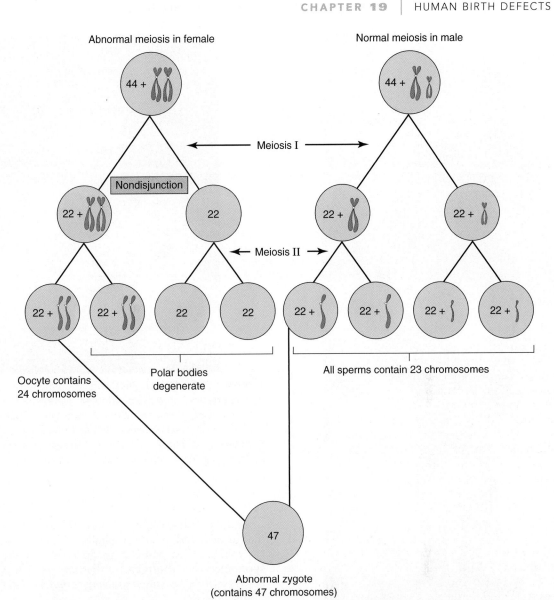

Figure 19–2 Nondisjunction of chromosomes during the first meiotic division of a primary oocyte, resulting in an abnormal oocyte with 24 chromosomes. Subsequent fertilization by a normal sperm produces a zygote with 47 chromosomes—**aneuploidy**—a deviation from the human diploid number of 46.

ANEUPLOIDY AND POLYPLOIDY

Changes in chromosome number result in either aneuploidy or polyploidy. **Aneuploidy** is any deviation from the human diploid number of 46 chromosomes. An *aneuploid* is an individual or a cell that has a chromosome number that is not an exact multiple of the haploid number of 23 (e.g., 45 or 47). The principal cause of aneuploidy is nondisjunction during cell division (Fig. 19-2), resulting in an unequal distribution of one pair of homologous chromosomes to the daughter cells.

One cell has two chromosomes, and the other has neither chromosome of the pair. As a result, the embryo's cells may be *hypodiploid* (45, X, or *Turner syndrome*) (Fig. 19-3) or *hyperdiploid* (usually 47, as in trisomy 21 or *Down syndrome*) (Fig. 19-4). Embryos with **monosomy**—missing a chromosome—usually die. Monosomy of an autosome is extremely uncommon, and approximately 99% of embryos lacking a sex chromosome (45, X) abort spontaneously.

Secondary sexual characteristics do not develop in 90% of girls with Turner syndrome, necessitating hormone replacement therapy.

The monosomy X chromosomal abnormality is the most common cytogenetic abnormality observed in live-born infants and fetuses that abort spontaneously; it accounts for approximately 18% of all spontaneous abortions caused by chromosomal abnormalities. In approximately 75% of cases it is the paternal X chromosome that is usually missing.

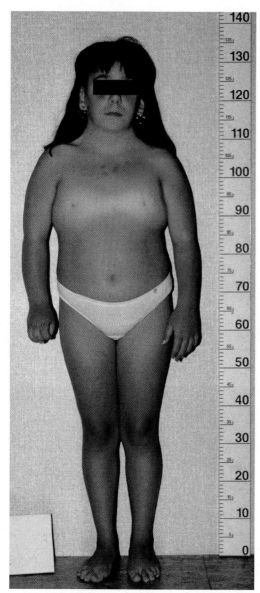

Figure 19–3 Turner syndrome in a 14-year-old girl. Note the classic features of the syndrome: short stature; webbed neck; absence of sexual maturation; broad shield-like chest with widely spaced nipples; and lymphedema of the hands and feet. *(Courtesy of Dr. F. Antoniazzi and Dr. V. Fanos, Department of Pediatrics, University of Verona, Verona, Italy.)*

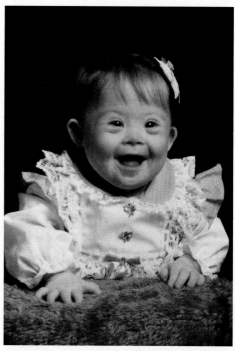

Figure 19–4 A child with Down syndrome (trisomy 21). Note the round face, up-slanted palpebral fissures, and short digits with in-curving of the fifth digit (clinodactyly). *(Courtesy of A.E. Chudley, M.D., Section of Genetics and Metabolism, Department of Pediatrics and Child Health, Children's Hospital and University of Manitoba, Winnipeg, Manitoba, Canada.)*

Infants with trisomy 13 and trisomy 18 are severely malformed and mentally challenged. They usually die early in infancy. More than 50% of trisomic embryos spontaneously abort early. *Trisomy of the autosomes occurs with increasing frequency as maternal age increases* (Table 19-2).

Mosaicism—two or more cell types containing different numbers of chromosomes (normal and abnormal)—leads to a less severe phenotype and the affected child may have a nearly normal IQ.

MOSAICISM

A person who has at least two cell lines with *two or more different genotypes* (genetic constitutions) is known as a **mosaic**. Either the autosomes or sex chromosomes may be involved. Usually, the birth defects are less serious than in persons with monosomy or trisomy (e.g., the features of the Turner syndrome are not as evident in 45 X/46, XX mosaic females as in the usual 45, X females). Mosaicism usually results from nondisjunction during early cleavage of the zygote (see Chapter 3). Mosaicism resulting from loss of a chromosome by *anaphase lagging* also occurs; the chromosomes separate normally, but one of them is delayed in its migration and is eventually lost.

Trisomy

If three chromosomes of one type are present instead of the usual pair, the abnormality is known as *trisomy*. Trisomies are the most common abnormalities of chromosome number. The usual cause of this numeric error is **meiotic nondisjunction of chromosomes** (Fig. 19-2), resulting in a gamete with 24 instead of 23 chromosomes and, subsequently, a zygote with 47 chromosomes.

Trisomy of the autosomes is associated mainly with three syndromes (Table 19-1):

● Trisomy 21, or Down syndrome (Fig. 19-4)
● Trisomy 18, or Edwards syndrome (Fig. 19-5)
● Trisomy 13, or Patau syndrome (Fig. 19-6)

Table 19–1 Trisomy of Autosomes

CHROMOSOMAL ABERRATION/SYNDROME	INCIDENCE	USUAL MORPHOLOGIC CHARACTERISTICS	FIGURE
Trisomy 21, or Down syndrome*	1:800	Mental deficiency; brachycephaly; flat nasal bridge; upward slant to palpebral fissures; protruding tongue; simian crease; clinodactyly of fifth digit; congenital heart defects	19-4
Trisomy 18 syndrome†	1:8000	Mental deficiency; growth retardation; prominent occiput; short sternum; ventricular septal defect; micrognathia; low-set, malformed ears; flexed digits; hypoplastic nails; rocker-bottom feet	19-5
Trisomy 13 syndrome†	1:25,000	Mental deficiency; severe central nervous system malformations; sloping forehead; malformed ears; scalp defects; microphthalmia; bilateral cleft lip or palate; polydactyly; posterior prominence of heels	19-6

*The importance of this disorder in the overall problem of mental deficiency (retardation) is indicated by the fact that persons with Down syndrome represent 10% to 15% of institutionalized, mentally defective individuals. The incidence of trisomy 21 at fertilization is greater than that at birth; however, 75% of affected embryos are spontaneously aborted and at least 20% are stillborn.
†Infants with this syndrome rarely survive beyond 6 months of age.

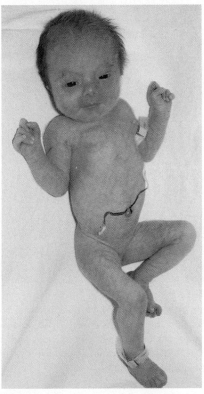

Figure 19–5 Female neonate with trisomy 18. Note the growth retardation, clenched fists with characteristic positioning of the fingers (second and fifth digits overlapping the third and fourth), short sternum, and narrow pelvis. *(Courtesy of A.E. Chudley, M.D., Section of Genetics and Metabolism, Department of Pediatrics and Child Health, Children's Hospital and University of Manitoba, Winnipeg, Manitoba, Canada.)*

Table 19–2 Incidence of Down Syndrome in Newborn Infants

MATERNAL AGE (YEARS)	INCIDENCE
20-24	1:1400
25-29	1:1100
30-34	1:700
35	1:350
37	1:225
39	1:140
41	1:85
43	1:50
45+	1:25

TRIPLOIDY

The most common type of polyploidy is **triploidy** (69 chromosomes). **Triploid fetuses** have severe **intrauterine growth restriction** (IUGR), with a disproportionately small trunk as well as other anomalies. Triploidy can result if the second polar body does not separate from the oocyte during the second meiotic division (see Chapter 2); more likely however, triploidy results when an oocyte is fertilized by two sperms (dispermy) almost simultaneously. Triploidy occurs in approximately 2% of embryos but most of them abort spontaneously. Triploid fetuses account for approximately 20% of chromosomally abnormal miscarriages.

TETRAPLOIDY

Doubling the diploid chromosome number to 92 (tetraploidy) probably occurs during the first cleavage division. Division of this abnormal zygote would subsequently result in an embryo with cells containing 92 chromosomes. **Tetraploid embryos** abort very early; often, all that is recovered is an empty chorionic sac.

Trisomy of the sex chromosomes is a common condition (Table 19-3); however, because no characteristic physical findings are seen in infants or children, this defect is not usually detected before puberty (Fig. 19-7). The diagnosis is best established by chromosomal and molecular analysis.

Table 19–3 Trisomy of Sex Chromosomes

CHROMOSOME COMPLEMENT*	SEX	INCIDENCE†	USUAL CHARACTERISTICS
47, XXX	Female	1:1,000	Normal appearance; usually fertile; 15% to 25% have mild mental deficiency
47, XXY	Male	1:1000	Klinefelter syndrome; small testes; hyalinization of seminiferous tubules; aspermatogenesis; often tall, with disproportionately long lower limbs; intelligence is less than in normal siblings; gynecomastia in approximately 40%
47, XYY	Male	1:1,000	Normal appearance; usually tall

*The numbers designate the total number of chromosomes, including the sex chromosomes (shown after the comma).
†Data from Nussbaum RL, McInnes RR, Willard HF: Thompson & Thompson Genetics in Medicine, 7th ed. Philadelphia, WB Saunders, 2007.

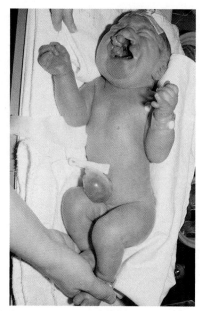

Figure 19–6   Female neonate with trisomy 13. Note the bilateral cleft lip, low-set, malformed ears, and polydactyly (extra digits). A small omphalocele (herniation of viscera into the umbilical cord) is also present. *(Courtesy of A.E. Chudley, M.D., Section of Genetics and Metabolism, Department of Pediatrics and Child Health, Children's Hospital and University of Manitoba, Winnipeg, Manitoba, Canada.)*

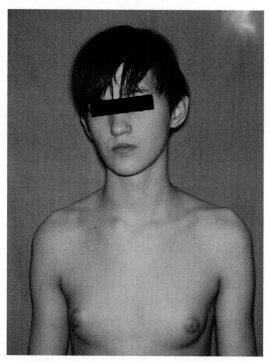

Figure 19–7   A teenage boy with Klinefelter syndrome (XXY trisomy). Note the presence of developed breasts; approximately 40% of males with this syndrome have gynecomastia (excessive development of the male mammary glands) and small testes. *(Courtesy of Children's Hospital and University of Manitoba, Winnipeg, Manitoba, Canada.)*

Structural Chromosomal Abnormalities

Most abnormalities of chromosome structure result from **chromosome breakage** followed by reconstitution in an abnormal combination (Fig. 19-8). **Chromosome breaks** may be induced by various environmental factors, such as irradiation, drugs, chemicals, and viruses. The resulting abnormality in chromosome structure depends on what happens to the broken pieces. The only two aberrations of chromosome structure that are likely to be transmitted from parent to child are structural rearrangements, such as inversion and translocation.

Translocation

Translocation is the transfer of a piece of one chromosome to a nonhomologous chromosome. If two nonhomologous chromosomes exchange pieces, it is called a

reciprocal translocation (Fig. 19-8A and G). Translocation does not necessarily cause abnormal development. Persons with a translocation between chromosome 21 and chromosome 14, for example (Fig. 19-8G), are phenotypically normal. Such persons are called *balanced translocation carriers*. They have a tendency, independent of age, to produce germ cells with an abnormal translocation chromosome. Between 3% and 4% of persons with Down syndrome have translocation trisomies; that is, the extra chromosome 21 is attached to another chromosome.

Deletion

When a chromosome breaks, a portion of it may be lost (Fig. 19-8B). A partial terminal deletion from the short arm of chromosome 5 causes **cri du chat syndrome**.

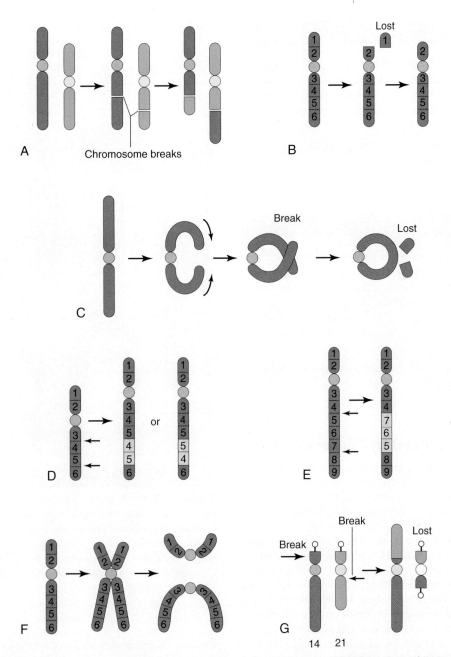

Figure 19–8 Various structural abnormalities of chromosomes. **A,** Reciprocal translocation. **B,** Terminal deletion. **C,** Ring chromosome. **D,** Duplication. **E,** Paracentric inversion. **F,** Isochromosome. **G,** Robertsonian translocation. *Arrows* indicate how the structural abnormalities are produced.

Affected infants have a weak, catlike cry at birth; growth delay with microcephaly (abnormally small head); hypertelorism (wide-set eyes); low-set ears; micrognathia (a small jaw); are severely mentally challenged (retardation); and have congenital heart disease.

A **ring chromosome** is a type of deletion chromosome from which both ends have been lost and the broken ends have rejoined to form a ring-shaped chromosome (Fig. 19-8C). Ring chromosomes are very rare, but they have been found for all chromosomes. These abnormal chromosomes have been described in persons with Turner syndrome, trisomy 18, and other abnormalities.

DUPLICATIONS

Duplications may be manifested as a duplicated part of a chromosome located within a chromosome (Fig. 19-8D), attached to a chromosome, or as a separate fragment. *Duplications are more common than deletion, and they are less harmful because no loss of genetic material occurs.* Duplication may involve part of a gene, a whole gene, or a series of genes.

INVERSION

Inversion is a chromosomal aberration in which a segment of a chromosome is reversed. *Paracentric inversion* is confined to a single arm of the chromosome (Fig. 19-8*E*), whereas pericentric inversion involves both arms and includes the centromere. Carriers of *pericentric inversions* are at risk for having offspring with birth defects because of unequal crossing over and malsegregation at meiosis.

ISOCHROMOSOMES

The abnormality resulting in isochromosomes occurs when the centromere divides transversely instead of longitudinally (Fig. 19-8*F*). An *isochromosome* is a chromosome in which one arm is missing and the other is duplicated. It appears to be the *most common structural abnormality of the X chromosome*. Persons with this chromosomal abnormality are often short in stature and have other stigmata of the Turner syndrome. These characteristics are related to the loss of an arm of an X chromosome.

Birth Defects Caused by Mutant Genes

Between 7% and 8% of birth defects are caused by gene defects (Fig. 19-1). A mutation usually involves a loss or a change in the function of a gene, and is any permanent, heritable change in the sequence of genomic DNA. Because a random change is unlikely to lead to an improvement in development, *most mutations are deleterious and some are lethal*. The mutation rate can be increased by a number of environmental agents, such as large doses of radiation. Birth defects resulting from gene mutations are inherited according to Mendelian laws; consequently, predictions can be made about the probability of their occurrence in the affected person's children and other relatives. An example of a *dominantly inherited birth defect* is **achondroplasia**—abnormality in conversion of cartilage to bone—(Fig. 19-9), which results from a *mutation of the complementary DNA in the fibroblast growth factor receptor 3 (FGFR-3) gene on chromosome 4p*. Other birth defects are attributable to *autosomal recessive inheritance*. Autosomal recessive genes manifest themselves only when homozygous; as a consequence, many carriers of these genes (heterozygous persons) are not identified.

Fragile X syndrome is the most common inherited cause of moderate mental disorders (Fig. 19-10). Fragile X syndrome has a frequency of 1 in 1500 male births and may account for much of the predominance of males in the mentally challenged population.

Several genetic disorders have been linked to the expansion of trinucleotides in specific genes. Examples include myotonic dystrophy, Huntington chorea, spino-bulbar atrophy (Kennedy disease), and Friedreich ataxia. X-linked recessive genes are usually manifested in affected

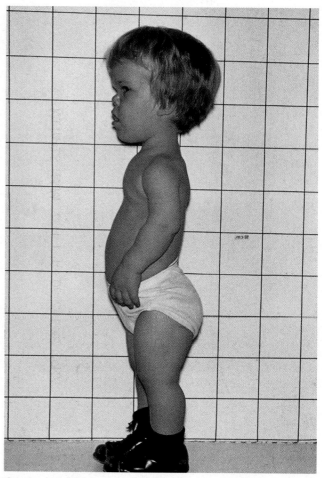

Figure 19–9 A young boy with achondroplasia. Note the short stature, short limbs and fingers, normal length of the trunk, relatively large head, prominent forehead, and depressed nasal bridge. (*Courtesy of A.E. Chudley, M.D., Section of Genetics and Metabolism, Department of Pediatrics and Child Health, Children's Hospital and University of Manitoba, Winnipeg, Manitoba, Canada.*)

(homozygous) males and occasionally in carrier (heterozygous) females (e.g., fragile X syndrome).

The **human genome** comprises an estimated 20,000 to 25,000 genes per haploid set, or 3 billion base pairs. Because of the *Human Genome Project* and international research collaboration, many disease- and birth defect–causing mutations in genes have been and will continue to be identified. Most genes will be sequenced and their specific function determined. Understanding the cause of birth defects will require an improvement in our understanding of gene expression during early development.

Most genes that are expressed in a cell are expressed in a wide variety of cells. These *housekeeping genes* are involved in basic cellular metabolic functions, such as nucleic acid and protein synthesis, cytoskeleton and organelle biogenesis, and nutrient transport and mechanisms. The *specialty genes* are expressed at specific times in specific cells and define the hundreds of different cell types that make up the human organism. An essential aspect of developmental biology is the regulation of gene

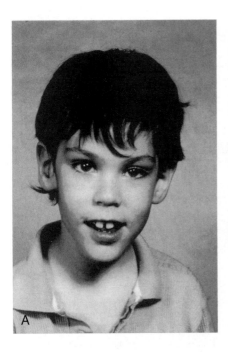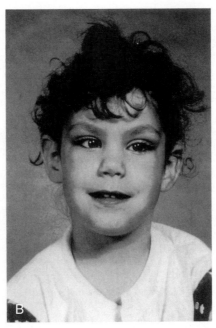

Figure 19–10 Fragile X syndrome. **A,** An 8-year-old, mentally deficient boy with this syndrome exhibiting a relatively normal appearance, with a long face and prominent ears. **B,** His 6-year-old sister also has this syndrome. She has a mild learning disability and similar features of long face and prominent ears. Note the strabismus (crossed right eye). *(Courtesy of A.E. Chudley, M.D., Section of Genetics and Metabolism, Department of Pediatrics and Child Health, Children's Hospital and University of Manitoba, Winnipeg, Manitoba, Canada.)*

expression. Regulation is often achieved by transcription factors, which bind to regulatory or promoter elements of specific genes.

Genomic imprinting is an epigenetic process whereby the female and male germ lines confer a sex-specific mark on a chromosome subregion, so that only the paternal or the maternal allele of a gene is active in the offspring. In other words, the sex of the transmitting parent influences the expression or nonexpression of certain genes in the offspring.

BIRTH DEFECTS CAUSED BY ENVIRONMENTAL FACTORS

Although the embryo is well protected in the uterus, certain environmental agents—**teratogens**—may cause developmental disruptions after maternal exposure to them (Table 19-4). *A teratogen is any agent that can produce a birth defect or increase the incidence of a defect in a population.* Environmental factors, such as infections and drugs, may simulate genetic conditions, such as when two or more children of normal parents are affected. *The important principle to remember is that not everything that is familial is genetic.*

The organs and parts of an embryo are most sensitive to teratogenic agents during periods of rapid differentiation (Fig. 19-11). Because molecular signaling and embryonic induction precede morphologic differentiation, the period during which structures are sensitive to interference by teratogens often precedes the stage of their visible development. Teratogens do not appear to be effective in causing birth defects until cellular differentiation has begun; however, their earlier actions may cause the death of an embryo. The exact mechanisms by which many drugs, chemicals and other environmental factors disrupt embryonic development and induce abnormalities are unclear.

Rapid progress in molecular biology is providing additional information on the genetic control of differentiation, as well as the cascade of molecular signals and factors controlling gene expression and pattern formation. Researchers are now directing increasing attention to the molecular mechanisms of abnormal development in an attempt to understand better the pathogenesis of birth defects.

Principles of Teratogenesis

When considering the possible teratogenicity of an agent, such as a drug or a chemical, three factors are important to consider:

- Critical periods of development
- Dose of the drug or chemical
- Genotype (genetic constitution) of the embryo

Critical Periods of Human Development

An embryo's susceptibility to a teratogen depends on its stage of development when an agent, such as a drug, is present (Fig. 19-11). The most critical period in development is when cell differentiation and morphogenesis are at their peak. *The most critical period for brain development is from 3 to 16 weeks,* but its development may be disrupted after this time because the brain is differentiating and growing rapidly at birth.

Teratogens (e.g., drugs) may cause limitation of mental development during the embryonic and fetal periods. *Tooth development continues long after birth* hence, the development of the permanent teeth may be disrupted by *tetracyclines* from 18 weeks (prenatal) to 16 years.

The skeletal system has a prolonged critical period of development, extending into childhood; hence, the growth of skeletal tissues provides a good gauge of general growth. Environmental disturbances during the first 2

Table 19–4 Some Teratogens Known to Cause Human Birth Defects

AGENTS	MOST COMMON CONGENITAL ANOMALIES
Drugs	
Alcohol	Fetal alcohol syndrome (FAS); intrauterine growth restriction (IUGR); mental deficiency; microcephaly; ocular anomalies; joint abnormalities; short palpebral fissures; fetal alcohol spectrum disorders (FASDs); cognitive and neurobehavioral disturbances
Androgens and high doses of progestogens	Varying degree of masculinization of female fetuses; ambiguous external genitalia (labial fusion and clitoral hypertrophy)
Methotrexate	IUGR; skeletal and renal defects
Cocaine	IUGR; prematurity; microcephaly; cerebral infarction; urogenital anomalies; neurobehavioral disturbances
Diethylstilbestrol	Abnormalities of uterus and vagina; cervical erosion and ridges
Isotretinoin (13-cis-retinoic acid)	Craniofacial abnormalities; neural tube defects such as spina bifida cystica; cardiovascular defects; cleft palate; thymic aplasia
Lithium carbonate	Various anomalies, usually involving the heart and great vessels
Methotrexate	Multiple anomalies, especially skeletal, involving the face, cranium, limbs, and vertebral column
Misoprostol	Abnormal development of the limbs, ocular defects, cranial nerve defects, and autism spectral disorders
Phenytoin (Dilantin)	Fetal hydantoin syndrome; IUGR; microcephaly; mental retardation; ridged metopic suture; inner epicanthal folds; eyelid ptosis; broad, depressed nasal bridge; phalangeal hypoplasia
Tetracycline	Stained teeth; hypoplasia of enamel
Thalidomide	Abnormal development of the limbs; meromelia (partial absence of limb) and amelia (complete absence of limb); facial anomalies; systemic anomalies (e.g., cardiac and kidney defects and ocular anomalies)
Trimethadione	Developmental delay; V-shaped eyebrows; low-set ears; cleft lip and/or palate
Valproic acid	Craniofacial anomalies; neural tube defects; often hydrocephalus; heart and skeletal defects; poor postnatal cognitive development
Warfarin	Nasal hypoplasia; stippled epiphyses; hypoplastic phalanges; eye anomalies; mental deficiency
Chemicals	
Methylmercury	Cerebral atrophy; spasticity; seizures; mental deficiency
Polychlorinated biphenyls	IUGR; skin discoloration
Infections	
Cytomegalovirus	Microcephaly; chorioretinitis; sensorineural loss; delayed psychomotor and mental development; hepatosplenomegaly; hydrocephaly; cerebral palsy; brain (periventricular) calcification
Herpes simplex virus	Skin vesicles and scarring; chorioretinitis; hepatomegaly; thrombocytopenia; petechiae; hemolytic anemia; hydranencephaly
Human parvovirus B19	Fetal anemia; nonimmune hydrops fetalis; fetal death
Rubella virus	IUGR; postnatal growth retardation; cardiac and great vessel abnormalities; microcephaly; sensorineural deafness; cataract; microphthalmos; glaucoma; pigmented retinopathy; mental deficiency; neonatal bleeding; hepatosplenomegaly; osteopathy; tooth defects
Toxoplasma gondii	Microcephaly; mental deficiency; microphthalmia; hydrocephaly; chorioretinitis; cerebral calcifications; hearing loss; neurologic disturbances
Treponema pallidum	Hydrocephalus; congenital deafness; mental deficiency; abnormal teeth and bones
Varicella virus	Cutaneous scars (dermatome distribution); neurologic anomalies (e.g., limb paresis, hydrocephaly, seizures); cataracts; microphthalmia; Horner syndrome; optic atrophy; nystagmus; chorioretinitis; microcephaly; mental deficiency; skeletal anomalies (e.g., hypoplasia of limbs, fingers, and toes); urogenital anomalies
High levels of ionizing radiation	Microcephaly; mental deficiency; skeletal anomalies; growth retardation; cataracts

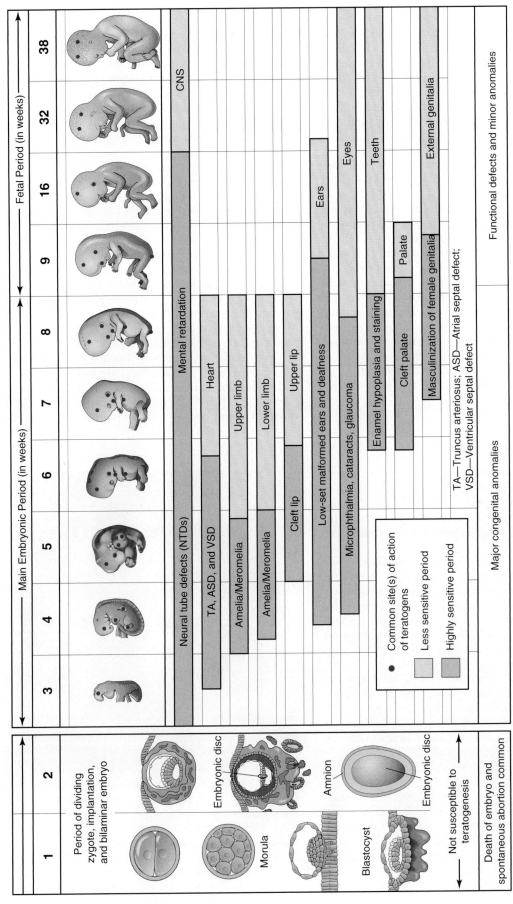

Figure 19-11 Critical periods in human prenatal development. During the first 2 weeks, the embryo is not usually susceptible to teratogens. At this point, a teratogen damages all or most of the cells, resulting in death of the embryo, or damages only a few cells, allowing the conceptus to recover and the embryo to develop without birth defects. The purple areas denote highly sensitive periods, when major defects may be produced (e.g., amelia, absence of limbs). The green sections indicate stages that are less sensitive to teratogens, when minor birth defects may be induced.

weeks after fertilization may interfere with cleavage of the zygote and implantation of the blastocyst, which may cause early death and spontaneous abortion of the embryo (Fig. 19-11).

Development of the embryo is most easily disrupted when the tissues and organs are forming (Fig. 19-11). During this **organogenetic period**, teratogenic agents may induce major birth defects. Physiologic defects—minor morphologic anomalies of the external ear, for example—and functional disturbances, such as limitation of mental development, are likely to result from disruption of development during the fetal period. *Each part, tissue, and organ of an embryo has a critical period during which its development may be disrupted* (Fig. 19-11). The type of birth defect produced depends on which parts, tissues, and organs are most susceptible at the time the teratogen is active.

Embryologic timetables, such as the one in Fig. 19-11, are helpful when considering the cause of birth defects. However, it is incorrect to assume that defects always result from a single event occurring during the critical period of development, or that it is possible to determine from these tables the day on which a defect was produced. What is known is that the teratogen would have to disrupt development of the tissue, part, or organ before the end of the critical period. *The critical period of limb development, for example, is 21 to 36 days after fertilization.*

Human Teratogens

Awareness that certain agents can disrupt prenatal development offers the opportunity to prevent some birth defects. For example, if women are made aware of the harmful effects of drugs, environmental chemicals and viruses, most pregnant women will avoid exposure to these teratogenic agents.

Drugs vary considerably in their teratogenicity. Some teratogens, such as thalidomide, cause severe disruption of development if administered during the organogenetic period of certain parts (e.g., the limbs) of the embryo (see Fig. 19-15). Other teratogens cause mental and growth restriction of embryos (Table 19-4). Drug consumption tends to be higher during the critical periods of development among heavy smokers and drinkers. Despite this, *fewer than 2% of birth defects are caused by drugs and chemicals.* Only a few drugs have been positively implicated as human teratogenic agents but new agents continue to be identified. It is best for women to avoid using all medication during the first trimester unless a strong medical reason exists for its use.

Cigarette Smoking

Maternal smoking during pregnancy is a well-established cause of **intrauterine growth restriction** (IUGR). Despite warnings that cigarette smoking is harmful to the fetus, more than 25% of women continue to smoke during pregnancy. In heavy cigarette smokers (20 per day), premature delivery is twice as frequent as in mothers who do not smoke. In addition, the infants of smokers weigh less than normal.

Nicotine constricts the uterine blood vessels, thereby causing a decrease in uterine blood flow and reducing the supply of oxygen and nutrients available to the embryo or fetus from the maternal blood in the intervillous space of the placenta. High levels of *carboxyhemoglobin*, resulting from cigarette smoking, appear in the maternal and fetal blood, and may alter the capacity of the blood to transport oxygen. As a result, chronic fetal hypoxia (a decrease in the oxygen level to below normal) may occur, affecting fetal growth and development.

Alcohol

Alcoholism is a drug abuse problem that affects 1% to 2% of women of childbearing age. Both moderate and high levels of alcohol intake during early pregnancy may result in alterations in the growth and morphogenesis of the fetus; the greater the intake, the more severe the signs. Infants born to mothers with chronic alcoholism exhibit a specific pattern of defects, including prenatal and postnatal growth and mental deficiency and other anomalies (Fig. 19-12). This pattern of anomalies, **fetal alcohol syndrome**, is detected in 1 to 2 infants per 1000 live births. *Maternal alcohol abuse is now believed to be the most common cause of mental deficiency.*

Even moderate maternal alcohol consumption (e.g., 1-2 oz daily) may produce **fetal alcohol effects**—children with behavioral and learning difficulties, for example—especially if the drinking is associated with malnutrition. **Binge drinking** (heavy consumption of alcohol for 1-3

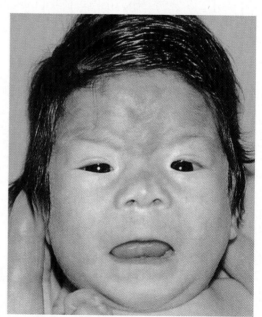

Figure 19–12 Infant with fetal alcohol syndrome. Note the thin upper lip, short palpebral fissures, flat nasal bridge, short nose, and elongated and poorly formed philtrum (vertical groove in the median part of the upper lip). Severe maternal alcohol abuse is believed to be the most common environmental cause of mental deficiency. *(Courtesy of A.E. Chudley, M.D., Section of Genetics and Metabolism, Department of Pediatrics and Child Health, Children's Hospital and University of Manitoba, Winnipeg, Manitoba, Canada.)*

days during pregnancy) is very likely to produce fetal alcohol effects. The susceptible period of brain development spans the major part of gestation; therefore, the safest advice is total abstinence from alcohol during pregnancy.

Androgens and Progestogens

Androgens and progestogens may affect the female fetus, producing masculinization of the external genitalia (Fig. 19-13). The preparations that should be avoided contain *progestins, ethisterone, or norethisterone.* From a practical standpoint, the teratogenic risk of these hormones is low. However, progestin exposure during the critical period of development is also associated with an increased prevalence of *cardiovascular abnormalities,* and exposure of male fetuses during this period may double the incidence of *hypospadias* in the offspring (see Chapter 13).

Oral contraceptive (birth control) *pills* containing progestogens and estrogens, when taken during the early stages of an unrecognized pregnancy, are believed to be teratogenic agents. Many infants of mothers who took *progestogen-estrogen birth control pills* during the critical period of development have been found to exhibit the VACTERL syndrome—Vertebral, Anal, Cardiac, Tracheal, Esophageal, Renal, and Limb anomalies.

Antibiotics

Tetracyclines cross the placental membrane and are deposited in the embryo's bones and teeth at sites of active calcification. As little as 1g daily of **tetracycline** during the third trimester of pregnancy can produce yellow staining of the primary, or deciduous, teeth.

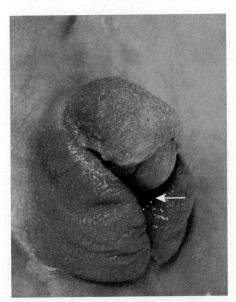

Figure 19–13 Masculinized external genitalia of a female infant with a 46, XX chromosome constitution. Observe the enlarged clitoris and fused labia majora. The *arrow* indicates the single orifice of a urogenital sinus. The virilization (mature masculine characteristics in a female) was caused by excessive androgens produced by the suprarenal glands during the fetal period (congenital adrenal hyperplasia). *(Courtesy of Dr. Heather Dean, Department of Pediatrics and Child Health and University of Manitoba, Winnipeg, Canada.)*

Tetracycline therapy during the fourth to ninth months of pregnancy may also cause tooth defects (e.g., enamel hypoplasia), yellow to brown **discoloration of the teeth,** and diminished growth of the long bones (see Fig. 18-10). Moreover, more than 30 cases of hearing deficit and CN VIII damage have been reported in infants exposed to **streptomycin** derivatives in utero. By contrast, *penicillin* has been used extensively during pregnancy and appears to be harmless to the human embryo and fetus.

Anticoagulants

All anticoagulants except heparin cross the placental membrane and may cause hemorrhage in the embryo or fetus. **Warfarin,** an anticoagulant, is definitely a teratogen. The period of greatest sensitivity is 6 to 12 weeks after fertilization, or 8 to 14 weeks after the last normal menstrual period. Second- and third-trimester exposure may result in mental deficiency, optic atrophy, and microcephaly. Heparin does not cross the placental membrane, and so is the drug of choice for pregnant women requiring anticoagulant therapy.

Anticonvulsants

Epilepsy affects approximately 1 in 200 pregnant women and these women require treatment with an anticonvulsant. Of the anticonvulsant drugs available, phenytoin has been definitively identified as a teratogen. **Fetal hydantoin syndrome** occurs in 5% to 10% of children born to mothers treated with phenytoins or hydantoin anticonvulsants (Fig. 19-14).

Valproic acid has been the drug of choice for the management of different types of epilepsy; however, its use by pregnant women has led to a pattern of anomalies consisting of poorer postnatal cognitive development and craniofacial, heart, and limb defects. There is also an increased risk of **neural tube defects.** Phenobarbital is considered a safe antiepileptic drug for use during pregnancy.

Antineoplastic Agents

Tumor-inhibiting chemicals are highly teratogenic. This is not surprising because these agents inhibit mitosis in rapidly dividing cells. It is recommended that they be avoided, especially during the first trimester of pregnancy. **Methotrexate,** *a folic acid antagonist* and a derivative of *aminopterin,* **is** a known potent teratogen that produces major congenital anomalies.

Angiotensin-Converting Enzyme Inhibitors

Exposure of the fetus to angiotensin-converting enzyme inhibitors, used as antihypertensive agents, causes oligohydramnios, fetal death, long-lasting hypoplasia of the bones of the calvaria, IUGR, and renal dysfunction.

Retinoic Acid (Vitamin A)

Isotretinoin (13-cis-retinoic acid), used for the oral treatment of severe cystic acne, is teratogenic in humans, even at very low doses. The critical period for exposure appears to be from the third week to the fifth week (5-7 weeks after the last normal menstrual period). The risk of spontaneous abortion and birth defects after exposure to **retinoic acid** is high. Postnatal follow-up studies of children

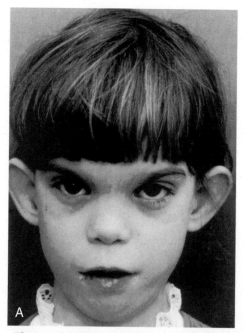
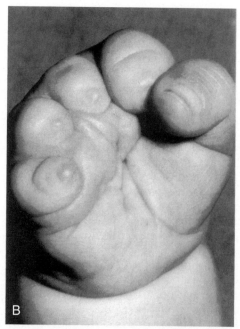

Figure 19–14   Fetal hydantoin syndrome. **A,** This young girl has a learning disability. Note the unusual ears, the wide spacing of the eyes, the epicanthal folds, the short nose, and the long philtrum. Her mother has epilepsy and took Dilantin throughout her pregnancy. **B,** Right hand of an infant with severe digital hypoplasia (short fingers), born to a mother who took Dilantin throughout her pregnancy. (**A,** Courtesy of A.E. Chudley, M.D., Section of Genetics and Metabolism, Department of Pediatrics and Child Health, Children's Hospital and University of Manitoba, Winnipeg, Manitoba, Canada. **B,** From Chodirker BN, Chudley AE, Persaud TVN: Possible prenatal hydantoin effect in child born to a nonepileptic mother. Am J Med Genet 27:373, copyright © 1987. Reprinted by permission of Wiley-Liss, a division of John Wiley and Sons, Inc.)

exposed to isotretinoin in utero showed significant **neuropsychological impairment**. Vitamin A is a valuable and necessary nutrient during pregnancy, but long-term exposure to large doses of vitamin A is unwise because of insufficient evidence to rule out a teratogenic risk.

Salicylates

Acetylsalicylic acid, or **aspirin,** is the most commonly ingested drug during pregnancy. Large doses are potentially harmful to the embryo or fetus. Studies indicate that low doses appear not to be teratogenic.

Thyroid Drugs

Iodides readily cross the placental membrane and interfere with thyroxin production. They may also cause thyroid enlargement and **cretinism** (arrested physical and mental development and dystrophy of bones and soft tissue). Maternal iodine deficiency may cause *congenital cretinism*. The administration of antithyroid drugs for the treatment of maternal thyroid disorders may cause *congenital goiter* if the dose administered exceeds that required to control the disease.

Tranquilizers

Thalidomide is a potent teratogen. Nearly 12,000 infants have been born with defects caused by this drug. The characteristic feature of thalidomide syndrome is

meromelia—*phocomelia,* or "seal limbs" (Fig. 19-15). It has been well established clinically that the period when thalidomide causes congenital anomalies is from 20 to 36 days after fertilization (34-50 days after the last normal menstrual period). *Thalidomide is absolutely contraindicated in women of childbearing age.*

Psychotropic Drugs

Lithium is the drug of choice for long-term maintenance therapy in people with the mental illness known as *bipolar disorder;* however, it has been known to cause birth defects, mainly of the heart and great vessels, in infants born to mothers given the drug early in pregnancy. Although lithium carbonate is a human teratogen, the Food and Drug Administration has stated that the agent may be used during pregnancy if "in the opinion of the physician the potential benefits outweigh the possible hazards." **Benzodiazepine** *derivatives* are psychoactive drugs that are frequently used by pregnant women. These include *diazepam* and *oxazepam*, which readily cross the placental membrane. The use of these drugs during the first trimester of pregnancy is associated with transient withdrawal symptoms and craniofacial anomalies in the neonate. **Selective serotonin reuptake inhibitors (SSRIs)** are used for the treatment of depression. Use of these drugs by the mother may lead to transient

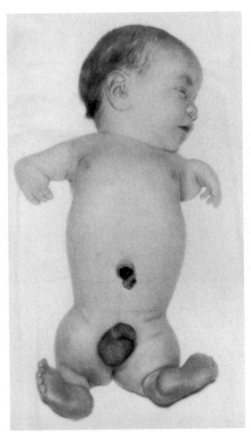

Figure 19–15 Newborn male infant with malformed limbs (meromelia—congenital absence of parts of the limbs) caused by maternal ingestion of thalidomide during the critical period of limb development. *(From Moore KL: The vulnerable embryo: Causes of malformation in man. Manitoba Med Rev 43:306, 1963.)*

neurobehavioral disturbances and persistent pulmonary hypertension in the neonate.

Illicit Drugs

Cocaine is one of the most commonly abused illicit drugs in North America, and its increasing use by women of childbearing age is of major concern. Many reports deal with the prenatal effects of cocaine; these include spontaneous abortion, prematurity, and diverse anomalies in the offspring.

Methadone, used for the treatment of heroin addiction, is considered a "behavioral teratogen," as is heroin. Infants born to narcotic-dependent women, lower birth weights, and receiving maintenance methadone therapy have been found to have *central nervous system dysfunction* and smaller head circumferences than nonexposed infants. There is also concern about the long-term postnatal developmental effects of methadone.

Environmental Chemicals as Teratogens

In recent years, there has been increasing concern about the possible teratogenicity of environmental, industrial, and agricultural chemicals, pollutants, and food additives.

Organic Mercury

Infants of mothers whose main diet during pregnancy consists of fish containing abnormally high levels of organic mercury acquire fetal **Minamata disease** and exhibit neurologic and behavioral disturbances resembling those associated with cerebral palsy. *Methylmercury is a teratogen* that causes cerebral atrophy, spasticity, seizures, and mental retardation.

Lead

Lead crosses the placental membrane and accumulates in fetal tissues. Prenatal exposure to lead is associated with an increased incidence of abortions, fetal anomalies, IUGR, and functional deficits.

Polychlorinated Biphenyls

Polychlorinated biphenyls (PCBs) are teratogenic chemicals that produce IUGR and skin discoloration in infants exposed to these agents in utero. The main dietary source of polychlorinated biphenyls in North America is probably sport fish caught in contaminated waters.

Infectious Agents as Teratogens

Rubella (German or Three-Day Measles)

The **rubella virus** crosses the placental membrane and infects the embryo or fetus. In cases of primary maternal infection during the first trimester of pregnancy, the overall risk of embryonic or fetal infection is approximately 20%. The clinical features of **congenital rubella syndrome** are *cataracts,* congenital glaucoma, *cardiac defects,* and *deafness* (Fig. 19-16). The earlier in pregnancy that maternal rubella infection occurs, the greater the danger that the embryo will be malformed.

Cytomegalovirus

Cytomegalovirus is the most common viral infection of the human fetus. Because the disease seems to be fatal when it affects the embryo, most pregnancies likely end in spontaneous abortion when the infection occurs during the first trimester. Later in pregnancy, *cytomegalovirus infection may result in IUGR and severe fetal anomalies.* Of particular concern are cases of asymptomatic cytomegalovirus infection, which are often associated with audiologic, neurologic, and neurobehavioral disturbances in infancy.

Herpes Simplex Virus

Maternal infection with **herpes simplex virus** in early pregnancy increases the abortion rate threefold, and infection after the 20th week is associated with an increased rate of prematurity as well as birth defects (e.g., microcephaly and mental deficiency). Infection of the fetus with herpes simplex virus usually occurs very late in pregnancy, probably most often during delivery.

Varicella (Chickenpox)

Varicella and herpes zoster (shingles) are caused by the same virus, **varicella-zoster virus.** There is convincing evidence that maternal varicella infection during the first 4 months of pregnancy causes several birth defects (such

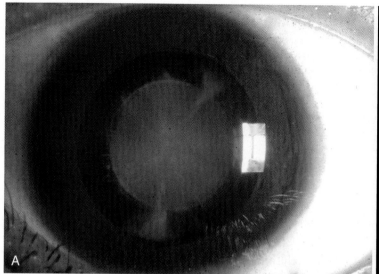
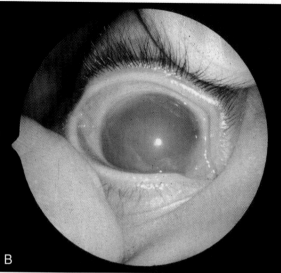

Figure 19–16 **A,** Typical appearance of a congenital cataract that may be caused by the rubella virus. Cardiac defects and deafness are other congenital defects common to this infection. **B,** Clouding of the cornea caused by congenital glaucoma. Corneal clouding may also result from infection, trauma, or metabolic disorders. *(Reprinted from Otolaryngologic Clinics of North America 40(1), Guercio J, Martyn L, Congenital malformations of the eye and orbit, 113–140, Copyright 2007, with permission from Elsevier.)*

as muscle atrophy and mental deficiency). There is a 20% incidence of these or other defects when the infection occurs during the critical period of development (Fig. 19-11).

Human Immunodeficiency Virus

Human immunodeficiency virus (HIV) is the retrovirus that causes *acquired immune deficiency syndrome* (AIDS). Infection of pregnant women with HIV is associated with serious health problems in the fetus. These include infection of the fetus, preterm delivery, low birth weight, IUGR, microcephaly, and craniofacial abnormalities. Transmission of the HIV virus to the fetus can occur during pregnancy, labor, or delivery.

Toxoplasmosis

Maternal infection with the intracellular parasite *Toxoplasma gondii* is usually through one of the following routes:

- Eating raw or poorly cooked meat (usually pork or lamb containing *Toxoplasma* cysts)
- Close contact with infected domestic animals (usually cats) or infected soil

The *T. gondii* organism crosses the placental membrane and infects the fetus, causing destructive changes in the brain that result in *mental deficiency* and other birth defects. Mothers of infants with congenital defects are often unaware of having had **toxoplasmosis.** Because animals (cats, dogs, rabbits, and other domestic and wild animals) may be infected with this parasite, pregnant women should avoid contact with them. In addition, unpasteurized milk should be avoided.

Congenital Syphilis

Syphilis infection affects approximately 3 in 10,000 live-born infants in the United States. *Treponema pallidum*, the small, spiral microorganism that causes syphilis, rapidly crosses the placental membrane as early as 9 to 10 weeks of gestation. The fetus can become infected at any stage of the disease or at any stage of pregnancy. **Primary maternal infections** (acquired during pregnancy and left untreated) nearly always cause serious fetal infection and birth defects. However, adequate treatment of the mother kills the organism. **Secondary maternal infections** (acquired before pregnancy) seldom result in fetal disease and anomalies. If the mother remains untreated, stillbirths occur in approximately 25% of cases.

Radiation as a Teratogen

Exposure to **high levels of ionizing radiation** may injure embryonic cells, resulting in cell death, chromosomal injury, and retardation of mental development and physical growth. The severity of the embryonic damage is related to the absorbed dose, the dose rate, and the stage of embryonic or fetal development when the exposure occurs. Accidental exposure of pregnant women to radiation is a common cause for anxiety.

No conclusive proof exists that human congenital anomalies have been caused by diagnostic levels of radiation. Scattered radiation from a radiographic examination of a part of the body that is not near the uterus (e.g., thorax, sinuses, teeth) produces a dose of only a few millirads, which is not teratogenic to the embryo. The recommended limit of maternal exposure of the whole body to radiation from all sources is 500 mrad (0.005 Gy) for the entire gestational period.

Maternal Factors as Teratogens

Poorly controlled **diabetes mellitus** in the mother with persisting hyperglycemia and ketosis, particularly during embryogenesis, is associated with a two- to three-fold higher incidence of birth defects. The infant of a diabetic mother is usually large (**macrosomia**). The common anomalies include *holoprosencephaly* (failure of the forebrain to divide into hemispheres), *meroencephaly* (partial absence of the brain), sacral agenesis, vertebral anomalies, congenital heart defects, and limb anomalies. If left untreated, women who are homozygous for phenylalanine hydroxylase deficiency—**phenylketonuria**—and those with **hyperphenylalaninemia** are at increased risk for having offspring with microcephaly, cardiac defects, mental retardation, and IUGR. The congenital anomalies can be prevented if the mother with phenylketonuria follows a phenylalanine-restricted diet before and during pregnancy.

Mechanical Factors as Teratogens

Clubfoot and congenital dislocation of the hip may be caused by mechanical forces, particularly in a malformed uterus. Such deformations may be caused by any factor that restricts the mobility of the fetus, thereby causing prolonged compression in an abnormal posture. A significantly reduced quantity of amniotic fluid (*oligohydramnios*) may result in mechanically induced deformation of the limbs such as hyperextension of the knee. Intrauterine amputations or other anomalies caused by local constriction during fetal growth may result from **amniotic bands** (see Fig. 8-14), rings formed as a result of rupture of the amnion during early pregnancy.

BIRTH DEFECTS CAUSED BY MULTIFACTORIAL INHERITANCE

Many common birth defects (e.g., cleft lip, with or without cleft palate) have familial distributions consistent with multifactorial inheritance (Fig. 19-1). Multifactorial inheritance may be represented by a model in which one's "liability" for a disorder is a continuous variable determined by a combination of genetic and environmental factors, with a developmental threshold dividing individuals with the anomaly from those without it. Multifactorial *traits are often single major defects,* such as cleft lip, isolated cleft palate, and neural tube defects. Some of these anomalies may also occur as part of the phenotype in syndromes determined by single-gene inheritance, chromosomal abnormality, or an environmental teratogen. The recurrence risks used for genetic counseling of families having birth defects that have been determined by multifactorial inheritance are *empirical risks* based on the frequency of the anomaly in the general population and in different categories of relatives. In individual families, such estimates may be inaccurate because they are usually averages for the population rather than precise probabilities for the individual family.

CLINICALLY ORIENTED QUESTIONS

1. If a pregnant woman takes aspirin in normal doses, will it cause congenital anomalies?

2. If a woman is a drug addict, will her child show signs of drug addiction?

3. Are all drugs tested for teratogenicity before they are marketed? If the answer is "yes," why are these teratogens still sold?

4. Is cigarette smoking during pregnancy harmful to the embryo or fetus? If the answer is "yes," would refraining from inhaling cigarette smoke be safer?

5. Are any drugs safe to take during pregnancy? If so, what are they?

The answers to these questions are at the back of the book.

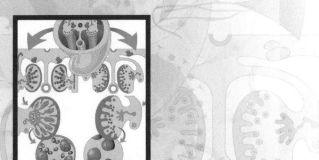

The Cellular and Molecular Basis of Development

Jeffrey T. Wigle and David D. Eisenstat

During embryonic development, undifferentiated precursor cells differentiate and organize into the complex structures found in functional adult tissues. This process requires cells to integrate many different cues, both intrinsic and extrinsic, for development to occur properly. These cues control the proliferation, differentiation, and migration of cells to determine the final size and shape of the developing organs. Disruption of these signaling pathways can result in human developmental disorders and birth defects. Interestingly, these key developmental signaling pathways may be co-opted in the adult by diseases such as cancer.

Although there are diverse changes that occur during embryogenesis, the differentiation of many different cell types is regulated through a relatively restricted set of molecular signaling pathways:

- **Intercellular communication.** Cells communicate with each other in several ways, including through gap junctions, ligand-receptor interactions and specific channels that permit the passage of ions, neurotransmitters, or proteins.

Table 20–1		International Nomenclature Standards for Genes and Proteins	
Gene	Human	Italics, all letters capitalized	*PAX6*
	Mouse	Italics, first letter capitalized	*Pax6*
Protein	Human	Roman, all letters capitalized	PAX6
	Mouse	Roman, all letters capitalized	PAX6

- **Morphogens.** These are diffusible molecules that specify which cell type will be generated at a specific anatomical location. Morphogens also direct the migration of cells and their processes to their final destination. These include retinoic acid, transforming growth factor β (TGF-β)/bone morphogenetic proteins (BMPs), and the hedgehog and Wnt protein families (see Table 20-1 for gene and protein nomenclature).
- **Receptor tyrosine kinases (RTKs).** Many growth factors signal by binding to and activating membrane-bound RTKs. These kinases are essential for the regulation of cellular proliferation, apoptosis, and migration as well, for example, growth of new blood vessels and axonal processes in the nervous system.
- **Notch/Delta.** This pathway often specifies the fate of precursor cells.
- **Transcription factors.** This set of evolutionarily conserved proteins activates or represses downstream genes that are essential for a number of cellular processes. Many transcription factors are members of the homeobox or helix-loop-helix (HLH) families. Their activity can be regulated by all of the other pathways described in this chapter.

Epigenetics relates to the ability of heritable properties of gene function that do not occur as a result of changes to the sequence of the DNA code. This can include variations in DNA packaging and DNA chemical modification.

INTERCELLULAR COMMUNICATION

Cells communicate with each other in several ways. **Gap junctions** are channels that permit ions and small molecules (less than 1 kD) to directly pass from one cell to another, known as gap junctional intercellular communication (GJIC). However, large proteins and nucleic acids do not transfer through gap junctions. Gap junctions are made from hemi-channels present on the surface of each cell known as *connexons*. Each connexon is made up of six *connexin* molecules that form hexamers. In early development, gap junctions are usually open, permitting exchange of small molecules in relatively large regions. However, as development proceeds, GJIC is more restricted, with establishment of boundaries, such as in the rhombomeres of the developing hindbrain. Gap junctions are particularly important for electrical coupling in the heart and brain. Mutations of specific connexin molecules, for example Cx43, are associated with human diseases, such as atherosclerosis.

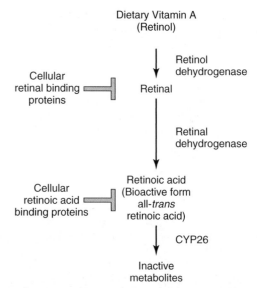

Figure 20–1 Regulation of retinoic acid metabolism and signaling. Dietary retinol (vitamin A) is converted to retinal via the action of retinol dehydrogenases. The concentration of free retinal is controlled by the action of cellular retinal-binding proteins. Similarly, retinal is converted to retinoic acid by retinal dehydrogenases, and its free level is modulated by sequestration by cellular retinoic acid–binding proteins and degradation by CYP26. The bioactive form of retinoic acid is all-*trans* retinoic acid.

MORPHOGENS

Extrinsic signaling by morphogens guide the differentiation and migration of cells during development, determining the morphology and function of developing tissues and organs (see Chapter 6). Many morphogens are found in concentration gradients in the embryo. Different morphogens can be expressed in opposing gradients in the dorsoventral, anteroposterior, and mediolateral axes. The fate of a specific cell can be determined by its location along these gradients. Cells can also be attracted or repelled by morphogens depending on the set of receptors expressed on the cell surface.

Retinoic Acid

The anteroposterior (AP) axis of the embryo is crucial for determining the correct location for structures such as limbs and for the patterning of the nervous system. For decades, it has been clinically evident that alterations in the level of vitamin A (retinol) in the diet (excessive or insufficient amounts) can lead to the development of congenital malformations (Chapter 19). The bioactive form of vitamin A is retinoic acid that is formed by enzymatic oxidation. Free levels of retinoic acid can be modulated by cellular retinoic acid–binding proteins that sequester retinoic acid. Retinoic acid can also be actively degraded into inactive metabolites by enzymes such as CYP26 (Fig. 20-1). Normally, retinoic acid acts to "posteriorize" the body plan and either excessive retinoic acid or inhibition of its degradation leads to a truncated body axis where structures have a more posterior nature. In contrast, insufficient retinoic acid or defects in the enzymes such as retinal aldehyde dehydrogenase will lead to a more anteriorized structure. At a molecular level, retinoic acid binds to its receptors (transcription factors) inside the cell and their activation will regulate the expression of down-stream genes. Hox genes are crucial targets of retinoic acid receptors in development. Because of their profound influence on early development, retinoids are powerful teratogens, especially during the first trimester.

Transforming Growth Factor β/Bone Morphogenetic Protein

Members of the TGF-β superfamily include TGF-β, BMPs, and activin. These molecules contribute to the establishment of dorsoventral patterning, cell fate decisions, and formation of specific organs and systems, including the kidneys, nervous system, the skeleton, and blood. In humans, there are three different forms of TGF-β (isoforms TGF-β_1, TGF-β_2, and TGF-β_3).

Binding of these ligands to transmembrane kinase receptors results in phosphorylation of intracellular receptor-associated Smad proteins (R-Smads) (Fig. 20-2). The Smad proteins are a large family of intercellular proteins that are divided into three classes: receptor-activated (R-Smads), common-partner (co-Smads, Smad4), and inhibitory Smads (I-Smads). R-Smad/Smad4 complexes regulate target gene transcription by interacting with other proteins or as transcription factors by directly binding to DNA. The diversity of TGF-β ligand, receptor, and R-Smad combinations contributes to particular developmental and cell-specific processes, often in combination with other signaling pathways.

Hedgehog

Sonic hedgehog (Shh) was the first mammalian ortholog of the *Drosophila* gene hedgehog to be identified. Shh and other related proteins, such as desert hedgehog and Indian hedgehog, are secreted morphogens critical to early patterning, cell migration, and differentiation of many cell types and organ systems. Cells have variable thresholds for response to the secreted Shh signal. The primary receptor for Shh is Patched (PTCH in human, PTC family in mouse), a transmembrane domain protein. In the absence of Shh, Patched inhibits transmembrane-domain, G-protein–linked protein (Smoothened [Smo]). This results in inhibitions of downstream signaling to the nucleus. However, in the presence of Shh, Ptc inhibition is blocked and downstream events follow, including transcriptional activation of target genes, such as Ptc–1, Engrailed, and others (Fig. 20-3).

Post-translational modification of Shh protein affects its association with the cell membrane, formation of Shh multimers, and the movement of Shh, which, in turn, alters its tissue distribution and concentration gradients.

One of the best explained activities of Shh in vertebrate development is its role in patterning the ventral neural tube. Shh is secreted at high levels by the notochord, and therefore the concentration of Shh is highest in the floor

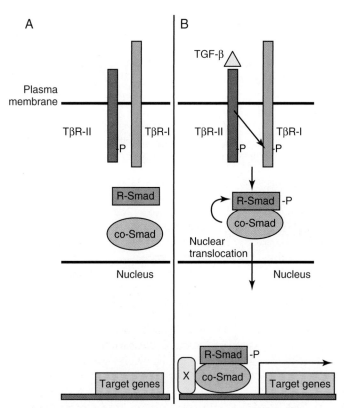

Figure 20–2 Transforming growth factor β (TGF-β)/Smad signaling pathway. **A,** The type II TGF-β receptor subunit (TβR-II) is constitutively active. **B,** Upon binding of ligand to TβR-II, a type I receptor subunit is recruited to form a heterodimeric receptor complex and the TβR-I kinase domain is transphosphorylated (-P). Signaling from the activated receptor complex phosphorylates R-Smads, which then bind to a co-Smad, translocate from the cytoplasm to the nucleus, and activate gene transcription with cofactor(s) (X).

plate of the neural tube and lowest in the roof plate, where members of the TGF-β family are highly expressed. The cell fates of ventral interneuron classes and motor neurons are determined by the relative Shh concentrations in the tissue and other factors.

The understanding of the requirement of Shh pathway signaling for many developmental processes has been enhanced by the discovery of human mutations of members of the Shh pathway. In addition, corresponding phenotypes of genetically modified mice, in which members of the Shh pathway are either inactivated (loss of function/knockout) or overexpressed (gain of function), have also added to this knowledge. Mutations of SHH and PTCH have been associated with holoprosencephaly in humans, a common congenital brain defect resulting in the fusion of the two cerebral hemispheres, dorsalization of forebrain structures, and anophthalmia or cyclopia (see Chapter 17). In sheep this same defect has been associated with exposure to the teratogen cyclopamine, which disrupts Shh signaling (see Fig. 20-3). Gorlin's syndrome, often due to germline PTCH mutations, is a constellation of congenital malformations mostly affecting the epidermis, craniofacial structures,

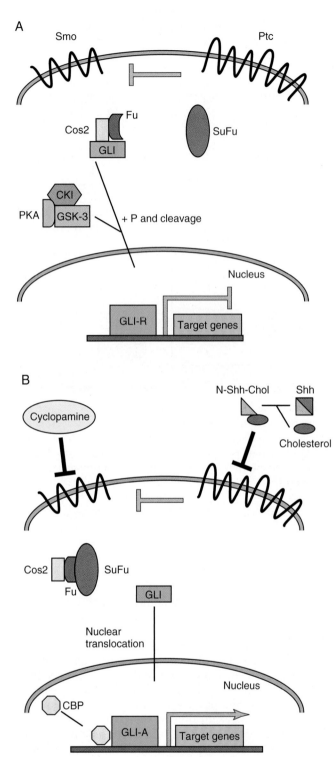

Figure 20–3 Sonic hedgehog/Patched signaling pathway. **A,** The Patched (Ptc) receptor inhibits signaling from the Smoothened (Smo) receptor. In a complex with Costal–2 (Cos2) and Fused (Fu), Gli is modified to become a transcriptional repressor, Gli-R. **B,** Sonic hedgehog (Shh) is cleaved, and cholesterol is added to its N-terminus. This modified Shh ligand inhibits the Ptc receptor, permitting Smo signaling, and ultimately activated Gli (Gli-A) translocates to the nucleus to activate target genes with CBP. *CBP,* cyclic AMP-binding protein; *CKI,* casein kinase I; *GSK–3,* glycogen synthase kinase–3; *P,* phosphate group; *PKA,* protein kinase A; *SuFu,* suppressor of Fused.

and nervous system. GLI3 mutations are associated with autosomal dominant polydactyly syndromes.

Wnt/β-Catenin Pathway

The Wnt-secreted glycoproteins are vertebrate orthologs of the *Drosophila* gene Wingless. Similar to the other morphogens, the nineteen Wnt family members control several processes during development, including establishment of cell polarity, proliferation, apoptosis, cell fate specification, and migration. Wnt signaling is a very complex process, and three signaling pathways have been elucidated to date; only the classic or "canonical" β-catenin-dependent pathway is discussed here (Fig. 20-4). Specific Wnts bind to 1 of 10 Frizzled (Fzd) seven-transmembrane domain, cell surface receptors, and with low-density, lipoprotein receptor–related protein (LRP5/LRP6) coreceptors, thereby activating downstream intracellular signaling events. In the absence of Wnt binding, cytoplasmic β-catenin is phosphorylated by glycogen synthase kinase (GSK–3) and targeted for degradation. In the presence of Wnts, GSK–3 is inactivated, and β-catenin is not phosphorylated and accumulates in the cytoplasm. The β-catenin translocates to the nucleus, where it activates target gene transcription, in a complex with T-cell factor (TCF) transcription factors. β-catenin/TCF target genes include vascular endothelial growth factor (VEGF) and matrix metalloproteinases.

Dysregulated Wnt signaling is a prominent feature in many developmental disorders such as Williams-Beuren syndrome (heart, neurodevelopmental, and facial defects) and cancer. LRP5 mutations are found in the osteoporosis-pseudoglioma syndrome (congenital blindness and juvenile osteoporosis). Similar to the Shh pathway, canonical Wnt pathway mutations have been described in children with medulloblastoma.

RECEPTOR TYROSINE KINASES

Common Features

Growth factors, such as insulin, epidermal growth factor, nerve growth factor, and other neurotrophins, and members of the platelet-derived growth factor family, bind to cell surface transmembrane receptors found on target cells. These receptors, members of the RTK superfamily, have three domains: (1) an extracellular ligand-binding domain, (2) a transmembrane domain (TMD), and (3) an intracellular kinase domain (Fig. 20-5). These receptors are found as monomers in the unbound state but become dimers upon ligand binding. This process of dimerization brings the two intracellular kinase domains into close proximity such that one kinase domain can phosphorylate and activate the other receptor. This process, transphosphorylation, is required to fully activate the receptors, which then initiate a series of intracellular signaling cascades. An inactivating mutation of one receptor subunit's kinase domain results in abolishment of signaling; such a mutation in the kinase domain of the VEGF receptor 3 (VEGFR–3) results in the autosomal dominantly inherited lymphatic disorder called Milroy disease.

A

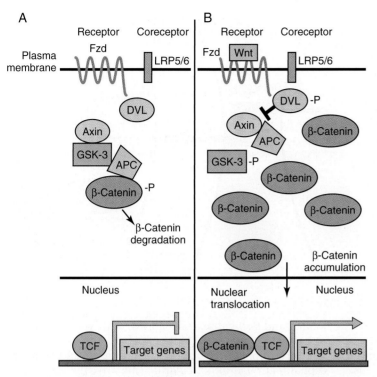

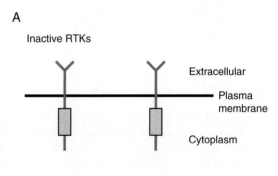

Figure 20–4 Wnt/β-catenin canonical signaling pathway. **A,** In the absence of Wnt ligand binding to Frizzled (Fzd) receptor, β-catenin is phosphorylated (-P) by a multiprotein complex and targeted for degradation. Target gene expression is repressed by T-cell factor (TCF). **B,** When Wnt binds to the Fzd receptor, LRP coreceptors are recruited, Disheveled (DVL) is phosphorylated and β-catenin then accumulates in the cytoplasm. Some β-catenin enters the nucleus to activate target gene transcription. APC, adenomatous polyposis coli; GSK–3, glycogen synthase kinase–3; LRP, lipoprotein receptor–related protein.

Regulation of Angiogenesis by Receptor Tyrosine Kinases

Growth factors generally promote cellular proliferation, migration, and survival (i.e., they are antiapoptotic). During embryogenesis, signaling through RTKs is crucial for normal development and affects many different processes such as the growth of new blood vessels (see Chapter 5), cellular migration, and neuronal axonal guidance.

Endothelial cells are derived from a progenitor cell (the hemangioblast) that can give rise to both the hematopoietic cell lineage and endothelial cells. The early endothelial cells proliferate and eventually coalesce to form the first primitive blood vessels. This process is termed vasculogenesis. After the first blood vessels are formed, they undergo intensive remodeling and maturation into the mature blood vessels in a process called angiogenesis. This maturation process involves the recruitment of vascular smooth muscle cells to the vessels that stabilize them. Vasculogenesis and angiogenesis are both dependent on the function of two distinct RTK classes, members of the VEGF and Tie receptor families. VEGF-A was shown to be essential for endothelial and blood cell development; VEGF-A knockout mice fail to develop blood or endothelial cells and die at early embryonic stages. A related molecule, VEGF-C, was shown to be crucial for the development of lymphatic endothelial cells. VEGF-A signals through two receptors, VEGFR–1 and VEGFR–2, that are expressed by endothelial cells but VEGFR–2 predominates in vasculogenesis in the embryo.

The process of angiogenic refinement depends on the function of the angiopoietin/Tie2 signaling pathway. Tie2 is a RTK that is specifically expressed by endothelial cells

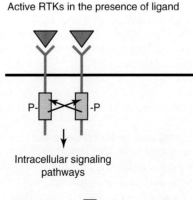

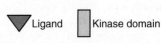

Figure 20–5 Receptor tyrosine kinase (RTK) signaling. **A,** In the absence of ligand, the receptors are monomers and are inactive. **B,** Upon binding of ligand, the receptors dimerize and transphosphorylation occurs, which activates downstream signaling cascades. P, phosphorylated.

Figure 20–6 Notch–Delta signaling pathway. In progenitor cells (right), activation of Notch signaling leads to cleavage of the Notch intracellular domain (NICD). NICD translocates to the nucleus, binds to a transcriptional complex, and activates target genes, such as the bHLH gene, Hes1, that inhibit differentiation. In differentiating cells (left), Notch signaling is not active.

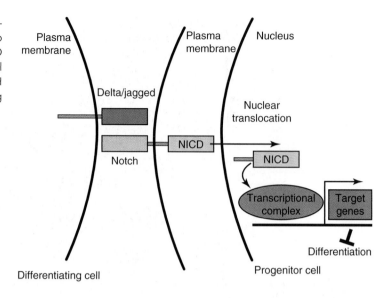

and angiopoietin 1 and angiopoietin 2 are its ligands that are expressed by the surrounding vascular smooth muscle cells. This represents a paracrine signaling system in which receptor and ligand are expressed in adjacent cells. Both the VEGF/VEGFR–2 and angiopoietin/Tie2 signaling pathways are co-opted by tumors to stimulate growth of new blood vessels, which stimulates their growth and metastasis. This demonstrates how normal signaling pathways in the embryo can be reused by disease processes, such as cancer.

NOTCH–DELTA PATHWAY

The Notch signaling pathway is integral for cell fate determination, including maintenance of stem-cell niches, proliferation, apoptosis, and differentiation. These processes are essential for all aspects of organ development through regulation of lateral and inductive cell-cell signaling. Notch proteins are single transmembrane receptors that interact with membrane-bound Notch ligands (e.g., Delta-like ligands and serrate-like ligands [Jagged]) on adjacent cells (Fig. 20-6). Ligand-receptor binding triggers proteolytic events leading to the release of the Notch intracellular domain (NICD). When the NICD translocates to the nucleus, a series of intranuclear events culminates in the induction of expression a transcription factor that maintains the progenitor state of the cell.

Lateral inhibition ensures in a population of cells with equivalent developmental potential, the correct number of two distinct cell types. In the initial cell–cell interaction, Notch receptor signaling maintains one cell as an uncommitted progenitor. The adjacent cell maintains reduced Notch signaling and undergoes differentiation. Inductive signaling with other surrounding cells expressing morphogens may overcome a cell's commitment to a default fate to an alternative cell fate. Understanding the function of the Notch–Delta signaling pathway in mammalian development has been assisted by loss-of-function studies in the mouse. Mutations Alagille syndrome (arteriohepatic dysplasia), with liver, kidney, cardiovascular,

ocular, and skeletal malformations, and NOTCH–3 gene mutations in the CADASIL (cerebral autosomal dominant arteriopathy with subcortical infarcts and leukoencephalopathy) adult vascular degenerative disease, with a tendency to early-age onset of stroke-like events, support the importance of the Notch signaling pathway in embryonic and postnatal development, respectively.

TRANSCRIPTION FACTORS

Transcription factors belong to a large class of proteins that regulate the expression of many target genes, either through activation or repression mechanisms. Typically, a transcription factor will bind to specific nucleotide sequences in the promoter/enhancer regions of target genes and regulate the rate of transcription of its target genes via interacting with accessory proteins. Transcription factors can both activate or repress target gene transcription depending on the cell in which they are expressed, the specific promoter, the chromatin context, and the developmental stage. Some transcription factors do not need to bind to DNA to regulate transcription: they may bind to other transcription factors already bound to the promoter DNA thereby regulating transcription or bind and sequester other transcription factors from their target genes, thus repressing their transcription. The transcription factor superfamily is composed of many different classes of proteins. Three examples of this diverse family of proteins are described: Hox/Homeobox, Pax, and bHLH transcription factors.

Hox/Homeobox Proteins

The Hox genes were first discovered in the fruit fly, *Drosophila melanogaster*. The order of the Hox genes along the AP axis is faithfully reproduced in their organization at the level of the chromosome. Mutations in these genes of the HOM-C complex lead to dramatic phenotypes (homeotic transformation) such as the Antennapedia gene in which legs instead of antennae sprout from the head of the fruit fly. In humans, the order of the Hox genes along the AP axis and chromosomal location is conserved as well. Defects in HOXA1 have been shown to impair human neural development, and mutations in HOXA13 and HOXD13 result in limb malformations.

All the Hox genes contain a 180-base-pair sequence, the homeobox, which encodes a 60-amino-acid homeodomain composed of three α helices. The third (recognition) helix binds to DNA sites that contain one or more binding motifs in the promoters of their target genes. The homeodomain is the most conserved region of the protein and is highly conserved across evolution, whereas other regions of the protein are not as well conserved. Mutations in the DNA-binding region of the homeobox gene NKX2.5 are associated with cardiac atrial-septal defects and mutations in ARX are associated with the central nervous system malformation syndrome lissencephaly.

Pax Genes

The Pax genes all contain conserved bipartite DNA-binding motifs called the Pax (or paired) domain, and most Pax family members also contain a homeodomain. PAX proteins have been shown to both activate and repress transcription of target genes. The *Drosophila melanogaster* ortholog of Pax6, eyeless, was shown to be essential for eye development because homozygous mutant flies had no eyes. Eyeless shares a high degree of sequence conservation with its human ortholog PAX6 and is associated with ocular malformations such as aniridia (absence of the iris) and Peter's anomaly. In human eye diseases, the level of PAX6 expression seems to be crucial because patients with only one functional copy (haploinsufficiency) have ocular defects and patients without PAX6 function are anophthalmic. This concept of haploinsufficiency is a recurring theme for many different transcription factors and corresponding human malformations.

PAX3 and PAX7 encode both homeodomain and Pax DNA-binding domains. The human childhood cancer alveolar rhabdomyosarcoma results from a translocation that results in the formation of a chimeric protein wherein PAX3 or PAX7 (including both DNA domains) is fused to the strong activating domains of the Forkhead family transcription factor FOXO1. The autosomal dominant human disease Waardenburg's syndrome type I has been demonstrated to result from mutations in the PAX3 gene. Patients with this syndrome have hearing deficits, ocular defects (dystopia canthorum), and pigmentation abnormalities best typified by a white forelock.

Basic Helix-Loop-Helix (bHLH) Transcription Factors

The bHLH genes are a class of transcription factors that regulate cell fate determination and differentiation in many different tissues during development. At a molecular level, bHLH proteins contain a basic (positively charged) DNA-binding region that is followed by two α helices that are separated by a loop. The α helices have a hydrophilic and a hydrophobic side (amphipathic). The

hydrophobic side of the helix is a motif for protein-protein interactions between different members of the bHLH family. This domain is the most conserved region of the bHLH proteins across different species. bHLH proteins often bind other bHLHs (heterodimerize) to regulate transcription. These heterodimers are composed of tissue-specific bHLH proteins bound to ubiquitously expressed bHLH proteins. The powerful prodifferentiation effect of bHLH genes can be repressed by several different mechanisms. For example, inhibitor of differentiation (Id) proteins are HLH proteins that lack the basic DNA-binding motif. When Id proteins heterodimerize with specific bHLH proteins, they prevent binding of these bHLH proteins to their target gene promoter sequences (called E-boxes).

Growth factors, which tend to inhibit differentiation, increase the level of Id proteins that sequester bHLH proteins from their target promoters. In addition, growth factors can stimulate the phosphorylation of the DNA-binding domain of bHLH proteins, which inhibits their ability to bind to DNA. bHLH genes are crucial for the development of tissues such as muscle (MyoD/Myogenin) and neurons (NeuroD/Neurogenin) in humans. MyoD expression was shown to be sufficient to transdifferentiate several different cell lines into muscle cells, demonstrating that it is a master regulator of muscle differentiation. Studies of knockout mice confirmed that MyoD and another bHLH, Myf5, are crucial for the differentiation of precursor cells into primitive muscle cells (myoblasts). Similarly, Mash1 and Neurogenin1 are proneural genes that regulate the formation of neuroblasts from the neuroepithelium. Mouse models have shown that these genes are crucial for the specification of different subpopulations of precursors in the developing central nervous system. For example, Mash1 knockout mice have defects in forebrain development, whereas Neurogenin1 knockout mice have defects in cranial sensory ganglia and ventral spinal cord neurons. Muscle and neuronal differentiation are controlled by a cascade of bHLH genes that function at early and at late stages of cellular differentiation. In addition, both differentiation pathways are inhibited via signaling through the Notch pathway.

EPIGENETICS

Epigenetics refers to inherited changes that affect gene expression as a result of mechanisms other than changes in the sequence of DNA. Examples include DNA methylation and chromatin modifications, such as acetylation of histones.

DNA Methylation

DNA is methylated at cytosine residues by DNA methyltransferases at CpG sites, where cytosine and guanine nucleotides are directly paired. CpG islands are DNA regions with high concentrations of CpG sites, and are often located in proximal promoter regions of genes. DNA methylation at CpG sites, in general, leads to a reduction of gene expression or gene silencing, whereas

DNA hypomethylation at CpG sites, conversely leads to gene overexpression. Silencing of tumor suppressor genes or overexpression of oncogenes may lead to cancer.

Acetylation

Histones are the positively charged nuclear proteins around which genomic DNA is coiled to tightly pack it within the nucleus. Modification of these proteins is a common pathway by which transcription factors regulate the activity of their target promoters. One such modification is acetylation. DNA is less tightly bound to acetylated histones, thus allowing for more open access of transcription factors and other proteins to the promoters of their target genes. Histone acetylation status is controlled by genes that add acetyl groups (histone transferase) or remove acetyl groups (histone deacetylases) (Fig. 20-7). Phosphorylation of histones also leads to an opening of the chromatin structure and activation of gene transcription. Disorders of chromatin remodeling include Rett, Rubinstein-Taybi, and alpha-thalassemia/X-linked mental retardation syndromes.

SUMMARY OF COMMON SIGNALING PATHWAYS USED DURING DEVELOPMENT

- There are marked differences among the various signaling pathways, but they share many common features: ligands, membrane-bound receptors and coreceptors, intracellular signaling domains, adapters, and effector molecules.
- Signaling pathways are co-opted at various times during development for stem cell renewal, cell proliferation, migration, apoptosis, and differentiation.
- Pathways have "default" settings that result in generation or maintenance of one cell fate rather than another.
- Many genes and signaling pathways are highly conserved throughout evolution.
- Knowledge of gene function has been acquired by reverse genetics using model systems with loss- or gain-of-function transgenic approaches and by forward genetics beginning with the description of abnormal

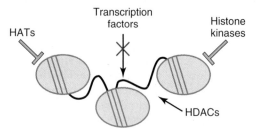

A

Transcriptionally inactive chromatin

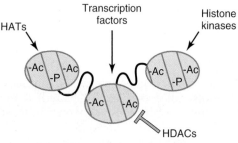

B

Transcriptionally active chromatin

Figure 20–7 Histone modifications alter transcriptional properties of chromatin. **A,** In areas of transcriptionally inactive chromatin, the DNA is tightly bound to the histone cores. The histones are not acetylated or phosphorylated. Histone deacetylases (HDACs) are active, whereas histone acetyl transferases (HATs) and histone kinases are inactive. **B,** In areas of transcriptionally active chromatin, the DNA is not as tightly bound to the histone cores. The histone proteins are acetylated (Ac) and phosphorylated (-P). HDACs are inactive, whereas HATs and histone kinases are active.

phenotypes arising spontaneously in mice and humans and then subsequent identification of the mutant gene.
- There is evidence of cross-talk among pathways. This communication among various signaling pathways facilitates our understanding of the far-reaching consequences of single gene mutations that result in malformation syndromes affecting the development of multiple organ systems or in cancers.

References and Suggested Reading

CHAPTER 1

Fritsch MK, Singer DB: Embryonic stem cell biology. Adv Pediatr 55:43, 2008.

Gasser R: Atlas of Human Embryos. Hagerstown, Harper & Row, 1975.

Gasser R: Virtual Human Embryo DREM Project. Baltimore, MD, NICHD, 2007.

Jirásel JE: An Atlas of Human Prenatal Developmental Mechanics. Anatomy and Staging. London and New York, Taylor & Francis, 2004.

Meyer AW: The Rise of Embryology. Stanford, CA, Stanford University Press, 1939.

National Institutes of Health: National Institutes of Health Guidelines on Human Stem Cell Research 2009. Available at http://stemcells. nih.gov/policy/2009guidelines.htm.

O'Rahilly R, Müller F: Developmental Stages in Human Embryos. Washington, DC, Carnegie Institution of Washington, 1987.

Rossant J: Stem cells and early lineage development. Cell 132:527, 2008.

Streeter GL: Developmental horizons in human embryos. Description of age group XI, 13 to 20 somites, and age group XII, 21 to 29 somites. Contrib Embryol Carnegie Inst 30:211, 1942.

Yamada S, Samtani RR, Lee ES, et al: Developmental atlas of the early first trimester embryo. Dev Dyn 239:1585, 2010.

CHAPTER 2

American Society for Reproductive Medicine: Revised guidelines for human embryology and andrology laboratories. Fertil Steril 90(Suppl):s45, 2008.

Barratt CLR, Kay V, Oxenham SK: The human spermatozoa—a stripped down but refined machine. J Biol 8:63, 2009.

Duggavathi R, Murphy BD: Ovulation signals. Science 324:890, 2009.

Moore KL, Dalley AF, Agur AMR: Clinically Oriented Anatomy, 6th ed. Philadelphia, Lippincott Williams & Wilkins, 2010.

Myers M, Pangas SA: Regulatory roles of transforming growth factor beta family members in folliculogenesis. WIREs Syst Biol Med 2:117, 2010.

CHAPTER 3

Gunby J, Bissonnette F, Librach C, et al: Assisted reproductive technologies (ART) in Canada: 2007 results from the Canadian ART Register. FertilSteril 95:542, 2011.

Harper J (ed): Preimplantation Genetic Diagnosis, 2nd ed. Cambridge, Cambridge University Press, 2009.

Kader AA, Choi A, Orief Y, et al: Factors affecting the outcome of human blastocyst. Reprod Biol Endocrin 7:99, 2009.

Pauli S, Berga SL, Shang W, et al: Current status of the approach to assisted reproduction. Pediatr Clin North Am 56:467, 2009.

Robertson SA: Immune regulation of embryo implantation—all about quality control. J Reprod Immun 81:113, 2009.

Rock J, Hertig AT: The human conceptus during the first two weeks of gestation. Am J Obstet Gynecol 55:6, 1948.

Sjoberg N-O, Hamberger L: Blastocyst development and early implantation. Hum Reprod 15(Suppl 6), 2000.

CHAPTER 4

Bianchi DW, Wilkins-Haug LE, Enders AC, et al: Origin of extraembryonic mesoderm in experimental animals: Relevance to chorionic mosaicism in humans. Am J Med Genet 46:542, 1993.

Hertig AT, Rock J, Adams EC: A description of 34 human ova within the first seventeen days of development. Am J Anat 98:435, 1956.

Kodaman PH, Taylor HS: Hormonal regulation of implantation. Obstet Gynecol Clin North Am 31: 745, 2004.

Lipscomb GH: Ectopic pregnancy. In Copeland LJ, Jarrell JF (eds): Textbook of Gynecology, 4th ed. Philadelphia, WB Saunders, 2000.

Luckett WP: Origin and differentiation of the yolk sac and extraembryonic mesoderm in presomite human and rhesus monkey embryos. Am J Anat 152:59, 1978.

Zorn AM, Wells JM: Vertebrate endoderm development and organ formation. Annu Rev Cell Dev Biol 25:221, 2009.

CHAPTER 5

Downs KM: The enigmatic primitive streak: prevailing notions and challenges concerning the body axis of mammals. Bioessays 31:892, 2009.

Flake AW: The fetus with sacrococcygeal teratoma. In Harrison MR, Evans MI, Adzick NS, Holzgrev W (eds): The Unborn Patient: The Art and Science of Fetal Therapy, 3rd ed. Philadelphia, WB Saunders, 2001.

Gasser RF: Evidence that some events of mammalian embryogenesis can result from differential growth, making migration unnecessary. Anat Rec (Part B New Anat) 289B:53, 2006.

Lewis J, Hanisch A, Holder M: Notch signaling, the segmentation clock, and the patterning of vertebrate somites. J Biol 8:44, 2009.

Powers SE, Taniguchi K, Yen W, et al: Tgif1 and Tgif2 regulate nodal signaling and are required for gastrulation. Development 137: 249, 2010.

Seckl MJ, Fisher RA, Salerno G, et al: Choriocarcinoma and partial hydatidiform moles. Lancet 356:36, 2000.

Tovar JA: The neural crest in pediatric surgery. J Ped Surg 42:915, 2007.

Wang Y, Steinbeisser H: Molecular basis of morphogenesis during vertebrate gastrulation. Cell Mol Life Sci 66:2263, 2009.

CHAPTER 6

Gasser R: Virtual Human Embryo DREM Project. New Orleans, Louisiana State University, 2007.

Jirásel JE: An Atlas of Human Prenatal Developmental Mechanics: Anatomy and Staging. London and New York, Taylor & Francis, 2004.

Kliegman RM: Intrauterine growth restriction. In Martin RJ, Fanaroff AA, Walsh MC (eds): Fanaroff and Martin's Neonatal-Perinatal Medicine: Diseases of the Fetus and Infant, 8th ed. Philadelphia, Mosby, 2006.

O'Rahilly R, Müller F: Development Stages in Human Embryos, Publication 637. Washington, DC, Carnegie Institution of Washington, 1987.

Persaud TVN, Hay JC: Normal embryonic and fetal development. In Reece EA, Hobbins JC (eds): Clinical Obstetrics: The Fetus and Mother, 3rd ed. Oxford, Blackwell Publishing, 2006.

Pooh RK, Shiota K, Kurjak A: Imaging of the human embryo with magnetic resonance imaging microscopy and high-resolution transvaginal 3-dimensional sonography: Human embryology in the 21st century. Am J ObstetGynecol 204:77.e1, 2011.

Steding G: The Anatomy of the Human Embryo: A Scanning Electron-Microscopic Atlas. Basel, Karger, 2009.

Yamada S, Samtani RR, Lee ES, et al: Developmental atlas of the early first trimester embryo. Dev Dyn 239:1585, 2010.

Whitworth M, Bricker L, Neilson JP, et al: Ultrasound for fetal assessment in early pregnancy. Cochrane Database Syst Rev 4:CD007058, 2010.

CHAPTER 7

Anderson MS, Hay WW: Intrauterine growth restriction and the small-for-gestational-age infant. In MacDonald MG, Seshia MMK, Mullett MD (eds): Avery's Neonatology: Pathophysiology & Management of the Newborn, 6th ed. Philadelphia, Lippincott Williams & Wilkins, 2005.

Chung R, Kasprian G, Brugger PC, et al: The current state and future of fetal imaging. Clin Perinatol 36:685, 2009.

Claris O, Beltrand J, Levy-Marchal C: Consequences of intrauterine growth and early neonatal catch-up growth. Semin Perinatol 34:207, 2010.

Cunningham FG, Leveno KJ, Bloom SL, et al: Williams Obstetrics, 23rd ed. New York, McGraw-Hill, 2009.

Deprest JA, Devlieger R, Srisupundit K, et al: Fetal surgery is a clinical reality. Semin Fetal Neonatal Med 15:58, 2010.

Durkin EF, Shaaban A: Commonly encountered surgical problems in the fetus and neonate. Pediatr Clin North Am 56:647, 2009.

Jirásel JE: An Atlas of Human Prenatal Developmental Mechanics: Anatomy and Staging. London and New York, Taylor & Francis, 2004.

Jobe AH: "Miracle" extremely low birth weight neonates. Obstet-Gynecol 116:1184, 2010.

Needlman RD: Fetal growth and development. In Behrman RE, Kliegman Jenson HB (eds): Nelson Textbook of Pediatrics, 17th ed. Philadelphia, Elsevier/Saunders, 2004.

Steding G: The Anatomy of the Human Embryo: A Scanning Electron-Microscopic Atlas. Basel, Karger, 2009.

Whitworth M, Bricker L, Neilson JP, et al: Ultrasound for fetal assessment in early pregnancy. Cochrane Database Syst Rev 4: CD007058, 2010.

CHAPTER 8

Alexander GR, Wingate MS, Salihu H, et al: Fetal and neonatal mortality risks of multiple births. Obstet Gynecol Clin North Am 32:1, 2005.

Brace RA: Amniotic fluid dynamics. In Creasy RK, Resnik R: Maternal-Fetal Medicine, 5th ed. Philadelphia, WB Saunders, 2004.

Callen PW (ed): Ultrasonography in Obstetrics and Gynecology, 5th ed. Philadelphia, Saunders/Elsevier, 2008.

Collins JH: Umbilical cord accidents: Human studies. Semin Perinatol 26:79, 2002.

Cunningham FG, Leveno KJ, Bloom SL, et al: Williams Obstetrics, 23rd ed. New York, McGraw-Hill, 2009.

Harman CR: Amniotic fluid abnormalities. Semin Perinatol 32:288, 2008.

Redline RW: Placental pathology. In Martin RJ, Fanaroff AA, Walsh MC (eds): Fanaroff and Martin's Neonatal-Perinatal Medicine: Diseases of the Fetus and Infant, 8th ed. Philadelphia, Mosby, 2006.

Robertson SA: Immune regulation of embryo implantation—all about quality control. J Reprod Immun 81:113, 2009.

Yagel S: The developmental role of natural killer cells at the fetal–maternal interface. Am J Obstet Gynecol 201:344, 2009.

CHAPTER 9

Cass DL: Fetal surgery for congenital diaphragmatic hernia: The North American Experience. Semin Perinatol 29:104, 2005.

Clugston RD, Zhang W, Alvarez S, et al: Understanding abnormal retinoid signaling as a causative mechanism in congenital diaphragmatic hernia. Am J Res Cell Mol Biol 42:276, 2010.

Kays DW: Congenital diaphragmatic hernia and neonatal lung lesions. Surg Clin North Am 86:329, 2006.

Rottier R, Tibboel D: Fetal lung and diaphragm development in congenital diaphragmatic hernia. Semin Perinatol 29:86, 2005.

Turell DC: Advances with surfactant. Emerg Med Clin North Am 26:921, 2008.

Wells LJ: Development of the human diaphragm and pleural sacs. Contrib Embryol Carnegie Inst 35:107, 1954.

CHAPTER 10

Berkovitz BKB, Holland GR, Moxham B: Oral Anatomy, Histology, and Embryology, 3rd ed. Philadelphia, Mosby, 2009.

Gross E, Sichel J-Y: Congenital neck lesions. Surg Clin North Am 86:383, 2006.

Hinrichsen K: The early development of morphology and patterns of the face in the human embryo. Adv Anat Embryol Cell Biol 98:1, 1985.

Jones KL: Smith's Recognizable Patterns of Human Malformation, 6th ed. Philadelphia, Elsevier/Saunders, 2005.

Mueller DT, Callanan VP: Congenital malformations of the oral cavity. Otolaryngeal Clin North Am 40:141, 2007.

Noden DM, Trainor PA: Relations and interactions between cranial mesoderm and neural crest populations. J Anat 207:575, 2005.

Rice DPC: Craniofacial anomalies: From development to molecular pathogenesis. Curr Mol Med 5:699, 2009.

Tovar JA: The neural crest in pediatric surgery. J Pediatr Surg 42:915, 2007.

Waldhausen JHT: Branchial cleft and arch anomalies in children. Semin Pediatr Surg 15:70, 2006.

Yatzey KE: DiGeorge syndrome, Tbx1, and retinoic acid signaling come full circle. Circ Res 106: 630, 2010.

CHAPTER 11

Abel R, Bush A, Chitty RS, et al: Congenital lung disease. In Chernick V, Boat T, Wilmott R, Bush A (eds): Kendig's Disorders of the Respiratory Tract in Children, 7th ed. Philadelphia, Saunders/Elsevier, 2006.

Brown E, James K: The lung primordium an outpunching from the foregut! Evidence-based dogma or myth. J Pediatr Surg 44:607, 2009.

Haddad GG, Fontán JJP: Development of the respiratory system. In Behrman RE, Kliegman Jenson HB (eds): Nelson Textbook of Pediatrics, 17th ed. Philadelphia, Elsevier/Saunders, 2004.

Jobe AH: Lung development and maturation. In Martin RJ, Fanaroff AA, Walsh MC (eds): Fanaroff and Martin's Neonatal-Perinatal Medicine: Diseases of the Fetus and Infant, 8th ed. Philadelphia, Mosby, 2006.

O'Rahilly R, Boyden E: The timing and sequence of events in the development of the human respiratory system during the embryonic period proper. Z Anat Entwicklungsresch 141:237, 1973.

Rawlins EL: The building blocks of mammalian lung development. DevDyn 240:403, 2011.

Shi W, Chen F, Cardoso WV: Mechanisms of lung development. Proc Am Thorac Soc 6:558, 2009.

Wells LJ, Boyden EA: The development of the bronchopulmonary segments in human embryos of horizons XVII and XIX. Am J Anat 95:163, 1954.

Whitsett JA, Wert SE: Molecular determinants of lung morphogenesis. In Chernick V, Boat T, Wilmott R, Bush A (ed): Kendig's Disorders of the Respiratory Tract in Children, 7th ed. Philadelphia, Elsevier/Saunders, 2006.

CHAPTER 12

Gosche JR, Vick L, Boulanger SC, et al: Midgut abnormalities. Surg Clin North Am 86:285, 2006.

Kapur RP: Practical pathology and genetics of Hirschsprung's disease. Semin Pediatr Surg 18:212, 2009.

Kluth D, Fiegel HC, Metzger R: Embryology of the hindgut. Semin-Pediatr Sur 20:152, 2011.

Lau ST, Caty MG: Hindgut abnormalities. Surg Clin North Am 86:285, 2006.

Ledbetter DJ: Gastroschisis and omphalocele. Surg Clin North Am 86:249, 2006.

Levitt MA, Pena A: Cloacal malformations: Lessons learned from 490 cases. Semin Pediatr Surg 9:118, 2010.

Mastroiacoovo P, Lisi A, Castilla A, et al: Gastroschisis and associated defects: An international study. Am J Med Genet 143:660, 2007.

Metzger R, Metzger U, Fiegel HC, et al: Embryology of the midgut. SeminPediatr Sur 20:145, 2011.

Mundt E, Bates MD: Genetics of Hirschsprung disease and anorectal malformations. Semin Pediatr Surg 19:107, 2010.

Naik-Mathuria B, Olutoye OO: Foregut abnormalities. Surg Clin North Am 86:261, 2006.

Stanchina L, Van de Putte T, Goosens M, et al: Genetic interaction between Sox10 and Zfhx1b during enteric nervous system development. Dev Biol 341:416, 2010.

Vakili K, Pomfret EA: Biliary anatomy and embryology. Surg Clin North Am 88:1159, 2008.

Van den Brink GR: Hedgehog signaling in development and homeostasis of the gastrointestinal tract. Physiol Rev 87:1343, 2007.

Van der Putte SCJ: The development of the human anorectum. Anat Rec 292:952, 2009.

Wyllie R: Pyloric stenosis and other congenital anomalies of the stomach; intestinal atresia, stenosis, and malformations; intestinal duplications, Meckel diverticulum, and other remnants of the omphalomesenteric duct. In Behrman RE, Kliegman RM, Jenson HB (eds): Nelson Textbook of Pediatrics, 17th ed. Philadelphia, WB Saunders, 2004.

CHAPTER 13

Haynes JH: Inguinal and scrotal disorders. Surg Clin North Am 86:371, 2006.

Lee PA, Houk CP, Ahmed SF, et al: Consensus statement on management of intersex disorders. Pediatrics 118:e4888, 2006.

Nishida H, Miyagawa S, Matsumaru D, et al: Gene expression analyses on embryonic external genitalia: identification of regulatory genes possibly involved in masculinization process. Congen Anom 48:63, 2008.

Palmert MR, Dahms WT: Abnormalities of sexual differentiation. In Martin RJ, Fanaroff AA, Walsh MC (eds): Fanaroff and Martin's Neonatal-Perinatal Medicine: Diseases of the Fetus and Infant, 8th ed. Philadelphia, Mosby, 2006.

Persaud TVN: Embryology of the female genital tract and gonads. In Copeland LJ, Jarrell J (eds): Textbook of Gynecology, 2nd ed. Philadelphia, WB Saunders, 2000.

Sobel V, Zhu Y-S, Imperato-McGinley J: Fetal hormones and sexual differentiation. Obstet Gynecol Clin North Am 31:837, 2004.

Wang MH, Baskin LS: Endocrine disruptors, genital development, and hypospadias. J Androl 29:499, 2008.

Woo LL, Thomas JC, Brock JW: Cloacal exstrophy: A comprehensive review of an uncommon problem. J Pediatr Urol 6:102, 2010.

CHAPTER 14

Adams SM, Good MW, DeFranco GM: Sudden infant death syndrome. Am Fam Physician 79:870, 2009.

Baschat AA: Examination of the fetal cardiovascular system. Semin Fetal Neonatal Med 16:2, 2011.

Bentham J, Bhattacharya S: Genetic mechanisms controlling cardiovascular development. Ann N Y Acad Sci 1123:10, 2008.

Bernstein E: The cardiovascular system. In Behrman RE, Kliegman RM, Jenson HB (eds): Nelson Textbook of Pediatrics, 17th ed. Philadelphia, WB Saunders, 2004.

Dyer LA, Kirby ML: The role of secondary heart field in cardiac development. Dev Dyn 336:137, 2009.

Hildreth V, Anderson RH, Henderson DJH: Autonomic innervations of the developing heart: Origins and function. Clin Anat 22:36, 2009.

Horsthuis T, Christoffels VM, Anderson RH, et al: Can recent insights into cardiac development improve our understanding of congenitally malformed heart. Clin Anat 22:4, 2009.

Kamedia Y: Hoxa3 and signaling molecules involved in aortic arch patterning and remodeling. Cell Tissue Res 336:165, 2010.

Loukas M, Groat C, Khangura R, et al: Cardiac veins: A review of the literature. Clin Anat 22:129, 2009.

Loukas M, Bilinsky C, Bilinski E, et al: The normal and abnormal anatomy of the coronary arteries. Clin Anat 22:114, 2009.

Männer J: The anatomy of cardiac looping: A step towards the understanding of the morphogenesis of several forms of congenital cardiac malformations. Clin Anat 22:21, 2009.

Solloway M, Harvey RP: Molecular pathways in myocardial development: A stem cell perspective. Cardiovasc Res 58:264, 2006.

Stoller JZ, Epstein JA: Cardiac neural crest. Semin Cell Dev Biol 16:704, 2005.

Watanabe M, Schaefer KS: Cardiac embryology. In Martin RJ, Fanaroff AA, Walsh MC (eds): Fanaroff and Martin's Neonatal-Perinatal Medicine: Diseases of the Fetus and Infant, 8th ed. Philadelphia, Mosby, 2006.

CHAPTER 15

Bamshad M, Van Heest AE, Pleasure D: Arthrogryposis: A review and update. J Bone Joint Surg Am 91(Suppl 4):40, 2009.

Buckingham M: Myogenic progenitor cells and skeletal myogenesis in vertebrates. Curr Opin Genet Dev 16:525, 2006.

Cole P, Kaufman Y, Hatef DA, et al: Embryology of the hand and upper extremity. J Craniofac Surg 20:992, 2009.

Cohen Jr MM: Perspectives on craniosynostosis: sutural biology, some well-known syndromes and some unusual syndromes. J Craniofac Surg 20:646, 2009.

Dallas SL, Bonewald LF: Dynamic of the transition from osteoblast to osteocyte. Ann N Y Acad Sci 1192:437, 2010.

Cooperman DR, Thompson GH: Musculoskeletal disorders. In Martin RJ, Fanaroff AA, Walsh MC (eds): Fanaroff and Martin's Neonatal-Perinatal Medicine: Diseases of the Fetus and Infant, 8th ed. Philadelphia, Mosby, 2006.

Dunwoodie SL: The role of Notch in patterning the human vertebral column. Curr Opin Genet Dev 19:329, 2009.

Franz-Odendaal TA, Hall, BK, Witten PE: Buried alive: How osteoblasts become osteocytes. Dev Dyn 235:176, 2006.

Hall BK: Bones and Cartilage: Developmental Skeletal Biology. Philadelphia, Elsevier, 2005.

Hinrichsen KV, Jacob HJ, Jacob M, et al: Principles of ontogenesis of leg and foot in man. Ann Anat 176:121, 1994.

Maldjian C, Hofkin S, Bonakdarpour A, et al: Abnormalities of the pediatric foot. Acad Radiol 6:191, 1999.

O'Rahilly R, Gardner E: The timing and sequence of events in the development of the limbs of the human embryo. Anat Embryol 148:1, 1975.

Towers M, Tickle C: Generation of pattern and form in the developing limb. Int J Dev Biol 53:805, 2009.

CHAPTER 16

De Wals P, Tairou F, Van Allen MI, et al: Reduction in neural-tube defects after folic acid fortification in Canada. N Engl J Med 357:135, 2007.

Diaz AL, Gleeson JG: The molecular and genetic mechanisms of neocortex development. Clin Perinatol 36:503, 2009.

Gressens P, Hüppi PS: Normal and abnormal brain development. In Martin RJ, Fanarof AA, Walsh MC (eds): Fanaroff and Martin's Neonatal-Perinatal Medicine: Diseases of the Fetus and Infant, 8th ed. Philadelphia, Mosby, 2006.

Haines DE: Neuroanatomy—An Atlas of Structures, Sections, and Systems, ed 8, Baltimore 2012, Lippincott Williams & Wilkins.

Johnston MV, Kinsman S: Congenital anomalies of the central nervous system. In Behrman RE, Kliegman Jenson HB (eds): Nelson Textbook of Pediatrics, 17th ed. Philadelphia, Elsevier/Saunders, 2004.

O'Rahilly R, Müller F: Embryonic Human Brain. An Atlas of Developmental Stages, 2nd ed. New York, Wiley-Liss, 1999.

ten Donkelaar HT, Lammens M: Development of the human cerebellum and its disorders. Clin Perinatol 36: 513, 2009.

Zhu X, Lin CR, Prefontaine GG, et al. Genetic control of pituitary development and hypopituitarism. Curr Opin Genet Dev 15:332, 2005.

CHAPTER 17

Barald KF, Kelley MW: From placodes to polarization: New tunes in inner ear development. Development 131:4119, 2004.

Barishak YR: Embryology of the Eye and Its Adnexa, 2nd ed. Basel, Karger, 2001.

Bauer PW, MacDonald CB, Melhem ER: Congenital inner ear malformation. Am J Otol 19:669, 1998.

FitzPatrick DR, van Heyningen V: Developmental eye disorders. Curr Opin Genet Dev 15:348, 2005.

Haddad Jr J: The Ear. In Behrman RE, Kliegman Jenson HB (eds): Nelson Textbook of Pediatrics, 17th ed. Philadelphia, Elsevier/Saunders, 2004.

Jason R, Guercio BS, Martyn LJ: Congenital malformations of the eye and orbit. Otolaryngol Clin North Am 40:113, 2007.

Jones KL: Smith's Recognizable Patterns of Human Malformation, 6th ed. Philadelphia, WB Saunders, 2005.

Mallo M: Formation of the middle ear: Recent progress on the developmental and molecular mechanisms. Dev Biol 231:410, 2001.

O'Rahilly R: The prenatal development of the human eye. Exp Eye Res 21:93, 1975.

Porter CJW, Tan SW: Congenital auricular anomalies: Topographic anatomy, embryology, classification, and treatment strategies. Plast Reconstr Surg 115:1701, 2005.

CHAPTER 18

Caton J, Tucker AS: Current knowledge of tooth development: patterning and mineralization of the murine dentition. J Anat 214: 407, 2009.

Coletta RD, McCoy EL, Burns V, et al: Characterization of the Six 1 homeobox gene in normal mammary gland morphogenesis. BMC Dev Biol 10:4, 2010.

Nanci A: Ten Cate's Oral Histology: Development, Structure, and Function, 7th ed. St. Louis, CV Mosby, 2008.

Behrman RE, Kliegman Jenson HB (eds): Nelson Textbook of Pediatrics, 17th ed. Philadelphia, Elsevier/Saunders, 2004.

Paller AS, Mancini AJ: Hurwitz Clinical Pediatric Dermatology: A Textbook of Skin Disorders of Childhood and Adolescence, 3rd ed. Philadelphia, WB Saunders, 2006.

Smolinski KN: Hemangiomas of infancy: Clinical and biological characteristics. Clin Pediatr 44:747, 2005.

Tompkins K: Molecular mechanisms of cytodifferentiation in mammalian tooth development. Connect Tissue Res 47:111, 2006.

Winter GB: Anomalies of tooth formation and eruption. In Welbury RR (ed): Paediatric Dentistry, 2nd ed. Oxford, Oxford University Press, 2001.

CHAPTER 19

Bale Jr JF: Fetal infections and brain development. Clin Perinatol 36:639, 2009.

Briggs GG, Freeman RK, Yaffe SJ: Drugs in Pregnancy and Lactation, 8th ed. Baltimore, Williams & Wilkins, 2008.

Centers for Disease Control and Prevention. Improved national prevalence estimates for selected major birth defects—United States, 1999–2001 (MMWR 54:1301, 2006). JAMA 295:618, 2006.

Hall JG: Chromosomal clinical abnormalities. In Behrman RE, Kliegman RM, Jenson HB (eds): Nelson Textbook of Pediatrics, 17th ed. Philadelphia, WB Saunders, 2004.

Hudgins L, Cassidy SB: Congenital anomalies. In Martin RJ, Fanaroff AA, Walsh MC (eds): Fanaroff and Martin's Neonatal-Perinatal Medicine: Diseases of the Fetus and Infant, 8th ed. Philadelphia, Mosby, 2006.

Jones KL: Smith's Recognizable Patterns of Human Malformation, 6th ed. Philadelphia, Elsevier/Saunders, 2006.

Medicode, Inc: Medicodes' Hospital and Payer: International Classification of Diseases, Clinical Modification, ICD-9-CM 2006, vols. 1–3, Salt Lake City, Medicode, 2006.

Nussbaum RL, McInnes RR, Willard HF: Thompson & Thompson Genetics in Medicine, 6 th ed., rev rep. Philadelphia, WB Saunders, 2004.

Rasmussen SA, Erickson JD, Reef SE, et al: Principles and practice of teratology for the obstetrician. Clin Obstet Gynecol 51:106, 2009.

Richardson GA, Goldschmidt L, Willford J: Continued effects of prenatal cocaine use: Preschool development. Neurotoxicol Teratol 31:325, 2009.

Weindling AM: Offspring of diabetic pregnancy: Short-term outcomes. Semin Fetal Neonatal Med 14:101, 2009.

Weiner CP: Drugs for Pregnant and Lactating Women, 2nd ed. Philadelphia, WB Saunders, 2009.

Yolton K, Khoury J, Xu Y, et al: Low-level prenatal exposure to nicotine and infant neurobehavior. Neurotoxicol Teratol 31:356, 2009.

CHAPTER 20

Appel B, Eisen JS: Retinoids run rampant: Multiple roles during spinal cord and motor neuron development. Neuron 40:461, 2003.

Bianchi S, Dotti MT, Federico A: Physiology and pathology of Notch signaling system. J Cell Physiol 207:300, 2006.

Cerdan C, Bhatia M: Novel roles for Notch, Wnt and Hedgehog in hematopoesis derived from human pluripotent cells. Int J Dev Biol 54:955, 2010.

Charron F, Tessier-Lavigne M: Novel brain wiring functions for classical morphogens: A role as graded positional cues in axon guidance. Development 132:2251, 2005.

Chizhikov VV, Millen KJ: Roof plate–dependent patterning of the vertebrate dorsal central nervous system. Dev Biol 277:287, 2005.

Clugston RD, Zhang W, Alvarez S, et al: Understanding abnormal retinoid signaling as a causative mechanism in congenital diaphragmatic hernia. Am J Res Cell Mol Biol 42:276, 2010.

Copp AJ, Greene NDE: Genetics and development of neural tube defects. J Pathol 220:217, 2010.

Coultas L, Chawengsaksophak K, Rossant J: Endothelial cells and VEGF in vascular development. Nature 438:937, 2006.

Dellovade T, Romer JT, Curran T, et al: The hedgehog pathway and neurological disorders. Annu Rev Neurosci 29:539, 2006.

Dunwoodie SL: The role of Notch in patterning the human vertebral column. Curr Opin Genet Dev 19:329, 2009.

Eisenberg LM, Eisenberg CA: Wnt signal transduction and the formation of the myocardium. Dev Biol 293:305, 2006.

Goetz SC, Anderson KV: The primary cilium: A signaling centre during vertebrate development. Nat Rev Genet 11:331, 2010.

Hooper JE, Scott MP: Communicating with hedgehogs. Nat Rev Mol Cell Biol 6:306, 2005.

Larsson J, Karlsson S: The role of Smad signaling in hematopoiesis. Oncogene 24:5676, 2005.

Lewis J, Hanisch A, Holder M: Notch signaling, the segmentation clock, and the patterning of vertebrate somites. J Biol 8:44, 2009.

Li F, Chong ZZ, Maiese K: Winding through the WNT pathway during cellular development and demise. Histol Histopathol 21:103, 2006.

Louvi A, Artavanis-Tsakonas S: Notch signaling in vertebrate neural development. Nat Rev Neurosci 7:93, 2006.

Lupo G, Harris WA, Lewis KE: Mechanisms of ventral patterning in the vertebrate nervous system. Nat Rev Neurosci 7:103, 2006.

MacLean JA, Wilkinson MF: The Rhox genes. Reproduction 140:195, 2010.

Parker MH, Seale P, Rudnicki MA: Looking back to the embryo: Defining transcriptional networks in adult myogenesis. Nat Rev Genet 4:497, 2003.

Pearson JC, Lemons D, McGinnis W: Modulating Hox gene functions during animal body patterning. Nat Rev Genet 6:893, 2005.

Port F, Basler K: Wnt trafficking: New insights into Wnt maturation, secretion and spreading. Traffic 11:1265, 2010.

Powers SE, Taniguchi K, Yen W, et al: Tgif1 and Tgif2 regulate nodal signaling and are required for gastrulation. Development 137: 249, 2010.

Staal FJT, Clevers HC: Wnt signaling and haematopoiesis: A Wnt–Wnt situation. Nat Rev Immunol 5:21, 2005.

Stanchina L, Van de Putte T, Goosens M, et al: Genetic interaction between Sox10 and Zfhx1b during enteric nervous system development. Dev Biol 341:416, 2010.

Tian T, Meng AM: Nodal signals pattern vertebrate embryos. Cell Mol Life Sci 63:672, 2006.

Wan M, Cao X: BMP signaling in skeletal development. Biochem Biophys Res Commun 328:651, 2005.

Wigle JT, Eisenstat DD: Homeobox genes in vertebrate forebrain development and disease. Clin Genet 73:212, 2008.

Yatzey KE: DiGeorge syndrome, Tbx1, and retinoic acid signaling come full circle. Circ Res 106: 630, 2010.

Yoon K, Gaiano N: Notch signaling in the mammalian central nervous system: Insights from mouse mutants. Nat Neurosci 8:709, 2005.

Zhu AJ, Scott MP: Incredible journey: How do developmental signals travel through tissue? Genes Dev 18:2985, 2004.

Answers to Clinically Oriented Questions

CHAPTER 1

1. The term *conceptus* refers to the embryo and its membranes (amnion, chorion, umbilical vesicle, and allantois). A conceptus refers to the products of conception; that is, everything that develops from the zygote. The embryo is the embryonic part of the conceptus.

2. Everyone, especially those in the health-care profession, should know about conception, contraception, and how the embryo develops, both normally and abnormally. Health-care professionals are expected to give intelligent answers to the questions people ask, such as, "When does the baby's heart start to beat?" "When does it move its limbs?" "When is the embryo most at risk for effects from alcohol?"

3. Physicians date pregnancies from the last normal menstrual period because this date is usually remembered by women. It is not possible to detect the precise time of ovulation or of fertilization (when development begins). Laboratory tests and ultrasound imaging can be performed to detect when ovulation is likely to occur and when pregnancy has occurred, but they are not routinely performed because of the costs involved.

CHAPTER 2

1. Pregnant women do not menstruate, even though there may be some bleeding at the usual time of menstruation. This blood may be leaking from the intervillous space because of partial separation of the placenta from the endometrium of the uterine wall. Because there is no shedding of the endometrium, this blood is not menstrual fluid; it is maternal blood that has escaped from the intervillous space in the placenta.

2. It depends on when she forgot to take the oral contraceptive. If it was at mid-cycle, ovulation might occur and pregnancy could result. Taking two doses the next day would not prevent ovulation.

3. Coitus interruptus refers to withdrawal of the penis from the vagina before ejaculation occurs. This method is not reliable. Often, a few sperms are expelled from the penis with the secretions of the auxiliary sex glands (e.g., seminal glands) before ejaculation occurs. One of these sperms may fertilize the oocyte.

4. Spermatogenesis refers to the complete process of sperm formation. Spermiogenesis is the transformation of a spermatid into a sperm. Therefore, spermiogenesis is the final stage of spermatogenesis.

5. A copper-releasing intrauterine device may inhibit the capacitation of sperms and their transport through the uterus to the fertilization site in the uterine tube; in this case, it would be a contraceptive device. A hormone-releasing intrauterine device (e.g., levonorgestrel) may cause changes that alter the morphologic features of the endometrium; as a result, the blastocyst does not implant. In this case, the intrauterine device would be a contraimplantation device.

CHAPTER 3

1. The ovarian and menstrual cycles typically cease between 48 and 55 years of age, with the average age being 51 years. Menopause results from the gradual cessation of gonadotropin production by the pituitary gland; however, it does not mean that the ovaries have exhausted their supply of oocytes. The risk of Down syndrome and other trisomies is increased in the children of women who are 35 years or older (see Chapter 19). Spermatogenesis also decreases after the age of 45 years, and the number of nonviable and abnormal sperms increases. Nevertheless, sperm production continues until old age. The risk of producing abnormal gametes is much less common in men than in women; however, older men may accumulate mutations that the child might inherit. Mutations may produce birth defects (see Chapter 19).

2. Considerable research on new contraceptive methods is being conducted, including the development of oral contraceptives for men. This research includes experimental work on hormonal and nonhormonal prevention of spermatogenesis and the stimulation of immune responses to sperms. Arresting the development of millions of sperms on a continuous basis has proven much more difficult than arresting the monthly development of a single oocyte monthly.

3. It is not known whether polar bodies are ever fertilized; however, it has been suggested that dispermic chimeras result from the fusion of a fertilized oocyte with a fertilized polar body. Chimeras are rare individuals who are composed of a mixture of cells from two zygotes. More likely, dispermic chimeras result

from the fusion of dizygotic twin zygotes early in development. Dizygotic twins are derived from two zygotes. If a polar body were fertilized and remained separate from the normal zygote, it could form an embryo.

4. The most common cause of spontaneous abortion during the first week of development is chromosomal abnormality, such as the abnormalities resulting from nondisjunction (see Chapter 2). Failure of the syncytiotrophoblast to produce an adequate amount of human chorionic gonadotrophin to maintain the corpus luteum in the ovary could also result in early spontaneous abortion.

5. Yes, it is possible; however, this phenomenon is extremely rare. The term superfecundation indicates fertilization (during separate acts of coitus) of two or more oocytes that are ovulated at approximately the same time.

6. Mitosis is the usual process of cell reproduction that results in the formation of daughter cells of the zygote. Cleavage is the series of mitotic cell divisions of the zygote. This process results in the formation of daughter cells, or blastomeres. The expressions *cleavage division* and *mitotic division* have the same meaning when referring to the dividing zygote.

7. The nutritional requirements of the dividing zygote are not great. The nutrients are derived mainly from the secretions of the uterine tubes.

8. Yes. One of the blastomeres could be removed, and a Y chromosome could be identified by fluorescence staining with quinacrine mustard or by molecular techniques (see Chapter 7). This technique could be made available to couples with a family history of sex-linked genetic diseases (e.g., hemophilia, muscular dystrophy) and to women who have already given birth to a child with such a disease and are reluctant to have more children. In these cases, only female embryos developing in vitro would be transferred to the uterus.

CHAPTER 4

1. Implantation bleeding refers to the loss of small amounts of blood from the implantation site of a blastocyst that occurs a few days after the expected time of menstruation. Women unfamiliar with this possible occurrence may interpret the bleeding as a light menstrual flow. In such cases, they may give the physician the wrong date for their last normal menstrual period. This blood is not menstrual fluid; it is blood from the intervillous space of the developing placenta. Blood loss could also result from the rupture of chorionic arteries, veins, or both (see Chapter 8).

2. Drugs or other agents may cause early abortion of an embryo, but they do not cause birth defects if taken during the first 2 weeks of development. A drug or other agent either damages all of the

embryonic cells, killing the embryo, or injures only a few cells, in which case the embryo recovers to develop normally.

3. Intrauterine devices are typically very effective at preventing pregnancy by altering sperm capacitation or motility or by altering, for instance, the morphologic features of the endometrium. However, an intrauterine device does not physically block a sperm from entering the uterine tube and fertilizing an oocyte, if one is present. Although the endometrium could be hostile to implantation, a blastocyst could develop and implant in the uterine tube (i.e., ectopic tubal pregnancy). If fertilization occurs in a woman who is using an intrauterine device, the risk of ectopic pregnancy is approximately 5%.

4. Abdominal pregnancies are very uncommon; but such a pregnancy may result from primary implantation of a blastocyst in the abdomen. In most cases, it is believed to result from ectopic implantation of a blastocyst that spontaneously aborts from the uterine tube and enters the peritoneal cavity. The risk of severe maternal bleeding and fetal mortality is high in cases of abdominal pregnancy. However, if the diagnosis is made late in pregnancy and the patient (mother) is free of symptoms, the pregnancy may be allowed to continue until the viability of the fetus is ensured (e.g., 32 weeks), at which time it would be delivered by cesarean section.

CHAPTER 5

1. Yes, certain drugs can produce birth defects if administered during the third week after the last normal menstrual period (see Chapter 19). For instance, antineoplastic agents (chemotherapy, or antitumor drugs) can produce severe skeletal and neural tube defects in the embryo, such as acrania and meroencephaly (partial absence of the brain), if administered during the third week.

2. Yes, risks to the mother 40 years or older and the embryo are increased. Advanced maternal age is a predisposing factor to certain medical conditions. Preeclampsia, a hypertensive disorder of pregnancy, characterized by increased blood pressure and edema, for example, occurs more frequently in older pregnant women than in younger ones. Advanced maternal age is also associated with a significantly increased risk to the embryo or fetus. The most common risks are birth defects associated with chromosomal abnormalities, such as Down syndrome and trisomy 13 (see Chapter 19); however, women older than 40 years may have normal children.

CHAPTER 6

1. Early in the eighth week, embryos have webbed toes and stubby, tail-like caudal eminences and look different from 9-week fetuses; however, by the end of the eighth week, embryos and early fetuses appear

similar. The name change is made to indicate that a new phase of development (rapid growth and differentiation) has begun and that the most critical period of development has been completed.

2. There are different opinions of when an embryo becomes a human being because opinions are often affected by religious and personal views. The scientific answer is that the embryo is a human being from the time of fertilization because of its human chromosomal constitution. The zygote is the beginning of a developing human.

3. No, it cannot. During the embryonic period, more similarities than differences exist in the external genitalia (see Chapter 13). It is impossible to tell by ultrasound examination whether the primordial sexual organ (genital tubercle at 5 weeks and phallus at 7 weeks) will become a penis or a clitoris. Sex differences are not clear until the early fetal period (10th–12th week). Sex chromatin patterns and chromosomal analysis (fluorescence in situ hybridization) of embryonic cells obtained during amniocentesis can show the chromosomal sex of the embryo (see Chapter 7).

◼ CHAPTER 7

1. Ultrasound examinations have shown that mature embryos (8 weeks) and young fetuses (9 weeks) show spontaneous movements, such as twitching (sudden jerking movements) of the trunk and limbs. Although the fetus begins to move its back and limbs during the 12th week, the mother cannot feel the fetus move until the 16th to 20th week. Women who have had several children usually detect this movement, called quickening, sooner than women who are pregnant for the first time because they know what fetal movements feel like. Quickening is often perceived as a faint flutter or a quivering motion.

2. Folic acid supplementation before conception and during early pregnancy is effective in reducing the incidence of neural tube defects (e.g., spina bifida). It has been shown that the risk of having a child with neural tube defect is significantly lower when a vitamin supplement containing 400 mg of folic acid is consumed daily. However, no consensus exists that vitamins are helpful in preventing these defects in most at-risk pregnancies.

3. Direct injury to the fetus from the needle during amniocentesis is very uncommon when ultrasound guidance is used to locate the position of the fetus and monitor needle insertion. The risk of inducing an abortion is slight (approximately 0.5%) in second-trimester pregnancies. Maternal or fetal infection is also an uncommon complication.

◼ CHAPTER 8

1. A stillbirth is the birth of an infant that was dead before delivery, weighs at least 500 g, and is at least 20 weeks old. The incidence of having a stillborn infant is approximately three times greater among mothers older than 40 years than among women 20 to 30 years. More male fetuses than female fetuses are stillborn. The reason for this is unknown.

2. Sometimes the umbilical cord is abnormally long and wraps around part of the fetus, such as the neck or a limb. This cord accident may obstruct the flow of high oxygen blood in the umbilical vein to the fetus and in the umbilical arteries from the fetus to the placenta. If this obstruction causes the fetus to receive insufficient oxygen and nutrients, then the fetus is likely to die. A true knot in the umbilical cord, formed when the fetus passes through a loop in the cord, also obstructs blood flow through the cord. Prolapse of the umbilical cord into the cervix at the level of a presenting part (often the head) may also be considered a cord accident. This creates pressure on the cord and prevents the fetus from receiving adequate oxygen. Entanglement of the cord around the fetus can also cause birth defects (e.g., absence of a forearm).

3. Most over-the-counter pregnancy tests are based on the detection of relatively large amounts of human chorionic gonadotrophin in the woman's urine. The results of such tests are positive a short time (approximately 1 week) after the first missed menstrual period (after embryo implantation). Human chorionic gonadotrophin is produced by the syncytiotrophoblast of the chorion. These tests usually give an accurate diagnosis of pregnancy; however, a physician should be consulted as soon as possible to confirm pregnancy because some tumors (choriocarcinomas) also produce this hormone.

4. The bag of waters is a colloquial term for the amniotic sac, which contains amniotic fluid (largely composed of water). Sometimes the amniochorionic sac ruptures before labor begins, allowing fluid to escape. Premature rupture of the membranes is the most common event leading to premature labor (birth). Premature rupture of the membranes may complicate the birth process or may allow a vaginal infection to spread to the fetus. Sometimes sterile saline is infused into the uterus by way of a catheter—amnioinfusion—to alleviate fetal distress. The term dry birth is used to describe a low volume of amniotic fluid.

5. Fetal distress is synonymous with fetal hypoxia, indicating decreased oxygenation to the fetus as a result of a general decrease of the maternal oxygen content of the blood, decreased oxygen-carrying capacity, or diminished blood flow. Fetal distress exists when the fetal heart rate is less than 100 beats per minute. Pressure on the umbilical cord may also cause fetal distress secondary to impairment of the blood supply to the fetus in approximately 1 in 200 deliveries. In these cases, the fetal body compresses the umbilical cord as it passes through the cervix and vagina.

6. The incidence of dizygotic twins increases with maternal age. Dizygotic twinning is an autosomal recessive trait that is carried by the daughters of

mothers of twins; hence, dizygotic twinning is hereditary. Monozygotic twinning, on the other hand, is a random occurrence that is not genetically controlled.

CHAPTER 9

1. Yes, it is. When an infant is born with a congenital diaphragmatic hernia, part of its stomach and liver may enter the thorax (chest); however, this is uncommon. Usually, the abnormally placed viscera are the intestines. The viscera enter the thorax through a posterolateral defect in the diaphragm, usually on the left side.

2. An infant born with a congenital diaphragmatic hernia may survive; however, the mortality rate may be high (approximately 76%). Treatment must be given immediately. A feeding tube is inserted into the stomach, and the air and the gastric contents are aspirated with continuous suction. Intubation of the airway, mechanical ventilation, and stabilization of the neonate are critical until surgery can be performed. The displaced viscera are replaced into the abdominal cavity, and the defect in the diaphragm is surgically repaired. Infants with large diaphragmatic hernias who are operated on within 24 hours after birth have survival rates of 40% to 70%. Intrauterine surgical repair of a congenital diaphragmatic hernia has been attempted; however, this intervention carries considerable risk to the fetus and mother. The developing use of minimally invasive surgical techniques may reduce this risk.

3. It depends on the degree of herniation of the abdominal viscera. With a moderate hernia, the lungs may be mature, but small. With a severe degree of herniation, lung development is impaired. Most infants with a congenital diaphragmatic hernia die, but not because of the defect in the diaphragm or viscera in the thorax; they die because the lung on the affected side is hypoplastic (underdeveloped).

4. Yes, it is possible to have a small congenital diaphragmatic hernia and not be aware of it. Some small hernias may remain asymptomatic into adulthood and may be discovered only during routine radiographic or ultrasound examination of the thorax. The lung on the affected side would probably develop normally because there would be little or no pressure on it during prenatal development.

CHAPTER 10

1. *Harelip,* a colloquial term, is the obsolete term for the clinical entity known as cleft lip. The term was adopted because the hare has a divided upper lip. It is not an accurate comparison, however, because the cleft in the hare's lip is in the median part of the upper lip, whereas most human clefts are lateral to the median plane. The term *harelip* can cause offence and should not be used.

2. No, both statements are inaccurate. All embryos have grooves in their upper lips where the maxillary prominences meet the merged medial nasal prominences; however, normal embryos do not have cleft lips. When lip development is abnormal, the tissue in the floor of the labial groove breaks down, forming a cleft lip.

3. The risk in this case is the same as in the general population, approximately 1 in 1000.

4. Although environmental factors may be involved, it is reasonable to assume that the son's cleft lip and cleft palate were hereditary and recessive in their expression. This would mean that the father also carried a concealed gene for cleft lip and that his family genetics were equally responsible for the son's anomalies.

5. Minor anomalies of the auricle of the external ear are common, and usually they are of no serious medical or cosmetic consequence. Approximately 14% of newborn infants have minor birth defects; fewer than 1% of them have other defects. The child's abnormal ears could be considered branchial anomalies because the six small auricular hillocks (swellings) of the first two pairs of pharyngeal arches contribute to the auricles; however, such minor abnormalities of ear shape would not normally be classified in this way.

CHAPTER 11

1. Multiple stimuli initiate breathing at birth. Slapping the buttocks used to be a common physical stimulus; however, this action is usually unnecessary. Under normal circumstances, the infant's breathing begins promptly, which suggests that it is a reflex response to the sensory stimuli of exposure to air and touching. The changes in blood gases after interruption of the placental circulation, such as the decrease in oxygen tension and pH and the increase in partial pressure of carbon dioxide, are also important in stimulating breathing.

2. Hyaline membrane disease, a common cause of the respiratory distress syndrome, occurs after the onset of breathing in infants with immature lungs and a deficiency of pulmonary surfactant. The incidence of respiratory distress syndrome is approximately 1% of all live births, and it is the leading cause of death in newborn infants. It occurs mainly in infants who are born prematurely. Hyaline membrane disease is caused mainly by surfactant deficiency.

3. A 22-week fetus is viable and, if born prematurely and given special care in a neonatal intensive care unit, may survive. The chances of survival, however, are poor for infants who weigh less than 600 g because the lungs are immature and incapable of

adequate alveolar-capillary gas exchange. Furthermore, the fetus's brain is not usually differentiated sufficiently to permit regular respiration.

CHAPTER 12

1. Undoubtedly, the infant had congenital hypertrophic pyloric stenosis, a diffuse hypertrophy (enlargement) and hyperplasia of smooth muscle in the pyloric part of the stomach. This condition produces a hard palpable mass; however, it is not a tumor. It is a benign enlargement and is definitely not a malignant tumor. The muscular enlargement causes narrowing of the exit canal (pyloric canal). In response to the outflow obstruction and vigorous peristalsis, the vomiting is projectile, as in the case of the infant described. Surgical relief of the pyloric obstruction is the usual treatment. The cause of pyloric stenosis is not known; however, it is believed to have a multifactorial pattern of inheritance (i.e., genetic and environmental factors are probably involved).

2. It is true that infants with Down syndrome have an increased incidence of duodenal atresia. They are also more likely to have imperforate anus and other birth defects (e.g., atrial septal defects). These birth defects are likely caused by their abnormal chromosomal constitution (i.e., three instead of two copies of chromosome 21). Duodenal atresia can be corrected surgically by bypassing the pyloric obstruction (duodenoduodenostomy).

3. In very uncommon cases, when the intestines return to the abdomen after physiologic umbilical herniation, they may rotate in a clockwise direction rather than in the usual counter-clockwise manner. As a result, the cecum and appendix are located on the left side, a condition called situs inversus abdominis. A left-sided cecum and appendix can also result from a mobile cecum. If the cecum is not fixed to the posterior abdominal wall during the fetal period, the cecum and appendix are freely movable and could migrate to the left side.

4. Undoubtedly, the individual described had an ileal (Meckel) diverticulum, a fingerlike outpouching of the ileum. This common anomaly is sometimes referred to as a second appendix, which is a misnomer. An ileal diverticulum produces symptoms that are similar to those of appendicitis. It is also possible, although rare, that the person had a duplication of the cecum, which would result in two appendices.

5. Hirschsprung disease, or congenital megacolon, is the most common cause of obstruction of the descending colon in newborn infants. The cause of the condition is failure of migration of neural crest cells into the wall of the intestine. The neural crest cells normally form neurons, so there is a deficiency of the nerve cells that innervate the muscular wall of the bowel—congenital aganglionosis. When the bowel wall collapses, obstruction occurs and constipation results. Bowel over distention and perforation may also occur.

6. If the infant had an umbilicoileal fistula, the abnormal canal connecting the ileum and the umbilicus could permit the passage of the contents of the ileum to the umbilicus. This occurrence would be an important diagnostic clue to the presence of this canal. The fistula results from the persistence of the intraabdominal part of the omphaloenteric duct.

CHAPTER 13

1. Most people with a horseshoe kidney have no urinary problems. The abnormal position of the fused kidneys is usually discovered at postmortem or during diagnostic imaging procedures. Nothing needs to be done with the abnormal kidney unless the person has an uncontrolled infection of the urinary tract. In some cases, the urologist may divide the kidney into two parts and fix them in positions that do not result in urinary stagnation.

2. His developing kidneys probably fused during the sixth to eighth weeks as they "migrated" from the pelvis. The fused kidneys then ascended toward the normal position on one side or the other. Usually, no problems are associated with fused kidneys; however, surgeons must be conscious of the possibility of this condition and recognize it for what it is. This abnormality is called crossed renal ectopia.

3. Affected individuals have both ovarian and testicular tissue. Although spermatogenesis is uncommon, ovulation is not. Pregnancy and childbirth have been observed in a few patients; however, this is very unusual.

4. By 48 hours after birth, a definite sex assignment can be made in most cases. The parents are told that their infant's genital development is incomplete and that tests are needed to determine whether the infant is a boy or a girl. They are usually advised against announcing their infant's birth to their friends until the appropriate sex has been assigned. Karyotyping (chromosomal staining, visualization, and counting) from whole blood lymphocytes is conducted as well as identification of the SRY gene (sex-determining region of the Y chromosome) by either fluorescence in situ hybridization (FISH) or polymerase chain reaction (PCR) amplification. Hormone studies may also be required.

5. Virilization (masculinization) of a female fetus as a result of congenital adrenal hyperplasia is the most common cause of ambiguous external genitalia. In other cases, androgens enter the fetal circulation after maternal ingestion of androgenic hormones. In unusual cases, these hormones are produced by a tumor on one of the mother's suprarenal glands. Partial or complete fusion of the urogenital folds or labioscrotal swellings is the result of exposure to androgens before the 12th week of development.

Clitoral enlargement occurs after this point; however, androgens do not cause sexual ambiguity because the other external genitalia are fully formed by this time.

CHAPTER 14

1. Heart murmurs are sounds transmitted to the thoracic wall from turbulence of blood in the heart or great arteries. Loud murmurs often represent stenosis of one of the semilunar valves (aortic or pulmonary valve). A ventricular septal defect or a patent oval foramen (foramen ovale) may also produce a murmur.

2. Congenital heart defects are common. They occur in 6 to 8 in 1000 newborn infants and represent approximately 10% of all congenital anomalies. Ventricular septal defects are the most common type of heart anomaly. They occur more frequently in males than in females, but the reason for this is unknown.

3. The cause of most congenital anomalies of the cardiovascular system is unknown. In approximately 8% of children with heart disease, a genetic basis is clear. Most of these anomalies are associated with obvious chromosomal abnormalities (e.g., trisomy 21) and deletion of parts of chromosomes. Down syndrome is associated with congenital heart disease in 50% of cases. Maternal ingestion of drugs, such as antimetabolites and warfarin (an anticoagulant), has been shown to be associated with a high incidence of cardiac defects. Heavy consumption of alcohol during pregnancy may cause heart defects.

4. Several viral infections are associated with congenital cardiac defects; however, only rubella virus (German measles) is known to cause cardiovascular disease (e.g., patent ductus arteriosus). Rubeola (common measles) does not cause cardiovascular defects. Rubella virus vaccine is available and is effective in preventing the development of rubella infection in a woman who has not had the disease and is planning to have a baby. It will subsequently prevent rubella syndrome from developing in her infant as well. Because of the potential hazard of the vaccine to the embryo, the vaccine is given only if there is assurance that there is no likelihood of pregnancy for the next 2 months.

5. This anomaly is called transposition of the great arteries because the positions of the great vessels (aorta and pulmonary trunk) are reversed. Survival after birth depends on mixing between the pulmonary and systemic circulations (e.g., through an atrial septal defect—patent oval foramen). Transposition of the great arteries occurs in slightly more than 1 in 5000 live births and is more common in male infants than in female infants (by almost 2 to 1). Most infants with this severe cardiac anomaly die during the first months of life; however, corrective surgery can be performed in those who survive for several months. Initially, an atrial septal defect may be created to increase mixing between the systemic and pulmonary circulations. Later, an arterial switch operation (reversing the aorta and the pulmonary trunk) can be performed. However, more commonly, a baffle (a device used to restrain the flow of blood) is inserted into the atrium to divert systemic venous blood through the mitral valve, left ventricle, and pulmonary artery to the lungs, and to divert pulmonary venous blood through the tricuspid valve, right ventricle, and aorta. This physiologically corrects the circulation.

6. Very likely, one twin has dextrocardia, which usually is of no clinical significance. The heart is simply displaced to the right. In the individual described, the heart presents a mirror image of the normal cardiac structure. This occurs during the fourth week of development, when the heart tube rotates to the left rather than to the right. Dextrocardia is a relatively common anomaly in monozygotic twins.

CHAPTER 15

1. An accessory rib associated with the seventh cervical vertebra is of clinical importance because it may compress the subclavian artery, the brachial plexus, or both, producing symptoms of artery and nerve compression. The most common type of accessory rib is a lumbar rib, but it usually causes no problems.

2. A hemivertebra can produce lateral curvature of the vertebral column (scoliosis). A hemivertebra is composed of one half of a body, a pedicle, and a lamina. This anomaly occurs when mesenchymal cells from the sclerotomes on one side do not form the primordium of half of a vertebra. As a result, more growth centers are found on one side of the vertebral column; this imbalance causes the vertebral column to bend laterally.

3. Craniosynostosis indicates premature closure of one or more of the cranial sutures. This developmental abnormality results in cranial malformations. Scaphocephaly, or dolichocephaly—a long, narrow cranium—results from premature closure of the sagittal suture. This type of craniosynostosis accounts for approximately 50% of cases of premature closure of cranial sutures and is more commonly seen in males.

4. The features of Klippel-Feil syndrome are a short neck, a low hairline, and restricted neck movements. In most cases, fewer than normal cervical vertebrae are present.

5. Prune-belly syndrome results from partial or complete absence of the abdominal musculature. Usually the abdominal wall is thin. This syndrome is usually associated with malformations of the urinary tract, especially the urinary bladder (e.g., exstrophy). In males, almost all patients have cryptorchidism (failure of one or both testes to descend into the scrotum).

6. Absence of the sternocostal part of the left pectoralis major muscle is usually the cause of an abnormally low nipple and areola. Despite its numerous and important actions, absence of all or part of the pectoralis major muscle usually causes no disability. The actions of other muscles associated with the shoulder joint compensate for the partial absence of this muscle.

7. The girl has a prominent sternocleidomastoid muscle. This muscle attaches the mastoid process to the clavicle and sternum; hence, continued growth of the side of the neck results in tilting and rotation of the head. This relatively common condition—congenital torticollis (wry neck)—may occur because of injury to the muscle during birth. Stretching and tearing of some muscle fibers may have occurred during delivery, resulting in bleeding into the muscle. Over several weeks, necrosis of some fibers occurs and the blood is replaced by fibrous tissue. This results in shortening of the muscle and pulling of the child's head to one side. If the condition is not corrected, the shortened muscle also could distort the shape of the face on the affected side.

8. The young athlete probably had an accessory soleus muscle. It is present in approximately 6% of people. This anomaly probably results from splitting of the primordium of the soleus muscle into two parts.

9. The ingestion of drugs did not cause the child's short limbs. The infant has a skeletal disorder known as achondroplasia. This type of short-limbed dwarfism has an incidence of 1 in 10,000 and shows an autosomal dominant inheritance. Approximately 80% of affected infants are born to normal parents and presumably, the condition results from fresh mutations (changes in the genetic material) in the parents' germ cells. Most people with achondroplasia have normal intelligence and lead normal lives within their physical capabilities. If the parents of an achondroplastic child have more children, the risk of having another child with this condition is slightly higher than the risk in the general population; however, the risk for the achondroplastic person's own children is 50%.

10. Brachydactyly is an autosomal dominant trait. If the woman (likely bb) marries the brachydactylous man (likely Bb), the risk is 50% for a brachydactylous child and 50% for a normal child. It would be best for her to discuss her obvious concern with a medical geneticist.

11. Bendectin, an antinauseant mixture of doxylamine, dicyclomine, and pyridoxine, does not produce limb defects in human embryos. Several epidemiologic studies have not shown an increased risk of birth defects after exposure to Bendectin or its separate ingredients during early pregnancy. In the case described, the mother took the drug more than 3 weeks after the end of the critical period of limb development (24–36 days after fertilization). Most limb reduction defects have a genetic basis.

12. Cutaneous syndactyly is the most common type of limb anomaly. It varies from cutaneous webbing between the digits to synostosis (union of the phalanges, the bones of the digits). This anomaly occurs when separate digital rays do not form in the fifth week or when the tissue between the developing digits does not undergo apoptosis. Simple cutaneous syndactyly is easy to correct surgically. The absence of the sternal head of the pectoralis major muscle caused the nipple to be lower than the other one.

13. The most common type of clubfoot is talipes equinovarus, occurring in approximately 1 in 1000 newborn infants. In this deformity, the soles of the feet are turned medially and the feet are plantar flexed. The feet are fixed in the tiptoe position, resembling the foot of a horse (Latin equinus, horse).

CHAPTER 16

1. Neural tube defects (NTDs) have a multifactorial inheritance pattern. Although only a few environmental factors have been shown to be directly related (such as folic acid), studies indicate that there are also genetic components. After the birth of one child with an NTD, the risk of a subsequent child having an NTD is much higher. The recurrence risk in the United Kingdom, where NTDs are common (7.6 per 1000 in South Wales and 8.6 per 1000 in Northern Ireland), is approximately 1 in 25. NTDs can be detected prenatally by a combination of ultrasound scanning and measurement of levels of alpha fetoprotein in the amniotic fluid and maternal serum.

2. Mental deficiency and growth restriction are the most serious aspects of fetal alcohol syndrome. Average IQ scores in affected children are 60 to 70. It has been estimated that the incidence of mental deficiency resulting from heavy drinking during pregnancy may be as high as 1 in 400 live births. Heavy drinkers are those who consume five or more drinks on one occasion, with a consistent daily average of 45 mL of absolute alcohol. Currently, no safe threshold for alcohol consumption during pregnancy is known. Physicians recommend complete abstinence from alcohol during pregnancy.

3. No conclusive evidence indicates that maternal smoking affects the mental development of a fetus; however, cigarette smoking compromises the oxygen supply to the fetus because blood flow to the placenta is decreased during smoking. Because it is well established that heavy maternal smoking seriously affects the physical growth of the fetus and is a major cause of intrauterine growth restriction, it is not wise for mothers to smoke during pregnancy. The reduced oxygen supply to the brain could affect fetal intellectual development, even though the effect may be undetectable. Abstinence gives the fetus the best chance for normal development.

4. Most laypeople use the term spina bifida in a general way. They are unaware that the common type, spina bifida occulta, is usually clinically insignificant. It is an isolated finding in up to 20% of radiographically examined vertebral columns. Most people are unaware that they have this vertebral defect because it produces no symptoms unless it is associated with a neural tube defect or abnormality of the spinal nerve roots. The various types of spina bifida cystica are of clinical significance. Meningomyelocele is a more severe defect than meningocele because neural tissue is included in the lesion. Because of this, the function of the abdominal and limb muscles may be affected. Meningoceles are usually covered with skin, and motor function in the limbs is usually normal unless associated developmental defects of the spinal cord or brain are present. Management of infants with spina bifida cystica is complex and involves several medical and surgical specialties. Spinal meningocele is easier to correct surgically than spinal meningomyelocele, and the prognosis is also better.

CHAPTER 17

1. The chance of significant damage to the embryo or fetus after rubella infection depends primarily on the timing of the viral infection. In cases of primary maternal infection during the first trimester of pregnancy, the overall risk of embryonic or fetal infection is approximately 20%. It is estimated that approximately 50% of such pregnancies end in spontaneous abortion, stillbirth, or congenital anomalies (deafness, cataract, glaucoma, and mental retardation). When infection occurs at the end of the first trimester, the probability of congenital anomalies is only slightly higher than that for an uncomplicated pregnancy. Certain infections occurring late in the first trimester, however, may result in severe eye infections (e.g., chorioretinitis), which may affect visual development. Deafness is the most common manifestation of late fetal rubella infection (i.e., during the second and third trimesters). If a pregnant woman is exposed to rubella, an antibody test can be performed. If she is determined to be immune, she can be reassured that her embryo or fetus will not be affected by the virus. Preventive measures are essential for the protection of the embryo. It is especially important for girls to obtain immunity to rubella (e.g., by active immunization) before they reach childbearing age.

2. The purposeful exposure of young girls to rubella (German measles) is not recommended. Although complications resulting from such infections are uncommon, neuritis and arthritis (inflammation of the nerves and the joints, respectively) occasionally occur. Encephalitis (inflammation of the brain) occurs in approximately 1 in 6000 cases. Rubella infection is often subclinical (difficult to detect), yet children with such infections represent an exposure risk to pregnant women. There is a chance of injury to embryos because the danger period is greatest when the eyes and ears are developing. This occurs early enough in pregnancy that some women might be unaware that they are pregnant. A much better way of providing immunization against rubella is the administration of live vaccine to children older than 15 months and to nonpregnant postpubertal females who can be reasonably relied on not to become pregnant within 3 months of immunization.

3. Congenital syphilis (fetal syphilis) results from transplacental transmission of the microorganism *Treponema pallidum*. Transfer of this microorganism from untreated pregnant women may occur throughout pregnancy; however, it usually takes place during the last trimester. Deafness and tooth deformities commonly develop in these children. These anomalies can be prevented by treating the mother early in pregnancy. The microorganism that causes syphilis is very sensitive to penicillin, an antibiotic that does not harm the fetus.

4. Several viruses in the herpes virus family can cause fetal blindness and deafness during infancy. Cytomegalovirus can cross the placenta, be transmitted to the infant during birth, and be passed to the infant in breast milk. Herpes simplex viruses (usually type 2, or genital herpes) are usually transmitted just before or during birth. The chances of normal development in infected infants are not good. Some infants have microcephaly, seizures, deafness, and blindness.

5. Methyl mercury is teratogenic in human embryos, especially to the developing brain. Because the eyes and internal ears develop as outgrowths from the brain, it is understandable that their development is also affected. Besides the methyl mercury that passes from the mother to the embryo or fetus through the placenta, the newborn infant may receive additional methyl mercury from breast milk. Sources of methyl mercury include fish from contaminated water, flour made from methyl mercury–treated seed grain, and meat from animals raised on contaminated food.

CHAPTER 18

1. Congenital absence of the skin is very uncommon. Patches of skin may be absent, most often from the scalp, or sometimes from the trunk and limbs. Affected infants usually survive because healing of the lesions is uneventful and takes 1 to 2 months. A hairless scar persists. The cause of congenital absence of hair, termed *aplasia cutis congenita*, is usually unknown. Most cases are sporadic; however, several well-documented pedigrees show autosomal dominant transmission of this skin defect.

2. The white patches of skin on a dark-skinned person result from partial albinism (piebaldism). This defect, which also affects light-skinned persons, is a heritable disorder transmitted by an autosomal dominant gene. Ultrastructural studies show an absence of

melanocytes in the depigmented areas of skin. Presumably, the cause is a genetic defect in the differentiation of melanoblasts. These skin and hair defects are not amenable to treatment; however, they can be covered with cosmetics and hair dyes.

3. The breasts, including the mammary glands within them, of males and females are similar at birth. Breast enlargement in a newborn infant is common and results from stimulation by maternal hormones that enter the infant's blood through the placenta. Therefore, enlarged breasts are a normal occurrence in young male infants and do not indicate abnormal sex development. Similarly, physiologic pubertal gynecomastia occurs in some males during their early teens as a result of decreased levels of testosterone. The breast enlargement is usually transitory. Familial gynecomastia is an X-linked, or autosomal dominant sex-linked, trait. Gynecomastia also occurs in approximately 50% of males with Klinefelter syndrome (described in Chapter 19). These boys and men are not intersexes because their external and internal genitalia are normal, except for their testes, which are very small because of degeneration of the seminiferous tubules.

4. An extra breast (polymastia) or nipple (polythelia) is common. The axillary breast may enlarge during puberty, or it may not be noticed until pregnancy occurs. The embryologic basis of extra breasts and nipples is the presence of mammary crests (ridges) that extend from the axillary to the inguinal regions. Usually, only one pair of breasts develops; however, breasts can develop anywhere along the mammary crests. The extra breast or nipple is usually just superior or inferior to the normal breast. An axillary breast or nipple is very uncommon.

5. Teeth that are present at birth are termed natal teeth and are observed in approximately 1 in 2000 newborn infants. Usually, two mandibular medial (central) incisors are present. The presence of natal teeth usually suggests that early eruption of other teeth may occur. Often, they fall out on their own. Because there is a danger that they may be aspirated, natal teeth are sometimes extracted.

CHAPTER 19

1. No evidence indicates that the occasional use of aspirin in recommended therapeutic dosages is harmful during pregnancy; however, large doses at subtoxic levels (e.g., for rheumatoid arthritis) have not been proven to be harmless to the embryo and fetus. All pregnant women should discuss the use of over-the-counter medications with their physicians.

2. A woman who is addicted to a habit-forming drug (e.g., heroin) and takes it during pregnancy is almost certain to give birth to a child who shows signs of drug addiction. The fetus's chances of survival until birth, however, are not good; mortality and premature birth rates are high among fetuses of drug-addicted mothers.

3. All drugs prescribed in North America are tested for teratogenicity before they are marketed. The thalidomide tragedy clearly showed the need for improved methods for detecting potential human teratogens. Thalidomide was not found to be teratogenic in pregnant mice and rats—yet it is a potent teratogen in humans during the fourth to sixth weeks of pregnancy. Because it is unethical to test the effects of drugs on human embryos, no way exists to guarantee that some drugs that may be human teratogens will not be marketed. Human teratologic evaluation depends on retrospective epidemiologic studies and the reports of astute physicians. This is the way that the teratogenicity of thalidomide was detected. Most new drugs contain a disclaimer in the accompanying package insert, such as, "This drug has not been proven safe for pregnant women." Some drugs may be used if, in the opinion of the physician, the potential benefits outweigh the possible hazards. All known teratogenic drugs that may be taken by a pregnant woman are available only through prescription by a physician.

4. Cigarette smoking during pregnancy is harmful to the embryo and fetus. Its most adverse effect is intrauterine growth restriction. Women who stop smoking during the first half of pregnancy have infants with birth weights closer to the birth weights of infants of nonsmokers. Decreased placental blood flow, believed to be a nicotine-mediated effect, is believed to cause decreased intrauterine blood flow. No conclusive evidence exists that maternal smoking causes birth defects. The growth of the fetus of a woman who smokes, but does not inhale is still endangered because nicotine, carbon monoxide, and other harmful substances are also absorbed into the maternal bloodstream through the mucous membranes of the mouth and throat. These substances are then transferred to the embryo or fetus through the placenta. Smoking in any manner during pregnancy is not advisable.

5. Ample evidence indicates that most drugs do not cause congenital anomalies in human embryos; however, a pregnant woman should take only drugs that are essential and are recommended by her physician. A pregnant woman with a severe lower respiratory infection, for example, would be unwise to refuse drugs recommended by her physician to cure her illness; her health and that of her embryo or fetus could be endangered by the infection. Most drugs, including sulfonamides, meclizine, penicillin, and antihistamines, are considered safe drugs. Similarly, local anesthetic agents, dead vaccines, and salicylates (e.g., aspirin) in low doses are not known to cause congenital anomalies.

Index

Page numbers followed by b, f, or t, denote boxes, figures, and tables, respectively.